Palliative Care for Infants, Children, and Adolescents

Palliative Care for Infants, Children, and Adolescents

A PRACTICAL HANDBOOK

Edited by

Brian S. Carter, M.D., F.A.A.P.

Associate Professor, Division of Neonatology
Department of Pediatrics, Vanderbilt University Medical Center
Nashville, Tennessee

AND

Marcia Levetown, M.D.

Program Director for Palliative Care
The Methodist Hospital
Houston, Texas

Foreword by Kathleen M. Foley, M.D.

The Johns Hopkins University Press

BALTIMORE AND LONDON

I dedicate this work to those patients, parents, families, and staff, both known and unknown, who have taught and humbled me, motivated and tempered me, and willingly given so much in our mutual journey. And to the memory of Benjamin, Bobbie Jean, Danny, Loyd, Art, and Tony—with gratitude for the love, insights, and lessons you provided.

> Brian S. Carter, M.D., F.A.A.P.

I dedicate this volume to my husband Philip Blum, M.D., who encouraged me to follow my heart regardless of the consequences; to my children, Alex and Lila, who have endured many sad stories and maternal absences over the years; to the patients I have had the privilege to care for and their families, who have demonstrated unparalleled bravery, shown me their needs and hopes, and allowed me to share some of the most intensely intimate moments of their lives; to my mentors, especially Kathleen Foley, M.D., Susan Block, M.D., Don Powell, M.D., and Leslie Strauss, M.S.W.; and to my colleagues, Brian Carter, M.D., Stacy Orloff, D.S.W., and Sue Huff, R.N., in addition to many others who have enabled and who continue to enable the field of pediatric palliative care to grow and flourish.

> Marcia Levetown, M.D.

Drug dosage: The authors and publisher have exerted every effort to ensure that the selection and dosage of drugs discussed in this text accord with recommendations and practice at the time of publication. However, in view of ongoing research, changes in governmental regulations, and the constant flow of information relating to drug therapy and drug reactions, the reader is urged to check the package insert of each drug for any change in indications and dosage and for warnings and precautions. This is particularly important when the recommended agent is a new or infrequently used drug.

This book was brought to publication with the generous assistance of a grant from the Initiative for Pediatric Palliative Care, Center for Applied Ethics and Professional Practice, Education Development Center, Inc., Newton, Massachusetts.

The Johns Hopkins University Press
2715 North Charles Street
Baltimore, Maryland 21218-4363
www.press.jhu.edu

Library of Congress Cataloging-in-Publication Data

Palliative care for infants, children, and adolescents : a practical handbook / edited by Brian S. Carter and Marcia Levetown ; foreword by Kathleen M. Foley.

    p. ;   cm.

    Includes bibliographical references and index.

    ISBN 0-8018-7969-8 (hardcover : alk. paper) — ISBN 0-8018-8005-X (pbk. : alk. paper)

    1. Terminally ill children—Care—Handbooks, manuals, etc. 2. Palliative treatment—Handbooks, manuals, etc. [DNLM: 1. Palliative Care—methods—Adolescent. 2. Palliative Care—methods—Child. 3. Palliative Care—methods—Infant. 4. Terminal Care—methods—Adolescent. 5. Terminal Care—methods—Child. 6. Terminal Care—methods—Infant. 7. Chronic Disease—Adolescent. 8. Chronic Disease—Child. 9. Chronic Disease—Infant. WS 200 P167 2004] I. Carter, Brian S., 1957– II. Levetown, Marcia, 1960–

    RJ249.P356 2004

    362.17′5′083—dc22   2004003175

A catalog record for this book is available from the British Library.

CONTENTS

FOREWORD

In 1993, a World Health Organization (WHO) committee drafted guidelines to ensure humane, compassionate care for children with life-limiting illness, specifically cancer. This WHO monograph, *Cancer Pain Relief and Palliative Care for Children,* called attention to the needs of children, infants, and adolescents with cancer for pain relief, symptom management, and treatment of their psychological distress. WHO advocated a three-pronged approach to facilitate the integration of palliative care into health care delivery systems and reform health care policies, to provide professional and public education, and to make available drugs for pain and palliative care.

Since then, increasing attention has focused on not only the needs of children with cancer but also the needs of all children with serious illnesses, ranging from HIV/AIDS to genetic and neurodegenerative diseases, from neonates to adolescents. Joining with WHO, international health care policy and medical organizations—including the Council of Europe, the European Union, and various European and American professional medical and nursing organizations—have adopted the proposition that pediatric palliative care needs to be an essential aspect of medical care services. This point was made most emphatically in the 2003 Institute of Medicine (IOM) report entitled "When Children Die." The IOM's interdisciplinary panel of pediatric experts framed their consensus about the need to improve care for children by stating that "children with fatal and potentially fatal conditions and their families fail to receive competent, compassionate and consistent care to meet their physical, emotional and spiritual needs." This evidence-based report emphasized that there is an existing body of knowledge that could, if applied, readily improve the care of children and their families. Like the WHO monograph, the IOM report called for professional education, policy reform, increased public awareness, and research focused on addressing the palliative care needs of children and their families, ranging from symptom management to grief and bereavement programs.

Yet significant barriers—attitudinal, educational, and institutional—prevent children from receiving the care that they deserve. This clinical handbook addresses the educational challenges set forth in the IOM report. It is a compendium of educational material uniquely edited to facilitate health care professionals' understanding of how to think about, talk with, and practice caring for the seriously ill child with competency and compassion. Each chapter weaves into the text a brief clinical scenario in a cogent, readable style, articulating the important issues and reviewing assessment and management strategies.

The chapters are rich in their emphasis on physician, patient, and family communication and even model useful dialogue. In contrast to other texts that present such material abstractly, this handbook contextualizes the information using a case-based method. This approach is effective in describing and differentiating what the facts are and in identifying the elements of a successful clinical encounter (namely, wisdom, judgment, empathy, and compassion). The handbook also fosters sophisticated thinking about the process of decision making.

The interdisciplinary teams of chapter authors frame the information in a pragmatic and integrative manner. Reading each of the chapters is like sitting with a master teacher. You hear the focused attention on the details of the case but you learn much more than the facts. You learn how to think about the issues, not merely the solution or the treatment protocol. What this handbook does so well is to emphasize the work of the interdisciplinary team in providing care and to recognize that the secret of caring for children is in caring for them, their parents, their siblings, their caregivers, and their health care professionals. This brilliant clinical handbook is an extraordinary resource, an educational tool that clinicians can use to educate themselves. Why is it so important that health care professionals who care for children learn pediatric palliative care? I learned the answer to this question from poignant interviews with parents whose children did not receive appropriate, humane palliative care. Parents entrust their seriously ill children to the care of a physician and an interdisciplinary team. They believe that the care their child receives will be the best care. We can assure these parents that this is so only if health care professionals have the skills and knowledge to integrate symptom management and psychological support into the difficult and emotionally wrenching situations of caring for a seriously ill dying child.

From a positive perspective, this clinical handbook is only one initiative in a series of ongoing efforts to advance palliative care for children. There are a growing number of pediatric health care professionals with special expertise in pediatric palliative care. The American Academy of Pediatrics, the National Hospice and Palliative Care Organization, the American Academy of Hospice and Palliative Medicine, the Hospice and Palliative Care Nursing Association, and the Association of Social Work Oncologists have developed initiatives to educate their members in the principles and practice of palliative care.

The challenge going forward is to create a seamless health care system, integrating the best in innovation with the best in palliation. In this way, we can assure children and their caregivers that we deserve their trust by meeting their needs for palliative care.

Kathleen M. Foley, M.D.
Professor of Neurology, Neurosurgery and Clinical Pharmacology
Weill Medical School of Cornell University;
Attending Neurologist, Pain and Palliative Care Service
Memorial Sloan-Kettering Cancer Center;
Director of Palliative Care Initiative, Open Society Institute

PREFACE

The practice of pediatric medicine, rich with the dynamic lives of infants, children, and adolescents and their individual dreams, goals, and experiences, is a privilege known by thousands of pediatricians and other child health professionals. Inherent in the practice is a hopefulness and a sense of potentiality. The daily lives of child health care professionals are filled with opportunities to encourage parents and children and to be encouraged themselves; to advocate for children's interests in private, public, and policy forums; and to educate children, their families, and society about pediatric and public health.

Less frequently, pediatric health care professionals must deal with a child who has a life-limiting or life-threatening condition. Children with complex chronic conditions may present to the clinic, emergency department, or delivery room with an acute health deterioration or may even be in the throes of death. In these situations, pediatric health professionals are called on to discern the best action, individualized to the patient and family within the context of current social and cultural values. A knowledge of the epidemiology, science, and natural history of such diseases, exquisite symptom assessment and management, effective and empathic communication skills, and the ability to negotiate critical collaborative decision making are essential to the appropriate delivery of care for such patients.

Indeed, optimal, essential, and compassionate care for children living with life-limiting or life-threatening conditions requires more than science. This handbook provides facts and figures, data, and relevant clinical instruction from numerous experienced clinicians from across the United States and abroad, to help the reader assist children and families in their most dire circumstances. A clinical handbook of this type has not previously been available. But the reader must be aware that, when dealing with critically ill children and their families, being a physician, a healer, also means being a fellow human—one who can share life's journey with each patient and family.

To be as available as our patients need us to be, pediatric health professionals need to be able to recognize and mitigate caregiver fatigue and burnout. We believe we can best reorient ourselves to this world's needy children by not viewing them as broken—for if we do, we will soon realize that we are unable to "fix" them all. Nor should we see each child or family as a "problem" needing to be solved—because we will not be able to solve them all. Rather, we should look at each child and family as affording an opportunity for us to provide service. The provision of this service (of whatever size or capacity) can enable each of us to go to bed fulfilled each night, knowing that we have done a meaningful good.

Finally, we believe that the presence, the virtue, and the power of love bring us to the bedside of the critically ill or dying child, or to the graveside of that child upon his or her death, just as love brings us to the clinic, the office, and the hospital each day. We would ask you, the readers of this handbook, to learn from the science and clinical content that follows, but also to take with you to each child's bedside your humanness, the posture of a servant, and the majesty of love—for the children, for their families, and for your colleagues.

CONTRIBUTORS

Marylene Audet, Montreal, Quebec, Canada

Anita Catlin, D.N.Sc., F.N.P., Associate Professor of Nursing, Sonoma State University, Rohnert Park, California

Susan Cohen, M.A., A.D.T.R., C.C.L.S., Supervisor, Child Life–Creative Arts Therapy, Tomorrow's Children Institute, Hackensack University Medical Center, Hackensack, New Jersey

Stephen R. Connor, Ph.D., Vice President, National Hospice and Palliative Care Organization, Alexandria, Virginia

Lynn Czarniecki, M.S.N., C.N.S., Advance Practice Nurse, Department of Pediatrics, New Jersey Medical School, Newark, New Jersey

Betty Davies, R.N., Ph.D., Professor and Chair, Department of Family Health Care Nursing, University of California at San Francisco, San Francisco, California

Deborah Dokken, M.P.A., Parent and Family Advocate, Chevy Chase, Maryland

Dale Evans, R.N., Ph.D., Vice President, Hospice and Community Services, Community Nursing Services, Salt Lake City, Utah

Chris Feudtner, M.D., Ph.D., M.P.H., Director of Research and Attending Physician for PACT (Palliative Care Team), Division of

General Pediatrics, Children's Hospital of Philadelphia, Philadelphia, Pennsylvania

W. Jeffrey Flowers, M.Div., Director of Pastoral Counseling, Medical College of Georgia Hospital and Clinics, Augusta, Georgia

Joel Frader, M.D., Professor of Pediatrics, Medical Ethics, and Humanities, Northwestern University, Children's Memorial Hospital, Chicago, Illinois

Gerri Frager, R.N., M.D., F.R.C.P.C., Medical Director, Pediatric Palliative Care Service, IWK Health Centre, Halifax, Nova Scotia, Canada

David R. Freyer, D.O., Associate Professor of Pediatrics and Human Development, Michigan State University College of Human Medicine; Division of Pediatric Hematology-Oncology and Bone Marrow Transplantation, DeVos Children's Hospital, Grand Rapids, Michigan

Sarah Friebert, M.D., Director, Division of Pediatric Palliative Care, Children's Hospital of Akron, Akron, Ohio

J. Russell Geyer, M.D., Professor of Pediatrics, Division of Hematology-Oncology, Children's Hospital and Regional Medical Center, Seattle, Washington

Mary Jo Gilmer, R.N., M.B.A., Ph.D., Associate Professor of Nursing, Vanderbilt University School of Nursing, Nashville, Tennessee

Sam Grubman, M.D., Pediatrician, Department of Pediatrics, Saint Vincent's Hospital, New York, New York

Maria Gudmundsdottir, R.N., Ph.D., Postgraduate Research Faculty, Department of Family Health Care Nursing, University of California at San Francisco School of Nursing, San Francisco, California

Richard Hain, M.B.B.S., M.D., M.Sc., M.R.C.P., F.R.C.P.C.H., Senior Lecturer in Paediatric Palliative Care, University of Wales College of Medicine, Llandough Hospital, Cardiff, Wales

Geraldine Haynes, R.N., B.S.N., Nursing and Palliative Care Consultant, Kirkland, Washington

Ross M. Hays, M.D., Professor, Departments of Rehabilitation Medicine and Pediatrics, University of Washington School of Medicine, and Director, Palliative Care Consulting Service, Children's Hospital and Medical Center, Seattle, Washington

Joanne M. Hilden, M.D., Chair, Department of Pediatric Hematology-Oncology, and Medical Director, Pediatric Palliative Care, The Children's Hospital at The Cleveland Clinic, Cleveland, Ohio

Bruce P. Himelstein, M.D., F.A.A.P., Pediatric Palliative Care Program Director, Children's Hospital of Wisconsin; Associate Professor, Division of Hematology-Oncology, Department of Pediatrics, Medical College of Wisconsin, Milwaukee, Wisconsin

Steven R. Leuthner, M.D., M.A., Associate Professor of Pediatrics and Bioethics, Medical College of Wisconsin, Milwaukee, Wisconsin

Tiffany Levinson, R.N., M.S., F.N.P., Stem Cell Transplant Nurse Practitioner, Children's Memorial Hospital, Chicago, Illinois

Stephen Liben, M.D., F.R.C.P., Director, Palliative Care Program, Montreal Children's Hospital, Montreal, Quebec, Canada

Yarrow McConnell, B.Sc., Student, Faculty of Medicine, Dalhousie University, Halifax, Nova Scotia, Canada

Elaine Morgan, M.D., Associate Professor of Pediatrics, Department of Hematology-Oncology, Children's Memorial Hospital, Northwestern University, Chicago, Illinois

Jason Morrow, M.D., Ph.D., University of Texas Medical Branch, Galveston, Texas

James Oleske, M.D., M.P.H., François-Xavier Bagnoud Professor of Pediatrics, and Director, Division of Pulmonary, Allergy, Immunology, and Infectious Diseases, Department of Pediatrics, New Jersey Medical School, Newark, New Jersey

Stacy F. Orloff, Ed.D., L.C.S.W., Manager, Child and Family Support Program, The Hospice of the Florida Suncoast, Largo, Florida

Anthony Perszyk, M.D., Geneticist and Pediatrician, Division of Genetics, Nemours Children's Clinic, Jacksonville, Florida

Sara Perszyk, R.N., B.S.N., Pediatric Palliative Care and Hospice Nurse, Child and Family Support Program, The Hospice of the Florida Suncoast, Largo, Florida

Kathleen Quance, M.S., C.C.L.S., Counselor, Child and Family Support Program, The Hospice of the Florida Suncoast, Largo, Florida

Cynda H. Rushton, D.N.Sc., R.N., F.A.A.N., Associate Professor of Nursing, Faculty, Phoebe Berman Bioethics Institute, and Coordinator, Harriet Lane Compassionate Care, Johns Hopkins University and Children's Center, Baltimore, Maryland

John M. Saroyan, M.D., Fellow, Pediatric Pain and Anesthesia, College of Physicians and Surgeons, Columbia University, New York, New York

Carson Strong, Ph.D., Professor of Human Values and Ethics, University of Tennessee Health Sciences Center, Memphis, Tennessee

Lizabeth Sumner, R.N., B.S.N., Director of the Children's Program, San Diego Hospice Corporation, San Diego, California

Suzanne Toce, M.D., Professor of Pediatrics, St. Louis University; Attending Neonatologist, Cardinal Glennon Children's Hospital, St. Louis, Missouri

Erwin Veale Jr., M.Div., Associate Director of Pastoral Care and Counseling, and Chaplain, Children's Medical Center, Medical College of Georgia Health, Inc., Augusta, Georgia

Sharon Weinstein, M.D., Director of Pain Medicine and Palliative Care, Huntsman Cancer Institute, University of Utah, Salt Lake City, Utah

Janice Wheeler, M.Ed., President and Founder, Project Joy and Hope for Texas, Pasadena, Texas

J. William Worden, M.Ed., Ph.D., Professor of Psychology, Rosemead Graduate School of Psychology, Laguna Niguel, California

PART I

SOCIETAL AND
INSTITUTIONAL ISSUES

Epidemiology and Health Services Research

Chris Feudtner, M.D., Ph.D., M.P.H., and Stephen R. Connor, Ph.D.

A team of pediatric health care providers—a social worker, a psychologist, a nurse, and a physician—convenes to design a new palliative and end-of-life care service for infants, children, and adolescents. Each member of the team has had extensive experience caring for youngsters living with life-limiting conditions. They realize, however, that their plans for this service will be best informed not by personal encounters but by a systematic review of the medical literature appraising several key issues. They ask themselves the following questions:

- How can we define and identify the children we seek to serve?
- What are the demographic characteristics of children who live with and ultimately die from life-limiting conditions?
- What medical conditions do they have?
- Where do they die?
- What kinds of health care services do they currently receive, and what might they and their families need that they do not currently get?
- How are the answers to these questions changing over time, so we can plan for the future?

The Problem of Case Definition

One of the first difficulties that the palliative care team encounters is that each member has a different notion of which children should be served and under what circumstances. The consensus among medical colleagues, hospital administrators, and third-party payers is that the need for a clear target population is urgent yet still elusive.

Who needs palliative care? Any systematic attempt to study or improve the provision of pediatric palliative care must grapple with this question. The most common answer is that children who "will die" need palliative care. Although this appears to be straightforward, in practice it is not, for four reasons.

The first reason arises from ambiguity in the phrase *will die.* We all will die; what is usually meant when one says that someone will die is that death is likely to occur within a certain time frame. These aspects of the terms *will die* and *dying*—time frame and probability—are not specified. Is a person who faces an 80 percent likelihood of death in the next four weeks "dying"? What if over the next six months the probability of death for that person were to climb to 97 percent, as could be the case if the person had relapsed cancer? What if the person had a 97 percent chance of death but only over the next ten years, as happens with neurodegenerative disorders: is this person dying? Finally, if a person has a persistently elevated risk of death because of a static injury or condition such as severe cerebral palsy with seizures and swallowing dysfunction, is this person dying? Each of these scenarios involves distinct and common patterns of how the risk of death varies over time, based on the underlying disease or injury (fig. 1.1). In each case, health care professionals would quite likely give different answers to the question of whether the person is dying, based on their experience and, more important, on their individual personalities, values, and beliefs. No consensus exists to clarify how high the probability of death needs to be, and over what time frame, for the term *dying* to be applied consistently.

The second reason stems from the ambiguity of the term *need.* Suppose it was known for sure that receipt of palliative care services would improve the quality of a child's remaining life by 20 percent. Would that child "need" palliative care? How much does a child have to benefit from a service before that service is seen as a need? This question is further complicated by potential trade-offs between the therapeutic goals of life extension and quality-of-life enhancement: under what circumstances does a person benefit more from improvement in quality of life if securing this benefit potentially entails a shorter life span?

The third reason is the uncertainty that surrounds all attempts to predict the future, particularly medical prognosis. Even for expert clinicians, prognostication is not an exact science. The probability that any particular person

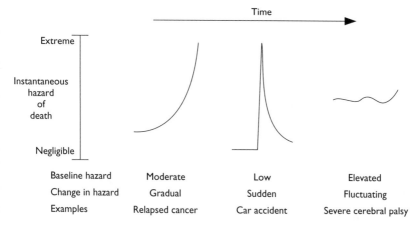

Figure 1.1. Hazard of death varies over time depending on underlying condition.

will die during a given time frame, let alone how much this person would benefit from palliative care services, is impossible to estimate with certainty. This uncertainty in both realms hinders many physicians from raising end-of-life issues with their patients and making suitable, individualized plans.

To provide a systematized answer to the question, "Who needs palliative care?" the ambiguous aspects of the terms *dying* and *need*—the probability of death and the benefit from palliative care—along with the attendant uncertainty must be addressed in a rigorous manner. These issues can be thought of as key dimensions of any case definition, as they are important, definable, and potentially measurable (fig. 1.2).

Several groups have championed the case definition of those in need of pediatric palliative care as children who are living with life-threatening conditions. This definition avoids the general reluctance in American culture to apply the word *dying* to any child and, more important, acknowledges the need to apply palliative care earlier than the phase of life considered to be the "dying" phase; nevertheless, the phrase "living with life-threatening conditions" has the same definitional ambiguities discussed above and will need further clarification.

The fourth reason that the statement "children who are dying need palliative care" can lead to problems in clinical practice emanates from the artificial boundaries separating palliative care from other forms of medical care, especially a mode of care called "curative" (fig. 1.3). Over the past decade,

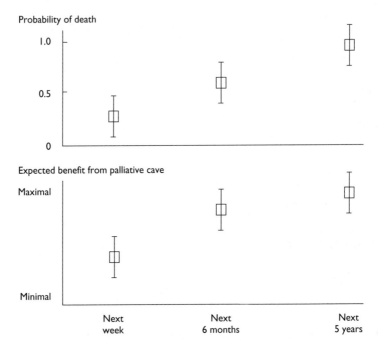

Figure 1.2. Case definition.

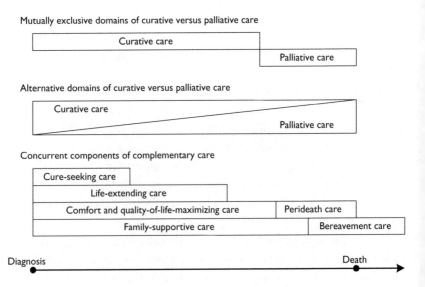

Figure 1.3. Models of care over the course of life-threatening illness.

health care professionals attuned to the needs of patients living with life-threatening conditions have emphasized that curative (or life-prolonging) and palliative care are not mutually exclusive; a gradual transition can be made over time to a greater proportion of care in the palliative mode.

For many children who die, however, cure—meaning the eradication of the disease or normalization of the underlying condition—was never possible or becomes impossible. Instead, medical care for these children consists largely or exclusively of life-extending therapy and of comfort or therapy that enhances the quality of life. Often, trade-offs have to be struck between these types of treatment, though some therapies that prolong life also promote comfort, as is the case with antibiotics used to treat people with severe lung disease from cystic fibrosis. Grappling successfully with therapeutic trade-offs and "double effects" (a bioethics phrase describing a situation in which a single action causes two things to happen, one desired and the other potentially not) is aided by a clearer sense of the goals of care, be they to eradicate disease, extend life, enhance comfort, promote quality of life in other realms, or support the family. Because these goals are not mutually exclusive, understanding of the care that can be provided is hindered if the model used is based on mutually exclusive curative and palliative modes of care.

These definitional difficulties pertain to efforts to prospectively identify children who will benefit from palliative care. Case definitions for retrospective studies have different but related challenges that affect both generalizability and accuracy. Typically, retrospective studies examine the experiences of children who have died owing to a specific cause, such as cancer, or in a particular place, such as a neonatal intensive care unit. Because of their focus on certain causes or places, these studies have been based on only a portion of the entire population of dying children and tend therefore to overrepresent the final stages of living with a life-threatening illness (since children living with life-threatening conditions who did not die during the study period were not included). Additionally, retrospective studies of the experiences of children before death—using either medical chart reviews or interviews with family and caregivers following the child's death—are hampered by incomplete or recall-biased information, which makes accurate determination of palliative care needs and even accurate description of goals difficult.

One methodological approach to surmounting the problems of generalizability is to extend the study to the broad population of children who have died, using data at the state or national level or within a varied assortment of children's hospitals. Much of the information presented in the remainder of this chapter is based on this approach, using data from vital records and administrative hospital discharge records. A generic definition of *complex chronic conditions* (CCC)—medical conditions that can be reasonably expected to last at least twelve months, unless death intervenes, and either to involve several different organ systems or to involve one organ system severely enough to require specialty pediatric care, with a likelihood of some period of hospitalization in a tertiary care center—led to the creation of a list of diagnoses used to identify children whose deaths might have been fore-seeable. While this method is limited by the incomplete information contained in large data sets, it offers a reasonable assessment of the epidemiology and health service use of children who die.

Deaths

While acknowledging the lack of a precise case definition, the team forges ahead with greater clarity regarding various aspects of the concept of pediatric palliative care. To envision the kinds of children who might be enrolled in their service, they decide first to examine the characteristics of children who have died over the past several years. In the United States in the year 2000, a total of 53,728 children and adolescents died between birth and 19 years of age (table 1.1). This count reflects a fairly steady annual decline, from 85,135 deaths in 1980 to 69,429 deaths in 1990. Several aspects of these mortality data have implications for pediatric palliative care.

AGE

The preponderance of deaths in 2000 occurred among infants (52.1% of all deaths during childhood). According to similar national data from 1997 (fig. 1.4), just over one-quarter of the deaths (26.6%) occurred within the first week of life (typically, within the first twenty-four hours of life), while another quarter (23.6%) occurred between the end of week 1 and the first birthday.

CONDITIONS

Child and adolescent deaths are caused by a wide variety of conditions. In 1997 cancer, which is perhaps the stereotypical condition associated with palliative care, accounted for 154 (0.5% of 28,045 total) infant deaths and 2,368 (8.5% of 27,834) deaths occurring past infancy. Cancer, however, constitutes only a fraction of potentially life-threatening conditions. Complex

Table 1.1. Causes of pediatric deaths, United States, 2000

Age	Cause	Number	Percentage	Rate[a]
Less than 1 year	Congenital and chromosomal anomalies	5,779	20.7	142.2
	Short gestation and low birth weight	4,299	15.4	105.8
	Sudden infant death syndrome	2,151	7.7	52.9
	Maternal complications of pregnancy	1,372	4.9	33.8
	Complications of placenta, cord, membranes	1,028	3.7	25.3
	Respiratory distress syndrome	1,018	3.6	25.0
	Accidents (unintentional injuries)	826	3.0	20.3
	Bacterial sepsis of newborn	723	2.6	17.8
	Intrauterine hypoxemia and birth asphyxia	642	2.3	15.8
	Diseases of the circulatory system	632	2.3	15.5
	Other	9,513	33.8	234.0
	TOTAL	27,983	100.0	688.4
1–4 years	Accidents (unintentional injuries)	1,780	36.0	11.7
	Congenital and chromosomal anomalies	471	9.5	3.1
	Malignant neoplasms	393	8.0	2.6
	Assault (homicide)	318	6.4	2.1
	Diseases of the heart	169	3.4	1.1
	Other	1,811	36.7	12.0
	TOTAL	4,942	100.0	32.6
5–9 years	Accidents (unintentional injuries)	1,341	41.1	6.8
	Malignant neoplasms	502	15.4	2.5
	Congenital and chromosomal anomalies	200	6.1	1.0
	Assault (homicide)	144	4.4	0.7
	Diseases of the heart	102	3.1	0.5
	Other	973	29.9	5.0
	TOTAL	3,262	100.0	16.5
10–14 years	Accidents (unintentional injuries)	1,538	37.7	7.7
	Malignant neoplasms	515	12.6	2.6
	Intentional self-harm (suicide)	292	7.2	1.5
	Assault (homicide)	221	5.4	1.1
	Congenital and chromosomal anomalies	187	4.6	0.9
	Other	1,325	32.5	6.7
	TOTAL	4,078	100.0	20.5

(continued)

Table 1.1. *(continued)*

Age	Cause	Number	Percentage	Rate[a]
15–19 years	Accidents (unintentional injuries)	6,573	48.8	33.1
	Assault (homicide)	1,861	13.8	9.4
	Intentional self-harm (suicide)	1,574	11.7	7.9
	Malignant neoplasms	725	5.4	3.6
	Diseases of the heart	372	2.8	1.9
	Other	2,358	17.5	11.8
	TOTAL	13,463	100.0	67.7

Source: Adapted from Hoyert et al. (2001, 1250, 1252).
[a] Infant rates are per 100,000 live births; for children 1 year or older, per 100,000 population in specified group.

	0–6 days	7–364 days	1–9 years	10–19 years	Total
Complex chronic conditions	3,523	3,719	2,835	2,866	12,943 (23.2%)
Other causes	11,336	9,467	6,311	15,822	42,936 (76.8%)
Total	14,859 (26.6%)	13,186 (23.6%)	9,146 (16.4%)	18,688 (33.4%)	55,879 (100%)

Figure 1.4. Pediatric deaths, by age and underlying cause, United States, 1997.
Source: Data from Feudtner et al. (2001).

chronic heart conditions, for instance, caused 2,386 (8.5%) infant and 1,132 (4.1%) child deaths, while neuromuscular conditions caused 1,038 (3.7%) infant and 1,244 (4.5%) child deaths. Altogether, approximately one-quarter (23.2%) of all childhood deaths in 1997 resulted from CCC (Feudtner et al. 2001).

Meanwhile, beyond infancy, trauma of various types (such as motor vehicle crashes, suicide, homicide, or drowning) was the major cause of death. While many traumatic deaths occur abruptly, not all do. Children who receive any medical care before dying from trauma are potential candidates for palliative care. Furthermore, all families whose children die from trauma warrant bereavement care, often requiring care of substantial intensity and duration.

MORTALITY RATES AND TRENDS OVER TIME

Improvements in child health and health care have, overall, decreased mortality rates associated with complex chronic conditions over the past few decades. Between 1979 and 1997, the annual rate of death owing to complex chronic conditions declined in varying degrees for almost every age group (ranging from a 7.1% decline for infants with cancer to a 49.9% decline for 1- to 4-year-olds dying from noncancer CCC). The notable exception regarded mortality attributed to noncancer CCC among 20- to 24-year-olds, for whom the rate of death was estimated to have increased by 11.6 percent over this eighteen-year interval (Feudtner et al. 2001). This observation fits the pattern of smaller declines in mortality over time seen in older age groups. One hypothesis to explain this finding is that advances in life-extending medical therapy is postponing what proves ultimately to be unavoidable early death. If this hypothesis is borne out, then pediatric palliative care may be applicable to children for longer periods of time or at older ages. Indeed, palliative care services will need to ensure that children living with life-threatening conditions who survive to adulthood do not fall between the cracks of the pediatric and adult worlds of medical care. For this reason, studies of pediatric deaths and palliative care should include experiences of young adults, into their twenties or thirties, who die from conditions with congenital or childhood onset.

ESTIMATED PREVALENCE AND TRENDS OVER TIME

For the United States, there are as yet no reliable data regarding the prevalence of children living with life-threatening conditions. The number of deaths

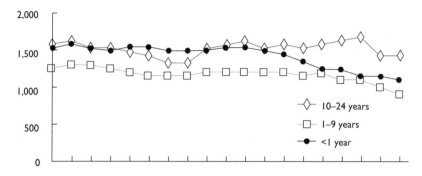

Noncancer deaths

—◇— 10–24 years
—□— 1–9 years
—●— <1 year

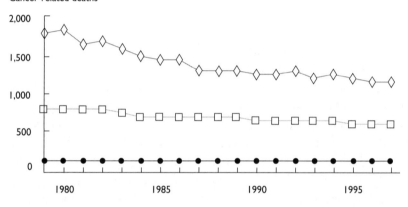

Cancer-related deaths

Figure 1.5. Average number of children within six months of death from complex chronic conditions, by cause of death, United States, 1979–1997.
Source: Data from Feudtner et al. (2001).

owing to these conditions does, however, provide a surrogate measure. Focusing on deaths caused by CCC, we can estimate the number of potential palliative care service days for children living with life-threatening conditions in the United States by retrospectively calculating the number of children who were living with such conditions on a particular day who subsequently died in the ensuing six-month period (fig. 1.5). Between 1979 and 1997, these numbers have generally trended downward, especially for deaths owing to cancer among the 10- to 24-year-old age group. By contrast, the numbers for deaths owing to noncancer CCC among this same group have remained fairly constant (Feudtner et al. 2001).

Another useful prevalence measure focuses on the deaths that occur within children's hospitals, as this allows one to determine how many children in a hospital would potentially benefit from skillful palliative care. A study of sixty children's hospitals for the years 1991, 1994, and 1997 finds hospitals reporting 50 to 99 deaths a year had, on a typical day, 3.5 patients (median value) who subsequently died; hospitals reporting 100 to 149 deaths a year had 5.0 terminally ill patients on a typical day; and in hospitals with 150 or more pediatric deaths a year, 7.0 patients on a typical day did not survive to discharge (Feudtner et al. 2002).

Location at the Time of Death

The team next considers whether their services should be designed to be mostly inpatient (following the model of many hospital-based adult palliative care services) or outpatient (following the model of hospice services) or both. They also wonder whether most of the hospitalized patients requiring palliative care are likely to be located in the intensive care units or elsewhere in the hospital. To assess these questions, they examine where children were when they died.

Few data exist regarding the location of children at the time of their death. A study in Washington State reveals that from 1980 to 1998, most deaths owing to CCC occurred in the hospital, overwhelmingly so for infants (fig. 1.6). Deaths in the emergency department or during transportation accounted for 2.1 percent of all infant deaths and 4.8 percent of all deaths of children between 1 and 25 years of age. Among older children who die of CCC, the proportion of patients dying at home rose during this period from 21 percent to 43 percent. Children residing in wealthier neighborhoods were significantly more likely to die at home (Feudtner, Silveira, and Christakis 2002).

Several case series reveal that location of children's deaths within hospitals varies by hospital. In one university teaching hospital in Chicago, 82 percent of children's deaths occurred in the pediatric intensive care unit, 13 percent in operating rooms, and 5 percent on the general wards (deaths occurring in the emergency department were not examined) (Lantos, Berger, and Zucker 1993). An Australian hospital reported that only 24 percent of its pediatric patients who died while in the hospital did so in the intensive care unit, while 36 percent died in the emergency department (Ashby et al. 1991). In a hospital in the Netherlands, by contrast, 71 percent of inpatient children's deaths

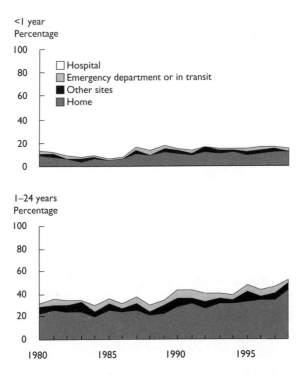

Figure 1.6. Location of pediatric deaths owing to complex chronic conditions, by age at time of death, Washington State, 1980–1998 (percentage).
Source: Data from Feudtner, Silveira, and Christakis (2002).

occurred in the pediatric intensive care unit, and 7 percent in the operating room (newborns and patients dying in the emergency department were excluded) (van der Wal et al. 1999). Eighty-three percent of children who died in one Canadian hospital died in the intensive care unit (McCallum, Byrne, and Bruera 2000).

Overall, then, among the populations studied, most children who died were in the hospital at the time of their death, and more often than not in the intensive care unit setting. With time and alterations in payments and service structures, these patterns may change.

Symptoms and Suffering

The relief of suffering and bothersome symptoms for children living with life-threatening conditions and their families is the team's primary mandate.

To prepare for this clinical mission, they wonder: What kinds of symptoms and which forms of suffering will their patients most likely have?

Several retrospective studies have sought to describe the epidemiology of symptoms and suffering among children who die. In one study, the parents of 89 percent of the 103 children who died from cancer after treatment in Boston, interviewed on average three years after the death, recalled that their children had suffered substantially from one or more symptoms during the last month of life, with pain, fatigue, dyspnea, and poor appetite being the most prevalent, followed by nausea, vomiting, constipation, and diarrhea, each of which affected 40 percent or more of these patients. Attempts to ameliorate symptoms, as judged retrospectively by the parents, were dramatically unsuccessful (Wolfe et al. 2000). A similar study interviewed bereaved parents of 44 children six months to two and a half years after the child's death, following treatment at a California pediatric tertiary care center for various conditions. These parents also emphasized the importance—and suboptimal achievement—of pain management (Contro et al. 2002). A hospice in England reviewed the records of 30 children who had died in the inpatient hospice setting. Although the overwhelming majority of these children died of neurologic conditions, during the last month of life most of the children still experienced pain, and a substantial minority experienced dyspnea, cough, excessive oral secretions, seizures, muscle spasms, anorexia, nausea or vomiting, and constipation (Hunt 1990).

Family members—parents and siblings—have been observed to suffer from a broad array of psychological and physical forms of distress. Parents report depression and feelings of grief, guilt, and anxiety as well as physical problems such as insomnia, headache, and musculoskeletal pain. Siblings struggle with fears, sensations of isolation, school and social difficulties, and resulting behavior problems (Mulhern, Lauer, and Hoffmann 1983; Sirkia, Saarinen-Pihkala, and Hovi 2000). Although data are limited, bereaved parents do not seem to divorce more often than the general population (Lansky et al. 1978).

Whether the impact of a child's death on parents and siblings differs between families whose child died in the hospital and families whose child died at home, in the context of special supportive care services, is still unclear. No randomized studies have been performed, so conclusions are at best tentative. One set of follow-up studies suggests that parents who provided home care for their dying child fared better, with subsequent healthier patterns of adjustment (Lauer et al. 1983, 1989; Mulhern, Lauer, and Hoffmann 1983).

Other investigators have found no substantial difference between these families and those whose children died in the hospital (Sirkia, Saarinen-Pihkala, and Hovi 2000).

Receipt of Health Care

With a clearer understanding of the demographic characteristics of dying children and their symptomatology (and of the problems confronted by the family), the team then turns to examine the kinds of health care that these children received before death. They believe that systematic review of the care that is typically provided will enhance the likelihood of the delivery of optimal palliative care services, as well as inform them of what services might be necessary.

Population-based studies of health care services received by children before death are scant. Data from Washington State for 1990 to 1996 reveal that 36 percent of infants and 11 percent of children and adolescents from 1 to 24 years of age who died were mechanically ventilated before death. For infants and for children and adolescents who died with underlying CCC, these proportions were, respectively, 50 percent and 19 percent. Chronically ill children and adolescents spent a median of eighteen days hospitalized during the year preceding their death, and a quarter of these cases spent nearly two months (fifty-two days or more) in the hospital (Feudtner, DiGiuseppe, and Neff 2003).

In Washington State children's hospitals during the 1990s, the mean length of stay for children who died in the hospital was 16.4 days. Looking more closely, 25 percent of the stays lasted 1 day or less, 50 percent lasted 4 days or less, 75 percent lasted 16 days or less, and 90 percent lasted 42 days or less. Among children who died without CCC, the mean length of stay was 8.7 days, whereas children with CCC had a mean length of stay of 21.4 days (Feudtner et al. 2002). The duration of terminal hospitalizations also varied across age groups (fig. 1.7), with a substantial increase for children with CCC. Mechanical ventilation was provided at some point during the hospitalization for 66 percent of neonates, 40 percent of infants, 36 percent of children, and 36 percent of adolescents. Patients with CCC were more likely than those without them to have been mechanically ventilated (across all age groups, 52% versus 46%) (Feudtner et al. 2002).

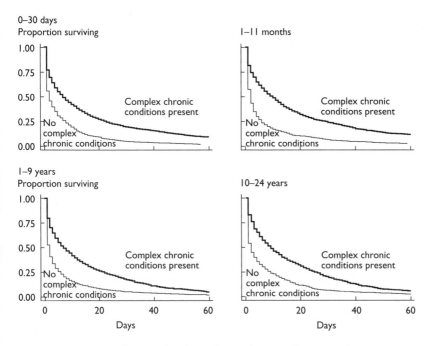

Figure 1.7. Duration of terminal pediatric hospitalizations, by age at admission, U.S. children's hospitals, 1990–1999 (percentage).
Source: Data from Feudtner et al. (2002).

Empirical health services studies may help us refine our ideas regarding modes of medical care for children with specific diseases. For example, a retrospective study of patients who died from cystic fibrosis underscored "the combination of preventive, therapeutic, and palliative care given at the end of life": three-fourths of the patients received intravenous antibiotics and oral vitamin or enzyme supplements on the day of their death (Robinson et al. 1997, 206).

Several studies have examined the proportion of children for whom medical interventions were either withheld or withdrawn before they died in hospital settings: approximately one-quarter were under do-not-resuscitate orders that limited therapy, and treatment for one-third was withdrawn (Lantos, Berger, and Zucker 1993; Vernon et al. 1993; Martinot et al. 1998; McCallum, Byrne, and Bruera 2000). Because these studies all focus on children whose death was imminent or who had already died, the true proportion of children who experience limited intervention is not known (since not all patients who have limitations of medical interventions die). A prospective survey of nurses and physicians in a pediatric intensive care unit has found that, for 63 (13%) of the 503 patients admitted over a six-month period, at least one of the providers thought that interventions (especially cardiopulmonary resuscitation and hemodialysis) should be limited. Do-not-resuscitate orders were actually written for 26 of these 63 patients, and 11 others died during their admission to the pediatric intensive care unit (Keenan et al. 2000).

Bereavement Care

Published evaluations of bereavement counseling programs for surviving parents and siblings are few in number and of limited methodological rigor. A survey of parents of infants who died after withdrawal of intervention in neonatal intensive care units in Scotland finds that follow-up meetings between attending physicians and parents within two months of the child's death occurred in only 46 percent of cases in one case series (McHaffie, Laing, and Lloyd 2001). Interviews with parents whose children had died traumatically assessed the overall benefit of a dinner meeting with staff members of a regional trauma center and fifteen "supporters" of the family; 77 percent of these parents believed that the meeting had been of continuing benefit (Oliver et al. 2001).

Conclusion

With their systematic review of the medical literature complete, the team continues the design of its palliative and end-of-life care services with a firmer sense of the characteristics of dying children and the health services they receive. They also have a keen awareness of how little is actually known in this realm.

A wise statistician once remarked that it is better to have an approximate answer to the right question than an exact answer to the wrong question (Salsburg 2001). This maxim (credited to John Tukey) could be the motto for this chapter, which recommends formulating the key questions first and then seeking the best available evidence, even though this evidence often provides only approximate answers at best.

Clearly, pediatric palliative care and end-of-life care are subjects that warrant more research. There ought to be better answers to the questions posed in this chapter. As health care providers seek information to guide the care of individual patients (using the concepts of clinical epidemiology), or to devise better systems of care at local or national levels (using population-based epidemiological or health services research), seven principles should be considered; if adhered to, these principles would, in the years to come, improve our answers to the right questions:

- *Orient on valued outcomes.* Ultimately, in our capacity as pediatric palliative care professionals we strive to improve the quality of life for children living with life-threatening conditions and the families of those children. Measures of the target population or of care processes (such as how many children died of specific conditions or were exposed to various types of medical treatments) are of value only insofar as this information is used to improve, in one way or another, outcomes that we value, such as reduction of pain or prevention of debilitating bereavement. Keeping this end in mind will quite likely enhance the impact of future epidemiological and health services research.

- *Assess costs thoroughly.* The costs involved in the evaluation of health care programs are often divided into direct costs (the money spent by the program) and indirect costs (the money spent outside of the program budget by patient and other participants, including the monetary equivalent for their time). In the evaluation of palliative care programs, the meticulous accounting of both direct and indirect costs will be crucial, as will be an understanding of how different programs impact the finances of families.

- *Evaluate rigorously.* As new techniques of individual patient-level pediatric palliative care are developed, assessment must proceed in the most rigorous manner possible—which usually means a randomized controlled trial. The same standards should apply to new systems for providing palliative and bereavement care, be they in hospital, home, or community settings.

- *Consider ethical implications.* Too often, advocates for services assert that randomized controlled trials are unethical, since the controls are not provided with the intervention that is being studied. The admirable passion of this view notwithstanding, rigorous evaluations will be the best means to determine what interventions or changes are truly beneficial for children and their families and also will be essential in convincing providers and payers to adopt new practices.

- *Keep the target population in view.* For the purposes of services planning, be it at the level of a hospital or community-based palliative care program or a national consortium examining workforce or reimbursement issues, the entire population of children living with life-threatening conditions ought to be considered, and all members given equal attention.
- *Use available data thoughtfully.* Although privacy must be scrupulously safeguarded, vital statistics records and administrative health care records offer useful data with which to define target populations, discern patterns of health care use, and identify changes in any of these parameters on an annual basis. Work in this area will also help guide the development of new and more perceptive data collection systems.
- *Reassess continuously.* The experience of children living with life-threatening conditions and their families is influenced by a broad array of interacting factors, from medical interventions through reimbursement arrangements. Because this encompassing system of "people care" is always changing, our assessment of what is occurring to whom, and with what impact, needs to be ongoing.

Authors rarely hope that their work becomes quickly obsolete; for us, this is not the case. We hope that within a decade, a cadre of investigators in pediatric palliative and end-of-life care, guided by these research principles, will have provided far superior answers to the questions posed in this chapter, to the betterment of the quality of life for children living with life-threatening conditions and for their families.

References

Ashby, M. A., R. J. Kosky, H. T. Laver, and E. B. Sims. 1991. An enquiry into death and dying at the Adelaide Children's Hospital: a useful model? *Med J Aust* 154:165–70.
Contro, N., J. Larson, S. Scofield, B. Sourkes, and H. Cohen. 2002. Family perspectives on the quality of pediatric palliative care. *Arch Pediatr Adolesc Med* 156:14–19.
Feudtner, C., D. A. Christakis, F. J. Zimmerman, J. H. Muldoon, J. M. Neff, and T. D. Koepsell. 2002. Characteristics of deaths occurring in children's hospitals: implications for supportive care services. *Pediatrics* 109:887–93.
Feudtner, C., D. L. DiGiuseppe, and J. M. Neff. 2003. Hospital care for children and young adults in the last year of life: a population-based study. *BMC Medicine* 1:3. www.biomedcentral.com/1741-7015/1/3.

Feudtner, C., R. M. Hays, G. Haynes, J. R. Geyer, J. M. Neff, and T. D. Koepsell. 2001. Deaths attributed to pediatric complex chronic conditions: national trends and implications for supportive care services. *Pediatrics* 107:e99–e103.

Feudtner, C., M. J. Silveira, and D. A. Christakis. 2002. Where do children with complex chronic conditions die? patterns in Washington State, 1980–1998. *Pediatrics* 109: 656–60.

Hoyert, D. L., M. A. Freedman, D. M. Strobino, and B. Guyer. 2001. Annual summary of vital statistics, 2000. *Pediatrics* 108:1241–55.

Hunt, A. M. 1990. A survey of signs, symptoms and symptom control in 30 terminally ill children. *Dev Med Child Neurol* 32:341–46.

Keenan, H. T., D. S. Diekema, P. P. O'Rourke, P. Cummings, and D. E. Woodrum. 2000. Attitudes toward limitation of support in a pediatric intensive care unit. *Crit Care Med* 28:1590–94.

Lansky, S. B., N. U. Cairns, R. Hassanein, J. Wehr, and J. T. Lowman. 1978. Childhood cancer: parental discord and divorce. *Pediatrics* 62:184–88.

Lantos, J. D., A. C. Berger, and A. R. Zucker. 1993. Do-not-resuscitate orders in a children's hospital. *Crit Care Med* 21:52–55.

Lauer, M. E., R. K. Mulhern, M. J. Schell, and B. M. Camitta. 1989. Long-term followup of parental adjustment following a child's death at home or hospital. *Cancer* 63:988–94.

Lauer, M. E., R. K. Mulhern, J. M. Wallskog, and B. M. Camitta. 1983. A comparison study of parental adaptation following a child's death at home or in the hospital. *Pediatrics* 71:107–12.

Martinot, A., B. Grandbastien, S. Leteurtre, A. Duhamel, and F. Leclerc. 1998. No resuscitation orders and withdrawal of therapy in French paediatric intensive care units. Groupe Francophone de Reanimation et d'Urgences Pediatriques. *Acta Paediatr* 87:769–73.

McCallum, D. E., P. Byrne, and E. Bruera. 2000. How children die in hospital. *J Pain Symptom Manage* 20:417–23.

McHaffie, H. E., I. A. Laing, and D. J. Lloyd. 2001. Follow up care of bereaved parents after treatment withdrawal from newborns. *Arch Dis Child Fetal Neonatal Ed* 84:F125–28.

Mulhern, R. K., M. E. Lauer, and R. G. Hoffmann. 1983. Death of a child at home or in the hospital: subsequent psychological adjustment of the family. *Pediatrics* 71:743–47.

Oliver, R. C., J. P. Sturtevant, J. P. Scheetz, and M. E. Fallat. 2001. Beneficial effects of a hospital bereavement intervention program after traumatic childhood death. *J Trauma* 50:440–48.

Robinson, W. M., S. Ravilly, C. Berde, and M. E. Wohl. 1997. End-of-life care in cystic fibrosis. *Pediatrics* 100:205–9.

Salsburg, D. 2001. *The lady tasting tea: how statistics revolutionized science in the twentieth century.* New York: Henry Holt.

Sirkia, K., U. M. Saarinen-Pihkala, and L. Hovi. 2000. Coping of parents and siblings with the death of a child with cancer: death after terminal care compared with death during active anticancer therapy. *Acta Paediatr* 89:717–21.

van der Wal, M. E., L. N. Renfurm, A. J. van Vught, and R. J. Gemke. 1999. Circumstances of dying in hospitalized children. *Eur J Pediatr* 158:560–65.

Vernon, D. D., J. M. Dean, O. D. Timmons, W. Banner, and E. M. Allen-Webb. 1993. Modes of death in the pediatric intensive care unit: withdrawal and limitation of supportive care. *Crit Care Med* 21:1798–802.

Wolfe, J., H. E. Grier, N. Klar, S. B. Levin, J. M. Ellenbogen, S. Salem-Schatz, E. J. Emanuel, and J. C. Weeks. 2000. Symptoms and suffering at the end of life in children with cancer. *N Engl J Med* 342:326–33.

2

Goals, Values, and Conflict Resolution

Carson Strong, Ph.D., Chris Feudtner, M.D., Ph.D., M.P.H.,
Brian S. Carter, M.D., F.A.A.P., and Cynda H. Rushton, D.N.Sc., R.N., F.A.A.N.

Few tasks in pediatrics are as challenging as caring for children with life-threatening or terminal illnesses. This challenge, unfolding over the course of a particular child's care, requires health care professionals to weave knowledge, skills, and values into an effective effort to promote the patient's quality of life and support the patient's family (table 2.1).

While this entire book strives to help us provide such care successfully, the specific aim of this chapter is to improve the way we address ethical questions related to palliative care. These questions include the following:

- When is the "right time" to discuss a poor prognosis with the patient and family?
- How should conflicts between parents and health professionals over goals of care be addressed?
- How should disagreements among health professionals about treatment decisions be handled?
- What are the obstacles to improved access to palliative care?

The Goals of Palliative Care

Pediatric palliative care is comprehensive care for infants and children who are not going to get better. Palliative care for these children is child centered yet attends to the needs of the child's entire family, striving to enhance with dignity the child's time on earth and to support the family's experience with empathy and culturally sensitive respect. Perhaps initially combined with cure-oriented or life-span-extending care, palliative care can intensify when these

Table 2.1. Steps in the provision of effective palliative care: Interplay of values, skills, and knowledge

Stage	Values	Skills	Knowledge
Understanding and appreciating the benefit of palliative care	• Respect for persons • Emphasis on quality of life • Beneficence	Training in palliative care	Understanding the causes of suffering
Recognizing patient's needs	• Patient-focused care • Beneficence	• Awareness of patient • Assessment of patient's needs and desires • Self-awareness	Signs and symptoms of suffering
Individual initiation of effort to provide palliative care	• Conviction • Fortitude	Forthright communication	Family context
Collaborative effort to provide palliative care	• Conviction • Respect for colleagues	• Forthright communication • Group facilitation • Conflict resolution • Values analysis	• Ethical principles • Colleagues potential contribution
Effective provision of palliative care	• Commitment to relief of suffering • Beneficence • Autonomy	• Assessment of the impact of care • Advocacy • Negotiation	Control of pain and symptoms

forms of care are no longer helpful or appropriate. A proactive and planned intervention, palliative care uses a team approach to prevent or relieve physical, psychological, social, emotional, and spiritual suffering while improving the quality of life for dying children and their families (World Health Organization 1990).

The provision of pediatric palliative care is necessarily interdisciplinary, because no single discipline in pediatric health care can provide all the support that the child and his or her family will require. Holistic care encompasses more than pain and symptom management; it addresses also the psychological and emotional needs of the child, at whatever stage of development, and the child's family. While palliative care may be applied within an inpatient treatment environment, its principles transcend the institutional setting and are applicable in home or outpatient care as well. Inpatient palliative care may be characterized by around-the-clock nursing assessment, physician management, and interdisciplinary support to manage symptoms that could occur in the dying child, such as pain, breathing difficulty, or seizures. These and other symptoms may persist and require attention at home by parents or other caregivers, but the holistic goals of palliative care remain the same.

Palliative care also attempts to address the spiritual needs of the family and, when applicable, the dying child. Spiritual concerns might include the interpretation of illness, dying, and death and the assignment of meaning to all that is happening. Some families approach these questions within a religious context; others seek answers outside of religion. Varied value systems, beliefs, traditions, and rituals will find their place in providing comfort for the dying child and his or her family. These spiritual dimensions also may ease the acceptance of death and the transition from life to death, with its attendant grief and process of bereavement by the family. Hospital chaplains or clergy of the family's choosing can be important members of the interdisciplinary team.

In summary, the goal of pediatric palliative care is to provide proactive, comprehensive, and holistic care to infants and children whose disease process is not amenable to cure-oriented interventions. In pursuing this goal, palliative care services support the child and family in all matters pertaining to the control of pain and other symptoms across care settings and provide necessary support in dealing with the psychosocial aspects of living with life-threatening illness, dying, and spiritual needs. Ultimately, the provision of the best quality of life for the child and family is sought.

Ethical Values in Palliative Care

The goals of palliative care are based on core values that form the basis of the relationship between the health care professional and the patient (Beauchamp and Childress 2001):

- *Beneficence:* the idea that health care professionals have a duty to promote the well-being of patients and to provide emotional support to patients' families. This gives rise to the duty to provide palliative care that addresses the well-being of the patient and family in a comprehensive way.
- *Nonmaleficence:* the principle that health care providers should avoid causing harm to others. This implies a duty to attempt to recognize when continued aggressive curative treatments are likely to cause more harm than benefit to the patient.
- *Autonomy:* the ideal that a person's self-rule be free from both the control of others and personal limitations that interfere with choice, such as lack of knowledge. The principle of autonomy implies that health care professionals have a duty to respect the autonomy of minor patients who are mentally competent to make their own decisions, to respect the moral right of parents to participate in medical decisions for their children who are not mentally competent, and, where appropriate, to respect the developing autonomy of minor patients who are not mentally competent by means such as seeking the child's assent to treatment.

Palliative care should be provided in a manner that is consistent with these autonomy-based duties. This means the inclusion of two other principles:

- *Respect for life:* The duty to preserve life is implicit in the principle of respect for life. However, it must sometimes be tempered by the duty to avoid causing harm to the patient. When curative efforts are likely to be unsuccessful and to cause more harm than benefit, the duty to avoid causing harm takes priority over the duty to prolong life. In this context, health professionals should recommend to the patient and family that caregiving be directed toward supportive care and palliation rather than measures that attempt to cure.
- *Respect for persons:* The essence of this overarching principle is that, to the extent possible, the ethical principles discussed above should be followed in dealing with terminally ill patients. Implicit in this

principle is the duty to attempt to recognize when palliative care is appropriate.

The duty to provide palliative care is thus an extension of the obligations already present in the relationship between health care professional and patient. A responsibility to provide palliative care when appropriate is inherent in the nature of the relationship.

The Nature of Ethical Problems in Palliative Care

A wide variety of situations encountered in modern health care are, in one way or another, ethically problematic. Some of these situations arise when different ethical values suggest conflicting courses of action and there is disagreement or uncertainty concerning which values should be given priority. Such cases include, for example, a situation in which the decision makers are uncertain about whether to resuscitate an infant with hypoxic brain injury who has a prognosis of severe cognitive deficit and is having episodes of bradycardia. Continued life support might cause more suffering than benefit for the child, thereby violating the principle "Do no harm." But the concern for protection of life suggests that one should err on the side of life support. Resolution of this type of ethical dilemma involves, in part, deciding which of the conflicting ethical values takes priority in the particular situation. Here, the conflict is between two competing goods—the ethical values of nonmaleficence and respect for life.

Ethical issues do not always involve a dilemma about how to prioritize values. Problems also arise when there is widespread agreement concerning what the appropriate norms of behavior are but a person or institution fails to act in accordance with those norms. Examples include treatment provided without consent, in a situation in which informed consent should and could have been obtained and a nurse who observes a physician failing to carry out a professional duty to relieve pain but feels too vulnerable to challenge the behavior. The ethical values are relevant in this case because they help to define the problem. For example, failure to obtain consent is a violation of the principle of autonomy, and failure to relieve pain is a violation of the principle of beneficence. Resolution of this second type of ethical problem often involves recognition and management of additional factors, such as power and authority (Feudtner, Christakis, and Schwartz 1996), as well as the ability to engage effectively in "difficult" conversations (Stone, Patton, and Heen 1999).

Ethical problems of both types arise in palliative care. Keeping these kinds of problems in mind can be helpful in identifying the factors that are present in various ethically problematic situations. When one is faced with an ethical problem, the values discussed above should be part of the thought process in deciding how to handle the situation.

The Main Types of Ethically Problematic Situations

The fictional clinical vignettes that follow illustrate various types of ethically problematic situations we have encountered while caring for children with life-threatening conditions. In each case, we attempt to clarify underlying values that may be in conflict and identify behaviors that are interfering with effective palliative care.

AVOIDANCE OR POSTPONEMENT OF BAD NEWS

Jason was devastatingly injured when a car struck him as he was riding his bicycle. For the past week, this teenager has developed one complication after another in the surgical intensive care unit. Because the physicians want to monitor his neurological status, they have been judicious in their use of opiates and other analgesic pain medications. Each day, outside the room, the surgical team discusses Jason's worsening prognosis in hushed tones. The attending physician, when discussing Jason's condition with the family, adopts a much more optimistic tone. He tells the team privately that "we can't take away hope from the parents" and that he will discuss withdrawal of life support when the time is right.

When is the time "right" to discuss a poor prognosis with the family?

When is it appropriate to raise the issue of reconsidering the goals of care, moving from a curative to a palliative framework?

Forthright communication given compassionately and skillful communication of bad news are of paramount importance.

The attending physician's concern about the well-being of the family derives from a beneficence-based duty to provide emotional support to the family. However, the physician's belief that giving bad news will "take away hope," and thereby constitute a failure to provide emotional support, causes him to overlook several other important ethical values. One is the parents' right to accurate information about their child's medical condition. Truthfulness is a requirement of respect for persons. If the parents are to participate in decisions about care, they need to understand the facts about the child's condition. Another value is the well-being of the patient. The delay in providing supportive care, particularly in providing adequate pain medication, may be causing the patient to suffer unnecessarily.

The physician's approach to this case is creating a conflict between these ethical values. His attempt to protect the parents from emotional distress is preventing them from receiving information to which they have a right, and it may be causing harm to the patient. This conflict need not occur. It can be argued that the attending physician's view about what needs to be done to provide emotional support is misguided. By keeping the family in the dark concerning the prognosis, the physician is setting them up for an even greater shock when the bad news is finally delivered. The family might be better able to cope if they are informed of the worsening prognosis as it develops. This will also help prepare them for a conversation about changing the goals of care, a topic that should be raised relatively soon.

Cases like Jason's are not unusual, because many physicians have not been trained in giving bad news and feel uncomfortable doing so. Many interpret such conversations as an admission of failure. The ability to communicate well and with compassion is an important part of providing good medical care. Physicians can improve their communication skills by consulting the growing body of articles and books, written by clinicians, that give advice about how best to deliver bad news (Buckman 1992). A few of the key points derived from that literature can be mentioned. The physical setting should be one that is conducive to such discussion. It should be a place that is relatively quiet, where the participants can sit down and be free from interruptions. The physician should set aside sufficient time for the meeting to allow information to be given, questions to be asked and answered, and emotional reactions of the parents to receive adequate response. In addition, clarity in conveying information is important. The physician should use terms the parents can understand and proceed at a pace that is conducive to their comprehension. Parents should be encouraged to ask questions. Moreover, there are certain things the physician can do to communicate concern and support. The physician should sit at the same level as the parents, rather than stand over them. Eye contact is important, and the physician should reassure the parents that the prognosis will not change the level of care and support for the patient and family (Creagan 1994).

When Polly's muscle biopsy results returned from the laboratory, the neurologist learned beyond a doubt that the 8-month-old girl, who had been admitted to the hospital because she was growing weaker, had Leigh syndrome. A rare and uniformly fatal disease, Leigh syndrome causes brain cells to die, and almost all patients die within a few months of diagnosis. Polly's physician notified the hospital team of the diagnosis and requested a care conference. Later that afternoon, the neurologist, along with a nurse, a social worker, and a physician-in-training, sat together with the parents in a conference room. The neurologist immediately blurted out, "Well, the test is back, and your daughter, I am afraid to say, has Leigh syndrome," then launched into a ten-minute explanation of the cause of the condition, a defect of mitochondrial metabolism. At the end of his disquisition, he asked the parents whether they had any questions; when they did not, he excused himself from the meeting, explaining that he would be happy to answer questions as they came up.

Clear and forthright communication is a sine qua non of the ethical delivery of bad news.

Cognitive clarity is only half the issue; attention to emotional support is equally important.

This is an example of the second type of ethically problematic situation discussed above—a case of a health care provider failing to act in accordance with accepted norms. The norms in question are a duty to provide information to the parents that will help them understand Polly's medical condition and a duty to provide emotional support to the family. Appropriate information includes the diagnosis and prognosis, presented in terms the parents can understand; symptoms that might be expected; types of palliative care that might be appropriate; and a discussion of any other implications of the disease for the patient and family. How much to tell at one time varies because persons differ in the amount of information they can absorb. The physician should be prepared to have more than one session to present information.

Although the provision of emotional support is an ongoing process, there are several things that can be done during a session in which bad news is delivered (Girgis and Sanson-Fisher 1995). The parents can be reassured that good care will continue without interruption and that the needs of the patient will be met. In addition, because many people cope with crisis situations by seeking information, the physician should strive to help the parents understand the information that is given to them. One should avoid devoting a great deal of time to medical details the parents do not understand. In addition, physicians in this type of situation should not hesitate to show their feelings, allowing the family to see that they are concerned about the interests of the patient and family. Body language can display warmth and sympathy. It is important to respond to expressions of grief. It may be acceptable to express concern by holding the parents' hands (though the physician should be aware of and sensitive to any cultural- or faith-specific dictums about the appropriateness or acceptance of touching). If the parents cry, expressions of sympathy followed by a period of silence might be appropriate, and facial tissue should be available.

At the end of the discussion, the physician should arrange a time in the near future to review the situation with the parents. During the interim, the physician should either be personally available or identify someone else who will be available to address any questions or concerns. The physician should ask the parents who they would like to tell about the situation and offer help in passing on the information. For example, a family meeting might be arranged.

DENIAL OF POOR PROGNOSIS

Two days ago, Alex nearly drowned. Intubated and mechanically ventilated, the 2-year-old boy is still in a profound coma. The attending physician in the pediatric intensive care unit approaches the parents, who are seated alone at Alex's bedside. She tells them about their son's medical status, pointing out that he still is deeply comatose and explaining that this is a bad prognostic sign, as virtually all children who are still comatose forty-eight hours after a near-drowning injury either never awaken or suffer severe brain damage. The parents, who have heard this information before, nod their heads slightly in apparent understanding. The attending physician then suggests that at this juncture, given the high likelihood that Alex will be permanently impaired, they should consider withdrawing ventilatory support. Stunned, the parents manage to say that no, they couldn't possibly "give up"; they are sure that their son is going to "beat the odds."

Parents' difficulty in accepting a grave prognosis and responding to it cognitively and emotionally can be crucial aspects of ethically problematic cases. Parents and professionals sometimes have a difficult time arriving at a common understanding and meaning of a child's prognosis. Health care professionals' assessment of a child's future is primarily grounded in the facts—evidence of accurate diagnosis and reliable data to support their assessment of prognosis. They expect the parents, once the information has been conveyed to them, to assign the same significance to those facts. But knowing the facts is not the same as understanding them. Parents generally understand their moral obligations as "good parents" to arise from their duty to protect the life of their child. Health care professionals can support parents in their efforts to understand the information and make sense of it by acknowledging the parents' advocacy for their child and by understanding their values and hopes concerning life, death, and disability.

THE MEANING OF HOPE

Parents' insistence on "not giving up" and their belief that their child will "beat the odds" reflect parental hope for a positive outcome despite the fact they have been told otherwise. Parental hope may appear disproportionate to the reality, yet parents need to sustain hope to endure an overwhelming situation. Hope allows resilience. To accept the reality of the child's imminent death is not to give up hope; hope may evolve as the situation unfolds. Ongoing counseling of the parents should continue to include information about prognosis but should also identify other things they can hope for, such as their child's freedom from suffering.

Alex's parents are facing the difficult task of adjusting to a changed reality and a changed future for their child and family. Parents are vulnerable during such periods, and their need for time to arrive at acceptance must be honored. Often, the health care professionals' need for closure drives them to expect that decisions will be made relatively soon. Shared decision making invites health care providers to honor the parents' need for a process that allows them to find their way to the decisions they make for their child. This approach is based on the beneficence-based duty to support the well-being of the family.

The language of "giving up" implies that beneficial interventions will not be provided. By presenting options for treatment that include a palliative focus, health care professionals have an important opportunity to clarify what can and will be done to ease the child's suffering. Options such as maintaining the current level of therapies while attending to pain, symptoms, and family needs may give families time to accept their child's new reality. When appropriate, discussion about writing a do-not-attempt-resuscitation order may begin a process of defining other limitations of treatment. In these discussions, parental values and hopes should be explored and honored.

Health care professionals in these cases must be mindful of the power imbalance between parents and professionals. As health care providers, we should attempt to avoid adversarial situations in which we feel compelled to invoke a futility policy or pursue legal action. Only rarely are such interventions necessary. Instead, health care professionals should ask themselves what is required to support this child and family during their difficult time and what measure of generosity and compassion will allow both parents and professionals to preserve their integrity.

ENTRENCHED POSITIONS

Jane, although only 3 years old, is known to everyone at the nearby children's hospital. Meconium aspiration at the time of her birth led to severe brain damage, leaving her unable to swallow anything safely, including her own saliva. Every month or two, she is readmitted to the hospital for yet another aspiration pneumonia. On two prior occasions, she became ill enough to require intubation and mechanical ventilation. These episodes, together with the injury that her lungs sustained as a newborn and the ongoing damage of chronic microaspiration, have left her with horrible lung disease. Now she is quite ill again. The staff in the pediatric intensive care unit believe that further mechanical ventilation is futile, and they are unwilling to reintubate her. When this position is explained to Jane's parents, they insist that "everything" be done for their daughter. "This isn't the first time we've been told by you doctors that she would die," they say, "and it won't be the last."

People's responses to new challenges presented by a child's evolving illness are shaped by their personal history of previous challenges, how they were handled, and what the outcomes were.

Fierce advocacy for the rights of children is one of the noblest behaviors parents exhibit.

This case represents a failure of shared decision making and the limits of professional prognostication. Jane is one of a growing number of babies who leave neonatal intensive care units to spend many years on a roller coaster of exacerbation, improvement, and near-death episodes. They often experience a chronic decline in function that may occur over a long period of time. Frequently, parents and health care professionals begin their journey together by agreeing on goals of care focused on improving the baby's chances for prolonged life. Over time, they can come to understand the meaning of "giving a child a chance for life" in different ways. Health care professionals may approach the uncertainty surrounding outcomes of these life-threatening events as evidence that further interventions should be curtailed. Alternatively, parents who have accompanied their child during these crises may see the current one as an opportunity to "beat the odds" once again. When health care professionals declare that a child will die, and turn out to have been wrong, their credibility is undermined, and this may lead to adversarial situations.

This case illustrates the importance of developing a palliative care plan from the beginning. Although Jane may live for an extended period, it is essential to establish a foundation for establishing goals, revising them, and monitoring the plan of care. Parents need to feel that they have sufficiently advocated for their child. They might believe that health care professionals are no longer committed to their child's life, focusing instead on limiting treatment and the negative aspects of the child's condition. Health care professionals often resort to this approach because they believe that parents do not understand the severity of the child's condition.

The challenge in such cases is to give a realistic assessment of the situation and at the same time respect the parent's advocacy. In cases in which persons can reasonably disagree over what is best for the child, health professionals have an autonomy-based duty to respect the parents' values. Health care professionals can share their concerns that a child might die without declaring that they *know* when a life will end. This difference in approach allows parents and professionals to remain committed to shared goals. Parents need guidance in interpreting how a current situation differs from past experiences, and they need to have their previous experiences validated and respected.

DISSENSION AMONG HEALTH CARE PROVIDERS

Rachel was born prematurely, arriving into this world at the beginning of the twenty-fifth week of gestation, weighing only six hundred grams. On the third day of her life, Rachel has suddenly become much more ill. A cranial ultrasound shows that she has had a severe hemorrhage in her brain. After discussing Rachel's prognosis and care options with the neonatologist, the parents decide to forgo further intensive care, and everyone agrees to embrace an entirely palliative mode of care. Plans are made to extubate Rachel later that day, after the family has had time to gather together and perform a meaningful ceremony. The attending physician writes the order for extubation, with a concomitant large dose of morphine to be given intravenously. The nurse, reading the order, informs the attending that she does not feel comfortable participating in euthanasia.

Does this disagreement over a medication relate more to poor communication regarding the goals of care, unacceptable intentions, or inappropriate dosing owing to a lack of knowledge?

How should disagreements between health care providers be handled?

This case raises issues about the importance of team communication and decision making. All members of the care team, particularly those who implement the decisions of others, must be engaged in clarifying the decision, the reasons supporting the decision, and the plan for implementing it. An essential part of this process is allowing team members to express their concerns and value conflicts in a respectful environment. Based on the ethical principle of autonomy, health care professionals have a right to refuse to participate in activities to which they object on grounds of conscience.

The language of euthanasia is generally used when individuals question the propriety of a decision, when they perceive that they are being asked to participate in an act they find morally objectionable, or when communication about the goals of care has been insufficient. The first step is to clarify what euthanasia means to the nurse and to understand the nature of her objection. It may be that she is unaware of the decision-making process or the ethical justification for treating pain and suffering at the end of life. Alternatively, she may be concerned about her role in the timing and circumstance of Rachel's death. She may believe that using such a large dose of narcotic gives the impression that the goal is to hasten death rather than to ease pain and suffering. This is a legitimate question that requires the team to examine its process for providing end-of-life care. The process should enable parents and professionals to be reassured about the goals of care.

If the primary goal is to relieve pain and suffering, it is ethically justifiable to accept the possibility that death might occur sooner. If Rachel has not had narcotics or is receiving a much smaller dose without evidence of discomfort, the nurse's concern may be justified. A process that incorporates an ongoing assessment of the infant's pain and suffering and uses titration of medications to achieve the desired effect might alleviate her concern. Moreover, implementing end-of-life care requires that the community of caregivers and family support one another and bear witness to the process. Embedded in the nurse's concern may be a fear of isolation and abandonment by other members of the team. While such concerns are not always articulated, end-of-life care requires attention to them.

It is possible that after clarifying the goals of care, the decision-making process, and the plan for implementing it, the nurse will continue to object on moral grounds. These objections must be taken seriously and handled in a respectful manner. The Joint Commission on Accreditation of Healthcare Organizations now requires that health care institutions have in place a process for responding to staff requests not to participate in actions they believe are morally objectionable.

GENUINE CONFUSION

Dan has mild mental retardation and a form of muscular dystrophy that in all cases causes the breathing muscles to fail sometime during early adulthood. Many people with this type of muscular dystrophy decide to have a tracheotomy and start mechanical ventilation, which can prolong life, though not indefinitely. This is what Dan's parents have envisioned happening. Now in his late adolescence, Dan is developing respiratory failure. When his doctors and parents talk to him about mechanical ventilation, however, Dan calmly yet firmly states that he does not want a "breathing tube" even though he knows that without mechanical ventilation he will die. His parents have always sought to respect Dan's autonomy, helping him make meaningful decisions for himself. In this instance, however, they believe that his anxiety regarding the "breathing tube" would be transient and that he would subsequently enjoy an acceptable quality of life for several more years if "forced" to start mechanical ventilation.

Sometimes, despite forthright dialogue, mutual goodwill, and clear communication, deciding the "right thing to do" is genuinely confusing.

In such instances, choosing among the therapeutic options under consideration often poses difficult trade-offs between ethical principles.

Clarifying these trade-offs explicitly can be helpful.

Creating new, possibly unusual, options may be pivotal.

Ethics committee consultation can be invaluable in these circumstances.

Dan's case poignantly illustrates how some circumstances create genuinely confusing ethical dilemmas. No one in this scenario is avoiding the implications of Dan's progressive illness or denying that he will someday die. Although each person who is involved has opinions regarding what should be done, no one is operating from an entrenched position, and "cooperative"— not "factious"—best describes the spirit of the conversation regarding what should be done. The problem encountered here is not rooted in personal or interpersonal behavior but rather in something else.

This "something else" is the standard bailiwick of bioethics, and this case represents a classic ethical dilemma: how can a respect for Dan's wishes regarding his care be balanced with a desire to protect what others consider his best interests? In Dan's case, this dilemma is compounded by one of the most difficult aspects of pediatric palliative care: how can we incorporate the preferences of our young or disabled patients into the decision-making process in a manner appropriate to their developmental level?

Like most genuinely confusing dilemmas, choosing among the therapeutic options being considered for Dan's care pits one set of legitimate concerns against another. If Dan's current wish is followed and no mechanical ventilation is provided, then he may die a few years sooner than he otherwise would, losing time and life experiences that he might have come to cherish. Conversely, if he is compelled by his parents and care providers to undergo a tracheotomy and start a course of mechanical ventilation, not only will his fragile autonomy have been overridden, he also may experience complications or diminishment in his quality of life that were not foreseen—and not of his choosing.

Spelling out the dilemma in clear terms—identifying not just what is at stake but how much is at stake—can help clarify where the confusion lies (Hammond, Keeney, and Raiffa 1999). The debate here does not simply boil down to autonomy versus beneficence. The dilemma hinges on a difficult question of balance and exchange: To what extent would Dan's preferences be violated in order to pursue what degree of benefit? That is, how much of Dan's autonomy would be sacrificed to secure how much longer, or better, a life? Clearly, more work can be done to clarify all of Dan's preferences regarding his care, as well as coming up with the best estimate of how life on mechanical ventilation would impact his life and that of his family.

Conscious effort to create new therapeutic options can also be pivotal. The confusing problem sometimes does not admit solution because a potential solution is not even being considered. These options may not be "standard operating procedure." For example, in Dan's case, his health care team may be unfamiliar with or simply has yet to use noninvasive mechanical ventilation, which does not require tracheotomy. A trial of noninvasive mechanical ventilation may be less threatening to Dan, so he might assent to this course of therapy. Proposal of this treatment option would respect his preferences and his autonomy while also enabling him to examine his preferences under new circumstances and perhaps come to understand them better.

There is no guarantee, however, that clarification of trade-offs or attempts to create new options will lead to resolution of the dilemma. Under such circumstances, consultation with an ethics committee can be invaluable. While asking for help from an ethics consultative service is almost never a bad idea, here it can add value in two key ways. First, the members of the committee may help to discover a "breakthrough" with the trade-off clarification or option creation process. Second, if the confusion still results in deadlock, the committee can help absorb the psychological weight of making such a difficult yet unavoidable decision, assisting all parties not simply to make the best possible decision but also to then live with it in peace.

ARTICULATE DISAGREEMENT

Sara is a newborn with hypoplastic left heart syndrome. This condition, if untreated, is always fatal. Surgery can be done to rebuild a functional heart from the existing malformed one, or a heart transplantation can be performed. Both of these surgical options entail extensive operations with prolonged hospitalization, an unknown amount of suffering, and a significant probability that the patient dies despite these efforts. Sara's parents, after learning about her condition and the treatment options from both the neonatologist and the pediatric cardiologist, decide that they want to take their daughter home and keep her as comfortable as possible until she dies. Deeply religious, they believe that the most important thing they can do for Sara is to surround her with the love of family and friends and then let God take her back, living without their daughter until they can finally rejoin her in the afterlife. The cardiologist, when informed of their decision, requests an ethics consultation, claiming that to decline potentially lifesaving cardiac surgery is tantamount to medical neglect.

Should surgery be provided, and who should make the decision? In this situation, all the parties want to do what is best for the patient, but they have differing views on what is best. Making a judgment about what is in the best interests of the infant involves a trade-off between improving the probability of long-term survival and avoiding reductions in quality of life. This case reflects the fact that reasonable people can disagree on how to weigh the duty to preserve life against the duty to avoid causing harm.

The disagreement in this case gives rise to two distinct ethical issues—a substantive issue and a procedural one. Substantive issues have to do with the question of what is the right action, such as whether or not surgical treatment should be provided. Procedural issues pertain to the question of who should make the decision when there is disagreement. Added complexity arises because these two issues, although distinct, cannot entirely be separated; the question of who should make the decision sometimes depends on what the right decision is. Normally, parents should be allowed to make medical decisions for their children, for several reasons. First, the presumption that parents want what is best for their children is reasonable because experience shows that in most cases it is true. In a given case, we should presume that it is true unless the parents' behavior indicates otherwise. Second, parents should be permitted a domain of autonomy in making decisions about how to raise their children, a domain that encompasses the making of medical decisions for their children.

Despite this presumption, conflicts between parental autonomy and the well-being of the child do arise; parents sometimes make medical decisions that are contrary to the child's interests. In such cases, it is considered ethical for the state to intervene to protect the child, and health care providers are justified in seeking a court order authorizing treatment. But it is rarely easy to distinguishing between cases in which intervention is justifiable and those in which it is not.

Ethical analysis can help resolve this situation by identifying factors to be considered in deciding whether to overrule the parents. These factors can vary from case to case. The ethical values central to this case are the well-being of the patient, the well-being of the family, and the autonomy of the parents.

Several factors are relevant to the well-being of the patient. One is the magnitude of harm that the treatment aims to prevent. Some cases involve life-threatening illnesses, other cases involve harms that are less severe. Another factor is the likelihood that the proposed treatment will be effective in preventing the harm in question. The more likely it is that the treatment would be effective, the stronger the argument for intervening. Other factors related to the patient's well-being are the likelihood that the treatment will have side effects and complications that would be harmful to the patient and the magnitude of such harm if it occurs. Factors related to the family's well-being include the likelihood that the family will experience emotional and psychological harm if the parents' wishes are overridden and the expected magnitude of such harm. When seriously ill children require prolonged treatment, families usually need sustained emotional support from the health care providers. Forcing treatment undermines the ability of the health care team to provide such support. One factor related to parental autonomy is the degree of intrusion into family life that would be required in imposing treatment over the objections of the parents.

The argument for intervening is relatively strong when the treatment is lifesaving, highly likely to be effective, and unlikely to have significant side effects and can be accomplished quickly so that there is minimal intrusion into the daily life of the family. Parental refusal of lifesaving blood transfusions for an otherwise healthy child would be an example in which these conditions for intervening are clearly satisfied (Ackerman 1980). By contrast, the strength of the argument diminishes when, as in the present case, the following factors are present:

- There is substantial uncertainty whether the treatment would be effective.
- The treatment would most likely involve complications that would significantly diminish the patient's quality of life.
- The parents would be required to cooperate with treatment they disagree with over a sustained period of time.

These considerations suggest that in this case the argument for intervening is not strong enough to justify overriding the parents' decision.

These are the sorts of considerations that should be taken into account by the ethics committee that is consulted in cases of articulate disagreement. In this case, these considerations support the view that the parents should be the ones who decide. The committee should attempt to explain to the cardiologist that the current case differs in several important ways from the sorts of cases in which overriding the parents' wishes is justifiable. When persons can reasonably disagree over what is best for the child, health care professionals should defer to parental autonomy and respect the parents' wishes.

Bobby, a 7-year-old boy, has relapsed with leukemia three months after receiving his bone marrow transplant. His parents and physicians, after considering Bobby's prognosis and the available treatment options, have agreed to focus on palliative care. Their goals are to enable Bobby to enjoy himself as much as possible, to maximize his comfort, and to keep him at home, which is far from the tertiary care center where he has received his cancer therapy. Unfortunately, the hospice and home nursing services in his rural home county, when contacted by the health care team, decline to accept him as a patient, saying that "we don't know how to take proper care of children."

Access to palliative care is a policy issue as well as a clinical issue. What are the obstacles to improving access to palliative care? And what can be done to overcome these obstacles? Our health care system currently gives inadequate attention to palliative care. This problem is manifest in a number of ways. Many physicians have not recognized the value of palliative care and lack the technical skills required for its provision. Medical schools and residency programs generally do not provide adequate training in palliative care. Insurance often does not cover or inadequately covers the costs of providing palliative care, and in many areas community resources, such as hospice programs or home nursing services, are insufficient.

Persuading more physicians of the importance of palliative care requires overcoming a number of obstacles. Many physicians regard palliative care as an alternative, rather than complement, to curative efforts. There is often a reluctance to "switch" to palliative care because to do so is perceived as "giving up" on curative approaches. Some physicians regard cessation of curative efforts as an acknowledgment of failure. But palliative care—or supportive care, to use another term—is often appropriate even as curative efforts are taking place (Sahler et al. 2000). Part of the problem, then, is teaching physicians this alternative way of looking at palliative care. Another obstacle is that many physicians are reluctant to use adequate pain medications for fear of being brought before their state licensing boards. They are concerned that they might be accused of causing addiction or collaborating with addicts if they write large numbers of prescriptions for high doses of opiates. In response, some states have passed legislation to reassure physicians that adequate treatment of pain will pose no threat to their license to practice.

In recent years, health maintenance organizations have not been especially responsive to consumer demands, and legislation might be required to bring about improved coverage. Several studies suggest that costs may indeed be reduced when palliative care is provided (Lonberger, Russell, and Burton 1997). Pragmatically speaking, further demonstrations of cost savings might be the most persuasive argument to motivate insurance companies to change their policies on reimbursement for services.

Ultimately, however, our medical system should not be governed by monetary considerations, as health care organizations are bound by ethical responsibilities similar to those that bind individual health care providers in a covenant with their patients (Reiser 1994; Spencer et al. 2000). For the same reasons that the provision of palliative care is a duty for health care providers, facilitating the provision of palliative care services is a duty for health care organizations and the society that encompasses them.

References

Ackerman, T. F. 1980. The limits of beneficence: Jehovah's Witnesses and childhood cancer. *Hastings Cent Rep* 10:13–18.

Beauchamp, T. L., and J. F. Childress. 2001. *Principles of biomedical ethics.* 5th ed. New York: Oxford University Press.

Buckman, R. 1992. *How to break bad news: a guide for health care professionals.* Baltimore: Johns Hopkins University Press.

Creagan, E. T. 1994. How to break bad news—and not devastate the patient. *Mayo Clin Proc* 69:1015–17.

Feudtner, C., D. A. Christakis, and P. Schwartz. 1996. Ethics and the art of confrontation: lessons from the John Conley Essays. *JAMA* 276:755–56.

Girgis, A., and R. W. Sanson-Fisher. 1995. Breaking bad news: consensus guidelines for medical practitioners. *J Clin Oncol* 13:2449–56.

Hammond, J. S., R. L. Keeney, and H. Raiffa. 1999. *Smart choices: a practical guide to making better decisions.* Boston: Harvard Business School Press.

Lonberger, E. A., C. L. Russell, and S. M. Burton. 1997. The effects of palliative care on patient charges. *J Nurs Admin* 27:23–26.

Reiser, S. J. 1994. The ethical life of health care organizations. *Hastings Cent Rep* 24:28–35.

Sahler, O. J. Z., G. Frager, M. Levetown, F. G. Cohn, and M. A. Lipson. 2000. Medical education about end-of-life care in the pediatric setting: principles, challenges, and opportunities. *Pediatrics* 105:575–84.

Spencer, E. M., A. E. Mills, M. V. Rorty, and P. H. Werhane. 2000. *Organization ethics in health care.* New York: Oxford University Press.

Stone, D. F., B. Patton, and S. Heen. 1999. *Difficult conversations: how to discuss what matters most.* New York: Penguin Books.

World Health Organization. 1990. *Cancer pain relief and palliative care.* Technical Report Series 804. Geneva: World Health Organization.

3

Barriers, Education, and Advocacy in Palliative Care

*Joel Frader, M.D., Elaine Morgan, M.D., Tiffany Levinson, R.N., M.S., F.N.P.,
Jason Morrow, M.D., Ph.D., John M. Saroyan, M.D.,
Mary Jo Gilmer, R.N., M.B.A., Ph.D., and Brian S. Carter, M.D., F.A.A.P.*

> Marcella, 3 years old, has received cancer treatment at a tertiary care
> children's hospital for disseminated neuroblastoma. After several
> attempts to provide curative treatment, the options for life-prolonging
> therapy have been exhausted. Her doctors recommend hospice care.
> The third child of Mexican immigrants, Marcella and her family live
> on the south side of Chicago. Her father works several jobs in the
> hospitality industry. His employers do not provide medical insurance.
> Her mother works at home, caring for the children. The preferred
> hospice agency for the children's hospital does not have adequate staff
> to provide coverage in the area where Marcella lives. Other hospices
> have refused referral for a variety of reasons: the family's limited under-
> standing of English, the physicians' and family's wish to continue to
> support Marcella with parenteral nutrition and blood products, lack
> of experience with palliative and hospice care for children and their
> families, and inadequate reimbursement from the state's Medicaid
> plan for hospice care.

This hypothetical case demonstrates some of the problems faced by pediatricians and other health care professionals who wish to provide state-of-
the-art palliative or hospice care (or both) for their patients and the patients'
families. Physicians, administrators, third-party payers, and policy makers
need to address a number of obstacles to appropriate end-of-life care if they
are to meet the palliative and hospice care needs of children and families in
a manner that approaches parity with services for adults.

These obstacles include social, psychological, financial, policy, and other barriers that interfere with the establishment and delivery of palliative and hospice care to children in the United States. The establishment of a Medicare "hospice benefit" has provided a major aid in the development of such services for adults, especially elderly persons. Why have policy makers in government and the private health care sectors not provided for equivalent hospice and palliative care for children?

Barriers to the Provision of Pediatric Palliative Care

The notion that children might require specialized hospice care is not new. St. Mary's Hospice for Children, the first pediatric hospice site, was founded by the Sisters of St. Mary of the Episcopal Church in 1870 (Wilson 1985). At least two books address various issues surrounding hospice care for children in the United States (Corr and Corr 1985; Armstrong-Dailey and Zarbock 2001). In addition, an issue of the National Hospice and Palliative Care Organization's magazine, *Hospice* (Cerquone 1995), and a special issue of the *Journal of Palliative Care* (Roy 1996) address aspects of pediatric palliative and hospice care. A highly organized approach to palliative care for children has considerable acceptance in England (Goldman and Heller 2000). Despite this recognition, hospice and palliative care for children in the United States lags decades behind the development of similar care for adults, especially the elderly. Several recent reports have noted the need for progress in providing palliative and hospice care within pediatrics (American Academy of Pediatrics 2000; Wolfe, Klar, et al. 2000; Hilden et al. 2001; Levetown 2001; Field and Behrman 2002). What stands in the way of developing parity between adult and pediatric end-of-life care?

Two general problems appear predominant: epidemiology and financing. Children die at much lower rates than do adults. Moreover, in contrast to adults, more than half the children who die in any period do so because of an acute event, such as an accident, homicide, suicide, or sudden, overwhelming illness. Goldman and Heller (2000) estimate that, in Britain, about 10 of every 100,000 children "die from a progressive disorder or a life-threatening condition of some sort." This figure does not include neonatal deaths or those resulting from rapidly developing conditions. Feudtner, Christakis, and Connell (2000) report 89.4 deaths per 100,000 children a year in Washington State, 24.3 percent of which result from a complex chronic condition, yielding an annual rate of 21.7 per 100,000. Differences in definitions and research methods probably account for the twofold frequency difference.

However, such national statistical details are largely of only academic interest. Pediatric health care providers will be more concerned with estimates of the number of children in a particular geographic area who could benefit from palliative and hospice care. Using publicly available data, we recently estimated that roughly 230 children died of selected chronic illnesses in the seven-county area including and surrounding Chicago during the calendar year 2000. Those patients, as well as an unknown number of newborns with prolonged stays in neonatal intensive care units, may well have had better deaths had palliative and hospice services been available to them and their families.

Even in a densely populated metropolitan area, the residences of the children who die of chronic conditions are dispersed across significant geographic distances. Since hospices in the United States typically provide care to limited localities, each agency might serve only a handful of children at a time. Similarly, the epidemiology of mortality from chronic illness means that primary care pediatricians will care for few dying children during their entire careers. These facts together have a clear implication: neither those providing primary care for children nor local hospice programs will care for a sufficient number of dying children to maintain the high level of technical and psychosocial skills needed to remain competent and comfortable in this emotionally taxing endeavor. In other words, the geographically distributed model of independent home hospice care used for adults cannot provide adequately for dying children. On the other hand, programs housed exclusively in a "central" location (for example, a tertiary care children's hospital) cannot hope to have personnel reach all families across a region quickly when a crisis arises, be it a death, out-of-control symptoms, or psychological and emotional emergencies of parents or siblings.

Reimbursement for hospice care for children also suffers by comparison with that for adults. This happens for two reasons. First, no nationally uniform payment scheme equivalent to the Medicare hospice benefit exists for children. Second, even when children qualify for hospice services, typical per diem payments do not adequately cover the kinds of services commonly provided to children living with life-threatening conditions. (Children in the end-stage renal disease program are generally the only pediatric patients who receive Medicare coverage.) Under the Medicare hospice benefit, which has been in place since 1986, a patient or his or her surrogate agrees to forgo "curative" (that is, life-prolonging) interventions in exchange for a package of services including nursing care, social work and volunteer services, and pastoral care aimed at easing the dying process. Treatment focuses on symptom management and addressing the psychological and spiritual needs of patients and loved ones. Hospice care usually involves many more in-home services than are provided in other circumstances, though care can also take place in specialized hospice inpatient units or even acute care hospitals, when warranted, to achieve specific goals, such as symptom control. Hospice agencies usually provide care for a single per diem payment expected to cover all services, including medications, personnel costs, and other interventions.

By contrast, the agreement to forgo all efforts involving disease-directed treatment has not worked in pediatrics. Families frequently will not give up interventions that may prolong life, such as chemotherapy for cancer or AIDS, nutrition supplementation, or use of blood products (red blood cells, platelets) in exchange for hospice care. At least two factors explain this. First, dying children often exhibit far less overall disability at the end of their lives than do adults, even with similar diagnoses, such as metastatic malignancies. A child with widespread cancer may be, literally, running around playing with friends and siblings just hours or days before death. Chemotherapy, transfusions, and "aggressive" nutrition may enhance the child's quality of life for substantial periods. Moreover, predicting the timing of death has proved much more difficult in pediatrics than in adult medicine. This makes suspension of life-prolonging efforts difficult for health care professionals, as well as for parents.

Second, at least in the developed world, the psychosocial impact of childhood death affects end-of-life decision making. The death of a child does not occur at the end of what we typically regard as a natural life span. Parents often feel responsible for the child's condition, no matter what the cause. Owing in part to inadequate knowledge of the benefits of symptom control and of a peaceful death, physicians and other health care providers may feel they have failed the child and family in some way when the patient dies, especially under circumstances in which some or many children with similar diagnoses experience cures or life-extension into adulthood. The impressive real progress in pediatric oncology, cystic fibrosis care, and other fields underscores common, if mistaken, beliefs that no given child has to succumb to his or her disease. Dashed expectations and hopes, bolstered by intense guilt, contribute to professionals' and parents' reluctance to discontinue therapy that might produce a "miracle" cure or buy time until research provides "the answer."

The determination to continue disease-directed treatment flies in the face of adult-oriented hospice care. Hospice personnel who care for adults find it hard to accept the radically different philosophy of palliative and hospice care as it has evolved in pediatrics. For some, the approach in pediatrics must appear primitive and unrealistic, even steeped in denial. For others, the problem is fiscal. The prospective per diem payments provided under most formal hospice benefits in both public and private insurance plans do not come close to meeting the costs of continued chemotherapy, blood products, or expensive nutritional interventions. In addition, hospice care for children involves inherently higher costs. Technical aspects of care for children often have a greater degree of difficulty (for example, restarting a peripheral intravenous line) than does similar care of adults. Pediatric hospice and palliative care often involves more time-intensive efforts, especially by nurses, than does hospice care for adults. This includes the use of additional specialized personnel (child-life, art, music, or other therapists) without increased reimbursement beyond standard per diem payments. Hospice care of children may also involve treatment of more people—parents, siblings, even grandparents, affected by the approaching death—followed by prolonged bereavement care needs, again without additional payment to cover the associated increased expense.

One other, rather different issue deserves mention. Despite progress in understanding the assessment and treatment of pain experienced by children, two myths about the effects of medication in children persist. The first involves a purported excess vulnerability of children to "addiction" to opioid analgesics. No data support this notion. Children do not become addicted more easily than adults. Many dying patients, including children, do become *dependent* on narcotics medications for symptom control. Some need quite large doses of morphine or other opiates. However, such physical dependence in dying patients poses no troubling questions and most certainly does not constitute addiction. The second myth involves a supposedly higher risk of death among children caused by appropriate analgesic doses of opioids. Again, no data support this idea, except perhaps in preterm infants or very young children with acidosis. Opioids have similar margins of safety (the ratio of analgesia to risk of respiratory depression) in children compared with adults. The persistence of these myths interferes with the provision of adequate pain control for children and underscores the need for professionals to become knowledgeable about, and comfortable with, palliative care for children. For these reasons—the relationship between quality and volume, philosophical differences from adult palliative care, and associated higher costs, as well as persistent misconceptions about medication effects in children—pediatric palliative and hospice care is not easily integrated into the existing "system" providing end-of-life care to adults in the United States.

Patients' and Families' Needs

Palliative and hospice care for children involves assessment and treatment of much more than the patient. Good palliative care for children also involves care for parents and siblings, as well. Other members of the extended family may live in the same household or have frequent, intimate involvement with the child and other members of the nuclear family. In many cases, other members of the child's community require intervention by the palliative and hospice care team, including schoolmates or children from an involved religious or other extracurricular community. This "extra" work may constitute an obstacle for short-staffed or economically struggling hospice programs; many hospices do not have personnel with the required expertise in child psychology and family dynamics to meet these needs. These needs may overwhelm personnel not prepared to confront their own feelings in the face of caring for dying children or those living with life-threatening conditions.

Health Care Providers' Needs

We have referred families to well-established hospices with little experience caring for dying children. In one dramatic situation, a social worker making a home visit broke down within a few minutes of beginning the encounter. She told the family she had not worked under these circumstances before and was not sure she could "handle it." Pediatric palliative and hospice care does present substantial psychological challenges. Even health care professionals with considerable experience caring for very sick children and their families may find the work overwhelmingly sad at times. Our modern, developed society does not expect children to die before their parents. Staff may find themselves identifying the patient and family members with their own children or grandchildren, making the work more difficult. Staff members need time and opportunity to support one another, to take breaks from the intense emotions, and to reflect on their experiences.

Pediatric palliative and hospice care also requires specialized knowledge. While children do not die more readily than adults when given opioids, drug dosing and idiosyncratic reactions to medications differ from those observed in adult medicine. Most important, pediatric health care professionals working with patients, siblings, and other family members need some understanding of child development. Personnel should anticipate and respond to the patients' and siblings' understanding and feelings about illness and death, which will vary with age and experience. This knowledge will guide both staff interaction with the children and counseling for the adults in their lives. Some persistent myths create problems in this arena, as well. Children generally know much more about death than adults appreciate. Dying children typically know much more about their situations than parents or others admit (Bluebond-Langner 1978). Obtaining appropriate knowledge of and experience in the medical and psychosocial aspects of palliative and hospice care for children is an obstacle for personnel used to caring for other populations.

Community Resources

Professionals in larger communities can often find appropriate consultative expertise about caring for children with life-limiting conditions within tertiary care hospitals providing services to children. Unfortunately, the expertise may not extend to specific needs for palliative care that children have as their disease progresses. Few children's hospitals have formally established palliative care programs. Palliative care services commonly involve only ad hoc or poorly organized arrangements. Other community resources that may help in providing care for dying children and their families include bereavement programs specializing in services for children. These agencies may help with the psychological and social issues. Other nursing agencies providing home care for children, including infusion services, have pediatric nurses with experience, if not formal training, in caring for dying children. However, willing and able nurses in these agencies may lack the leadership and support necessary to sustain their efforts. For instance, home visits for children no longer needing the originally prescribed therapies will not be paid for, nor will the nurse have authority to administer appropriate symptom-relieving medications.

Few, if any, geographic areas have a sufficient population density to maintain full-time interdisciplinary teams dedicated solely to providing pediatric hospice care. Providing good hospice care in the home requires rapid response times (no more than twenty or thirty minutes) in emergencies, including at the time of death. Therefore, a midtown Manhattan hospice with a pediatrics program cannot reasonably serve the Bronx, nor can a northern suburban Chicago hospice serve a family in the expanding western suburbs or southern neighborhoods of the city itself. The current hospital-based regionalized model for providing pediatric tertiary care services for children has no doubt improved treatment (and outcomes) and aided progress in pediatrics. However, it does not work well for home-based palliative and hospice care for children.

The failure of both community-based and hospital-centered models implies the need to find alternative, innovative approaches. Agencies could designate a limited number of interested employees to spend part of their time working with children and families. Agencies could employ child-focused individuals on a part-time basis. Alternatively, interested institutions (hospitals with tertiary care services for children, hospices) could form coalitions or umbrella organizations that find unique solutions based upon the circumstances in that area. No doubt, local variations in the pools of available professionals, insurance arrangements, and politics will require unique arrangements crafted to match community resources with community needs.

Providing appropriate care for dying children must become and remain a policy priority at the institutional, local, state, and federal levels. Just as the field of pediatrics as a whole and, subsequently, subspecialties of pediatrics had to establish separate identities from their counterparts in adult medicine, so palliative and hospice care for children has to gain acceptance as a distinctive entity judged and paid for independently from care for adults. Failure to provide adequate care for dying children and their families in the United States is morally and medically unconscionable.

Education in Pediatric Palliative Care

While educating adults may not change fundamental attitudes and values, structured learning experiences can assist motivated professionals to provide compassionate care and overcome bad habits or misinformation acquired in technically oriented training. Such is the aim of education in palliative and hospice care. Pediatric palliative care education strives to integrate modern knowledge and skills with ancient values and attitudes, such as compassion and mercy, to enable professionals to provide competent, humanistic care for children living with life-threatening conditions and their families.

OBSTACLES

Some professional barriers derive, as mentioned earlier in this chapter, from therapeutic optimism associated with the technical successes in biomedicine in the past century. The focus on biomedical aspects of disease has resulted in relative inattention to the psychosocial dimensions of the doctor-patient relationship (Billings and Block 1997). Striving to cure at all costs obstructs opportunities to engage patients and loved ones in meaningful discussions about such difficult issues as treatment "failure" or the substantial hazards that therapies may entail. Professionals may lose the opportunity to discuss patients' and family members' values and goals for care, including the possibility of focusing on support and comfort rather than cure (MacDonald 1999). The poor representation of palliative care issues in textbooks, medical school courses, residency program curriculums, and board and licensing examinations reflects this professional shortsightedness, as does the paucity of fellowship programs in pediatric palliative care (Weissman et al. 1997; Kaneja and Milrod 1998). Health care professionals who will devote significant portions of their activity to the care of children living with life-limiting conditions need to learn how to advocate for the pediatric palliative and hospice care appropriate for their patients (Sahler et al. 2000). Thus residency programs in pediatrics and family medicine should include didactic and direct experience with end-of-life care for children, as should educational programs for advance practice nurses in pediatrics, neonatal and pediatric intensive care, and related occupations. Fellowship programs in subspecialty pediatrics and pediatric surgery should include responsibility for end-of-life care, supervised by those with pediatric palliative and hospice care expertise. Orientation programs for nurses who will work on inpatient services for children should include information about and, where possible, experience in working with dying children and their families. Similarly, pediatric palliative and hospice care should appear in orientation materials for social workers and hospital chaplains who will provide for seriously ill children. Care for dying children needs a routine and prominent place in the education and training of professionals providing health care for children.

At the personal level, education must address the emotionally taxing aspects of caring for children with life-threatening conditions and their families. Caregivers may develop feelings of inadequacy, helplessness, and grief, especially in a biomedical culture that views death as medical failure (Hafferty and Franks 1994). Clinicians must struggle with prognostic uncertainties, ambiguities in quality-of-life assessments, and the inadequacies of standard medical practice to address many of the common problems that patients experience (Sahler et al. 2000). While normal psychological defenses can mitigate these caregiver burdens, educational programs have a role in helping clinicians acknowledge and discuss their feelings and in preventing emotions from unduly influencing clinical decisions (Katz 1984; Charlton 1996).

Academic health centers can create environments that help shape the priorities of current and future clinicians (MacDonald 1999). These institutions should make explicit and concrete commitments to providing palliative care for children and encourage clinicians to appreciate the value of these services to their patients (Weissman et al. 1997). In addition, readily accessible counseling and other supportive services (for example, forums for discussion of feelings stirred up by caring for dying patients) for students, residents, and practicing clinicians will help professionals more effectively explore end-of-life issues with patients (Kaneja and Milrod 1998).

OBJECTIVES

Pediatric palliative care requires, first, a strong desire to be of service to children with life-threatening conditions and their families and, second, a willingness to accept that death is not only part of the life of every clinician's patient, young or old, but also part of each of our own lives. Pediatric palliative care education strives to assist clinicians who possess compassionate dispositions by providing the support of educators in addressing the pragmatic and psychological concerns of students at various levels of training.

Andrew, an 8-year-old boy with high-risk acute lymphocytic leukemia, has been readmitted for a relapse detected when he returned from a trip with severe headache. His white blood cell count was 400,000, and his potassium was dangerously elevated. The morning after admission, he sits in his hospital bed, fearful and sullen. After the house-staff finish discussing tumor-lysis syndrome and electrolyte abnormalities with the attending pediatric oncologist, the team enters his room for morning rounds. The oncologist, seeing Andrew's distress, sits down at the bedside, and asks "How are you this morning, Andrew?" Andrew says nothing. The attending waits for some time, then asks, "What are you afraid of?" Andrew whispers, "I don't know." A long silence ensues. Neither Andrew nor his mother speaks. The house-staff members stare at the floor. Observing the trainees and the frightened family, the oncologist puts his hand on the boy's shoulder. After a few more minutes, the physician says, "I want to talk to you and your mother more later. Is that okay?" Andrew nods.

In this hypothetical case, the oncologist demonstrates the empathy and skill that younger clinicians must learn. He shows the importance of sitting down, enduring silence, noticing what is happening with both learners and the family, and knowing when not to press his patient. These actions model a multidimensional approach to pediatric palliative care education. The following remarks emphasize practical suggestions for teaching these principles in the clinical setting.

In their discussion of empathy and whether it can be taught, Spiro and colleagues (1993) suggest that the secret to teaching empathy is "keeping it there"—modeling it in the presence of students. If empathic individuals are selected for medical training, then medical educators have the responsibility of not socializing it out of students. This means that education about caring for dying children and their families must also involve extending empathy for trainees experiencing stress and sadness while participating in the process of providing end-of-life care.

As the discipline of palliative care has evolved, core content objectives best presented in a didactic format have emerged. The American Academy of Pediatrics (2000) recommends a set of objectives that broadens the focus of pediatric palliative care education beyond symptom management and incorporates effective communication and empathic understanding. The organization lists the content objectives of pediatric palliative care education as communication skills, understanding of grief and loss, management of prognostic uncertainty, decisions to forgo life-sustaining medical treatment, the spiritual dimensions of life and illness, and alternative medicine (exhibit 3.1).

Papadatou (1997) offers objectives that address the particular concerns of children living with life-threatening illnesses. He recommends seven didactic units in pediatric palliative care education, focusing on developmental psychology, crisis intervention and counseling skills, and applications of systems theory to families facing illness and death:

- Pediatric hospice philosophy and principles of care
- Individual and family coping with chronic and life-threatening illness in childhood
- Symptom control and management during the terminal phase

- Psychosocial and spiritual care of dying children and their family members
- Symbolic and creative interaction with dying and bereaved children
- Parental and sibling grief process, including cultural aspects of bereavement
- Stress management and prevention of burnout in professionals caring for a dying child and grieving families

Successful integration of the core components of pediatric palliative care education requires an institutional commitment to providing palliative services as well as educators' capacity to address the needs of clinicians at different stages of training. Palliative care can be integrated into medical school curriculums by incorporating the core objectives into preclinical courses, such as pharmacology, medical ethics, and behavioral medicine. In residency and fellowship, didactic components can take their place in routinely provided conferences spread throughout the programs. For established clinicians, pediatric palliative care education probably deserves specialized continuing medical education courses.

METHODS

There is little published about current practices in pediatric palliative care education in health-related professional schools and pediatric residencies. Contro and colleagues (2002) address the insensitive delivery of bad news, which can complicate family members' grief for many years. Patterson (1995) notes that clinicians are key to empowering families during times of stress. Faculty can encourage residents to reinforce positive parental behavior, such as complimenting a father on his calming presence during a procedure. Similarly, educators should facilitate trainees' efforts to find out about a patient's community resources (whether based in religious organizations, local agencies,

Exhibit 3.1. AAP parameter content objectives of pediatric palliative care education

- Communication skills
- Grief and loss
- Managing prognostic uncertainty
- Decisions to forgo life-sustaining medical treatment
- Spiritual dimensions of life and illness
- Alternative medicine

or networks maintained around the family's social, ethnic, political, or other affiliation).

BEHAVIORAL DIMENSIONS

In response to pediatric residents' discomfort with communicating with families under stressful situations, Morgan and Winter (1996) have designed a course with didactic and role-play-based learning. The first half of the course includes didactic presentations and a panel discussion about principles of communication and empathic techniques for delivering bad news. Residents then participate in role-playing that involves delivering bad news and responding to angry parents. The second half of the course includes psychologists, social workers, parents, and adolescent patients who address topics such as talking with children about their illnesses and death and dying.

Papadatou (1997) and Corr (1995) suggest four dimensions of pediatric palliative care education: cognitive (acquisition of information and knowledge), behavioral (development of specific skills), affective (acknowledgment and exploration of personal feelings), social (actual provision of health services in a specific sociocultural context), and valuational (identification, articulation, and affirmation of personal values). Educational efforts should attend to intellectual and skill-based faculties and to these four dimensions (Papadatou 1997). The latter factors can effectively change practice outcomes (Boakes et al. 2000). The affective and behavioral components of pediatric palliative care education can be incorporated into didactic, small-group, and other interactive formats, as well as pretests, posttests, and subsequent clinical opportunities to practice the relevant objectives (Weissman et al. 1997).

OPPORTUNITIES FOR AFFECTIVE, BEHAVIORAL, SOCIAL, AND VALUATIONAL DIMENSIONS OF LEARNING

Case scenarios can supplement traditional didactic techniques in preclinical courses. Teaching evaluations have shown that participants respond best to cases reflecting day-to-day conflicts (Weissman 1993; Diekhma and Shugerman 1997).

> Susan, a second-year resident in pediatrics, is on call in the neonatal intensive care unit. She has just unsuccessfully attempted to resuscitate a twenty-four-week-gestation newborn. The delivery was by "crash" caesarean section, indicated by fetal distress. She and the neonatology attending physician have told the parents (with the aid of a Spanish

translator) that the baby, Manuel, has died, despite their best efforts. Following this discussion, Susan and the nurse return to the room with the baby. The father stands at the bedside, probably in shock. Thirty minutes later, the mother hands Manuel back to Susan, still crying. The nurse asks the father if he wants to hold his son. His whole body is shaking. He says, "No, I can't."

The Papadatou and Corr perspective might explore the valuational, affective, and social dimensions by asking the following questions: Would taking the baby and leaving after the father's response be in keeping with your personal beliefs? What steps might Susan take to attend to her own emotional needs, considering both the unsuccessful resuscitation and the family's grief? How might she find out how the family's background and culture might inform the best steps to take now?

As much as possible, teaching formats should involve active participation and include creative nondidactic components. Role-playing and case studies, when carefully planned and reflected on, are especially useful. These techniques allow trainees to go beyond the intellectual content of the material and explore their own biases (Weissman 1993). The following example describes this sort of role-playing (Allmond, Tanner, and Gofman 1999).

Attending pediatric intensivist: You are on call in the pediatric intensive care unit. If a particular five-month-old patient dies overnight, your colleagues expect you to obtain consent for autopsy. The child had been discharged from the hospital four days after a previous admission. At the time, the baby was found to have enterovirus meningitis. The baby returned two days later with overwhelming Pseudomonas sepsis. She had not responded well to treatments offered, despite aggressive therapy with antibiotics, inotropic agents, and mechanical ventilation. Consultants suspect an underlying metabolic or immune disorder.

Father of patient: You are furious that your infant was sent home with "just a virus" and returned with overwhelming bacterial infection. You have threatened to sue. When the doctors indicate that they expected your baby to die and would have approached you for permission for an autopsy, you become enraged at the idea of putting your child through more procedures by "cutting him open."

Mother of patient: Despite being grief stricken, you are quite composed
during the interaction and try to mediate the disagreement between your husband and the physician. You worry that your
baby has a condition that might affect future children.

Facilitator (to discussion group before role-play): A very sick child
has died unexpectedly shortly after being discharged with viral
meningitis and being readmitted in bacterial sepsis. The intensivist will now attempt to obtain consent for autopsy from the
parents.

The scenario presents opportunities to assess behavioral, affective, and
valuational dimensions of pediatric palliative care. In behavioral terms, the
person playing the intensivist will most likely avoid addressing the father's
anger directly. Most commonly, he or she will repeatedly try to explain the
medical reasons for the autopsy. It may help to stop the action for this role-
player to work on acknowledging the father's anger and expressing empathy.
The affective dimension can be addressed by discussing the emotional challenges posed by the need to ask the family for permission to perform an autopsy.
In particular, efforts to avoid taking litigious threats personally should be
explored. The valuational element could be brought to the fore by discussing
whether seeking autopsy permission in this case might violate a professional's
personal values.

SOCIAL DIMENSION

Pediatric palliative and hospice care usually demands thinking beyond the
confines of the acute care setting. Students and more advanced trainees can
derive substantial educational value from participating in home care visits
with members of the hospice team. Familiarity with these health care professionals and services may ease collaboration during discharge planning.
Moreover, home visits provide an opportunity to see how families adapt in
the surroundings they know and control best, albeit without many of the
resources available in the hospital. Such experiences may also enable physicians
in training to better understand the conditions that make a "good death"—
as defined by patients and loved ones—possible (Charlton 1996).

Faculty can also encourage interested students to become hospice volunteers or to work at a camp for children living with cancer or human immunodeficiency virus (HIV). These experiences can provide insight into children's

abilities to enjoy life until shortly before they die. Being in the patient's home or observing child-patients at camp can help students learn about the patient's ability to fully participate in his or her life and to carry on relationships with peers and community.

Finally, faculty should ensure that students and residents have permission and the time needed to attend funerals. Participation in socially and culturally important ceremonies allows professionals to acknowledge their own feelings. Families usually appreciate this extension of the relationship beyond the point of technical intervention, and the value of emotional connections in the professional-patient-family relationship is thereby reinforced (Kaneja and Milrod 1998).

ROLE-MODELING AS AN EDUCATIONAL INTERVENTION

Weissman and colleagues (1997) describe the value of one role-model program to promote institutional change to better manage acute and chronic cancer pain. Senior nurses are invited to a regional medical center to learn better approaches to the treatment of pain. The program includes didactic conferences, observation of others applying the lessons in clinical settings, hands-on use of the new knowledge and skills by attendees complete with critiques by program faculty, and a follow-up meeting to address challenges participants faced after they returned to their home institutions.

NARRATIVES OF THE EXPERIENCE OF ILLNESS

Educators may derive considerable value from using actual or fictional accounts of patients' and family members' experiences with life-threatening illnesses. Such stories can help trainees overcome the tendency to focus excessively on treating disease rather than confronting the entire human experience of serious illness and death. Indeed, one prominent practitioner and scholar has advised, "It is necessary to make the patient's and the family's narrative of the illness experience more central in the educational process" (Kleinman 1988, 255).

Stories can provide a vital and revealing perspective on doctor-patient communications and the complexities of decision making under conditions of ambiguity, uncertainty, and ambivalence. Such accounts draw attention "to the processes by which patients, families, and health care providers find personal meaning in illness, and how personal meanings influence the experience and outcome of care" (Barnard et al. 2000, 7). Reading and reflecting on illness narratives can increase the professionals' sensitivity to nontechnical aspects of care and help them anticipate, elicit, and respond to the concerns and fears of patients and family members.

AUDITING AND ACCREDITATION

Educators should advocate regular auditing of existing practices to help ensure that they reflect current standards of palliative care. Regular auditing "is important for education and training because the structured review allows analysis, comparison, and evaluation of individual performance; promotes adherence to local clinical policies; and offers an opportunity for publication of the results" (Hearn and Higginson 1999). Implementing recommendations arising from audits of palliative and hospice care should become part of the process of fulfilling hospital accreditation requirements, just as occurs in other domains of hospital care (MacDonald 1999).

SUMMARY OF EDUCATIONAL RECOMMENDATIONS

Introducing palliative care into the preclinical classroom and the community experience of students sends the important message that care of and for the dying has as much value as care aimed at cure. Incorporating palliative care education into the clinical years of medical and nursing school training makes sense: having responsibility for only a few patients presents opportunities to teach holistic compassionate care of children living with life-threatening disorders. Small-group discussion and role-playing can supplement didactic sessions focused on content and help learners prepare for the emotional challenges inherent in providing end-of-life care; these techniques also have value for pediatric palliative care education in residency and for continuing medical education. No matter what the target educational audience, pediatric palliative care education needs to address the many kinds of knowledge, relational skills, and attention to feelings necessary for providing high-quality palliative and end-of-life care for children and their families.

Advocacy in Palliative Care

As indicated throughout this text, enhancing the quality of life for children with terminal conditions requires the coordinated effort of numerous providers from varied disciplines. Effective advocacy to improve pediatric palliative and hospice care will involve families, health care providers, administrators, and even policy makers. The following comments suggest a number of steps health care professionals and concerned laypersons may take to work toward parity between pediatric and adult palliative and hospice care.

INDIVIDUAL PATIENTS AND THEIR FAMILIES

Those interested in bringing the benefits of palliative and hospice care to patients and their families will find themselves needing to remind their health care colleagues to consider the following:

- the developmental level of the child
- the child's previous experiences with death
- the child's usual strategies for coping with pain and sadness
- the family's cultural and religious beliefs about death
- the expected circumstances of death

Primary treatment teams should be helped to enlist the assistance of psychologists and other mental health professionals, spiritual counselors, and trained volunteers in planning end-of-life care. Where appropriate, advocates can educate and enlist the help of teachers, school principals and nurses, and others in the community who play important roles in the lives of patients and their siblings. Palliative and hospice care consultants can advocate for patients and families when community resources (including schools) or the health care system seem unwilling to recognize or address end-of-life issues.

Child health professionals can help families maintain their attention and focus in the face of overwhelming needs. Effective advocacy for the family can involve assisting them to get needed emotional, financial, and physical support (James and Johnson 1997), including respite care, home-delivered meals, child care services for siblings, and involvement with support groups. Retreat services and camp experiences for both children and families offer opportunities to share common ground with others immersed in a similar process.

Support groups for patients and families may play an important role in preparing families to face the final phase of a child's life. Perhaps more important, members of support groups can suggest to families successful ways to advocate with insurance companies and agencies that pay for medical services for payment of appropriate palliative and hospice care services for their children.

INSTITUTIONS

Administrators can advocate for children with life-threatening conditions by ensuring that resources are available and effectively used. Partnerships between acute care facilities and hospice organizations can enable sharing of expertise specific to the settings. Personnel in acute care facilities may benefit from hospice professionals' expertise in clinical palliative care. At the same time, many hospice programs have little experience in caring for children; thus hospice personnel may benefit from additional education about the unique needs of the pediatric patient. In this way, a conjoint effort may benefit children in either facility.

Support groups, professional organizations, and hospital public relations offices can and should begin mounting a serious effort to educate the public. Such groups could initiate lobbying activities for state and federal legislation and regulation to require insurance coverage for pediatric palliative and hospice care at least equivalent to that provided for adults. Ideally, new regulations and insurance arrangements will recognize the added costs of these services for children and their families and provide coverage for the extra expenses, including those associated with the need for prolonged services (Wolfe, Grier, et al. 2000).

Public engagement may include arranging local news media interviews of parents and professionals about the needs of dying children and sponsorship of local performances of dramatic works (plays, films, readings of fiction, poetry, and personal essays) telling the stories of dying children. While some health care institutions may be reluctant to have their names associated with childhood death rather than "miraculous" cures, it seems likely that hospitals would benefit by demonstrating an interest in providing compassionate, holistic care through all stages of disease. Moreover, those institutions that provide continuity of care for children living with life-threatening conditions, regardless of the site of care, have a palatable message that they are enhancing the quality of life for these fragile patients and their families, from diagnosis through bereavement.

Within tertiary care facilities, those interested in palliative and hospice care should consider working toward establishing two systemic changes: the integration of palliative care into clinical programs providing care for children with life-threatening disorders (Frager 1996) and the development of palliative care consultation services (Pierucci, Kirby, and Leuthner 2001). Of course, given the high degree of interest families have in caring for dying children at home, without appropriate home hospice services in-hospital consultation services may only raise expectations without the possibility of adequate follow-through.

BEYOND INSTITUTIONS

The Medicare model of hospice care addresses the needs of adult patients, especially those with cancer, and provides benefits to individuals with a life expectancy of no more than six months. Given the difficulty in predicting life expectancy in children, the model does not work well in pediatrics, as children are not little adults. Accurate criteria and indexes for predicting impending death in children are needed to assist health care professionals in anticipating the likely course of illness and the treatment needs that may arise (Horn et al. 2001). Unfortunately, states have followed the Medicare model for most Medicaid hospice benefits, including those provided for children. Advocates need to educate policy makers about the different and more extensive needs of children living with life-threatening conditions and their families, such as antibiotics for children with cystic fibrosis to prevent unremitting coughing and shortness of breath, that are currently prohibitively expensive for hospice programs (American Academy of Pediatrics 2000)—and convince them of the value of more funding than current models allow.

RESEARCH

Although Bluebond-Langner (1978) demonstrated a quarter of a century ago that dying children know much more about what is happening to them than adults often care to admit, there are still no well-developed protocols for including children in end-of-life decision making. Substantially more research is needed into questions such as the influence of age, duration of illness, maturity, cognitive function, and family and community cultural and religious practices in the context of health care decision making, before sophisticated approaches to consulting with children and gaining their assent can be designed. These same issues need clarification as those with adequate decisional capacity to give informed consent consider enrolling in hospice care programs or limiting further "curative" interventions.

A related and important component of advocacy for adequate palliative and hospice care for children involves fostering a general increase in research in the field. This should include such topics as systematic studies of pharmacologic interventions for symptom control, cost-effectiveness studies of alternative modes of hospice care delivery, and the impact of supportive measures (blood component therapy, nutritional therapies, maintenance of chemotherapy, and so on) on quality of life. Given the relatively small number of patients in each institution, professionals will need to overcome "turf" concerns and develop regional and national cooperative study groups to make the most scientifically sound and efficient progress in pediatric palliative and hospice care research.

Conclusion

Caring for children living with life-threatening conditions and for their families is a daunting task. For competent and compassionate care to be broadly available to such families, clinicians must confront and overcome social, educational, and financial barriers. Current educational models are inadequate to meet the needs of terminally ill children: means of providing effective symptom control and philosophically valuing successes in these arenas are not included in the training of health professionals at the present time, particularly in pediatric professionals' education. Education must address not only such technical issues but also the psychosocial needs of the individuals receiving care and of those providing it. Several suggestions to achieve such education are presented in this chapter.

Many of the systems in place at present to manage terminal illness are effective in meeting the needs of adults but are inadequate for children, given their less-frequent death, geographical dispersion, and the variety of circumstances and conditions leading to child mortality. Meaningful change will occur only through collaborative efforts of caregivers, institutions, and families to educate the public, legislators, the research community, and third-party payers about the critical needs of patients, families, and caregivers facing one of the most difficult modern challenges today—how to enable a child with a life-threatening condition to live well, die peacefully, and leave a family grieving but not resentful and devastated for the reminder of their days.

References

Allmond, B. W., J. L. Tanner, and H. F. Gofman. 1999. *The family is the patient: using family interviews in children's medical care.* Baltimore: Wilkins and Wilkins.

American Academy of Pediatrics, Committee on Bioethics and Committee on Hospital Care. 2000. Palliative care for children. *Pediatrics* 106:351–57.

Armstrong-Dailey, A., and S. Zarbock, eds. 2001. *Hospice care for children.* 2d ed. New York: Oxford University Press.

Barnard, D., A. Towers, P. Boston, and Y. Lambrinidou. 2000. *Crossing over: narratives of palliative care*. Oxford, U.K.: Oxford University Press.

Billings, J. A., and S. Block. 1997. Palliative care in undergraduate medical education: status report and future directions. *JAMA* 278:733–38.

Bluebond-Langner, M. 1978. *The private worlds of dying children*. Princeton: Princeton University Press.

Boakes, J., D. Gardner, K. Yuen, and S. Doyle. 2000. General practitioner training in palliative care: an experiential approach. *J Palliat Care* 16:11–19.

Cerquone, J., ed. 1995. *Hospice* 6:2–36.

Charlton, R. 1996. Medical education: addressing the needs of the dying child. *Palliat Med* 10:240–46.

Contro, N., J. Larson, S. Scofield, B. Sourkes, and H. Cohen. 2002. Family perspectives on the quality of pediatric palliative care. *Arch Pediatr Adolesc Med* 156:14–19.

Corr, C. A. 1995. Death education for adults. In *A challenge for living: dying, death, and bereavement*, ed. I. B. Corless, B. B. Germino, and M. A. Pittman. Boston: Jones and Bartlett.

Corr, C. A., and D. M. Corr, eds. 1985. *Hospice approaches to pediatric care*. New York: Springer.

Diekhma, D. S., and R. P. Shugerman. 1997. An ethics curriculum for the pediatric residency program: confronting barriers to implementation. *Arch Pediatr Adolesc Med* 151:609–14.

Feudtner, C., D. A. Christakis, and F. A. Connell. 2000. Pediatric deaths attributable to complex chronic conditions: a population-based study of Washington State, 1980–1997. *Pediatrics* 106:205–9.

Field, M. J., and R. E. Behrman. 2002. *When children die: improving palliative and end-of-life care for children and their families*. Institute of Medicine Report. Washington, D.C.: National Academies Press.

Frager, G. 1996. Pediatric palliative care: building the model, bridging the gaps. *J Palliat Care* 12:9–12.

Goldman, A., and K. S. Heller. 2000. Integrating palliative and curative approaches in the care of children with life-threatening illnesses. *J Palliat Med* 3:353–59.

Hafferty, F. W., and R. Franks. 1994. Medical culture, medical ethics, and the medical school curriculum. *Acad Med* 69:861–71.

Hearn, J., and I. J. Higginson. 2000. Development of a core outcome measure for palliative care: the palliative care outcome scale. *Qual Health Care* 8:219–27.

Hilden, J. M., B. P. Himelstein, D. R. Freyer, S. Friebert, and J. R. Kane. 2001. End-of-life care: special issues in pediatric oncology. In *Improving palliative care for cancer*, ed. K. M. Foley and H. Gelband. Washington, D.C.: National Academies Press.

Horn, S., A. Torres, D. Willson, J. M. Dean, J. Gassaway, and R. Smout. 2001. Development of a pediatric age- and disease-specific severity measure. Unpublished manuscript.

James, L., and B. Johnson. 1997. The needs of parents of pediatric oncology patients during the palliative care phase. *J Pediatr Oncol Nurs* 14:83–95.

Kaneja, S., and B. Milrod. 1998. Educational needs among pediatricians regarding caring for terminally ill children. *Arch Pediatr Adolesc Med* 152:909–14.

Katz, J. 1984. *The silent world of doctor and patient.* New York: Free Press.

Kleinman, A. 1988. *The illness narratives: suffering, healing, and the human condition.* New York: Basic.

Levetown, M. 2001. A call for change: recommendations to improve the care of children living with life-threatening conditions. Alexandria, Va.: National Hospice and Palliative Care Organization. www.nhpco.org/files/public/ChIPPSCallfor Change.pdf (accessed February 19, 2004).

MacDonald, N. 1999. Palliative care education: a global imperative. *Cancer Treat Rev* 100:185–201.

Morgan, E. R., and R. J. Winter. 1996. Teaching communication skills: an essential part of residency training. *Arch Pediatr Adolesc Med* 150:638–42.

Papadatou, D. 1997. Training health professionals in caring for dying children and grieving families. *Death Studies* 21:575–600.

Patterson, J. M. 1995. Conceptualizing family adaptation to stress: children, families, and stress. In *Children, families, and stress: report of the twenty-fifth Ross Roundtable on Critical Approaches to Common Pediatric Problems in collaboration with the Ambulatory Pediatric Association,* ed. J. L. Tanner, 11–22. Columbus, Ohio: Ross Products Division.

Pierucci, R. L., R. S. Kirby, and S. R. Leuthner. 2001. End-of-life care for neonates and infants: the experience and effects of a palliative care consultation service. *Pediatrics* 108:653–60.

Roy, D. J., ed. 1996. When children have to die. *J Palliat Care* 12:3–59.

Sahler, O. J. Z., G. Frager, M. Levetown, F. G. Cohn, and M. A. Lipson. 2000. Medical education about end-of-life care in the pediatric setting: principles, challenges, and opportunities. *Pediatrics* 105:575–84.

Spiro, H., M. McCrea Curnen, E. Peshcel, and D. St. James. 1993. *Empathy in the practice of medicine.* New Haven: Yale University Press.

Weissman, D. E. 1993. Preclinical palliative medicine education at the Medical College of Wisconsin. *J Cancer Educ* 8:191–95.

Weissman, D. E., J. Griffie, D. B. Gordon, and J. L. Dahl. 1997. A role model program to promote institutional changes for management of acute and cancer pain. *J Pain Symptom Manage* 77:274–79.

Wilson, D. C. 1985. Developing a hospice program for children. In *Hospice approaches to pediatric care,* ed. C. A. Corr and D. M. Corr. New York: Springer.

Wolfe, J., H. E. Grier, N. Klar, S. B. Levin, and J. M. Ellenbogen. 2000. Symptoms and suffering at the end of life in children with cancer. *N Engl J Med* 342:326–33.

Wolfe, J., N. Klar, H. E. Grier, J. Duncan, S. Salem-Schatz, E. J. Emanuel, and J. C. Weeks. 2000. Understanding of prognosis among parents of children who died of cancer. *JAMA* 284:2469–75.

PART II

THE CYCLE OF CARE

4

Decision Making in Pediatric Palliative Care

Yarrow McConnell, B.Sc., Gerri Frager, R.N., M.D., F.R.C.P.C., and Marcia Levetown, M.D.

Stevie, a 3½-year-old boy with a neurodegenerative disorder of unknown etiology, was hospitalized thirty-nine times in his brief life. All the admissions were for either aspiration pneumonitis with bronchospasm or status epilepticus. Not surprisingly, Stevie's whole family was affected by his illness. His parents were divorced because of it; his mother was so overwhelmed by his care that she could not work, maintain friendships, care for her other children or herself, or go to worship. His sister had run away from home, and his brother was failing in school owing to an undiagnosed hearing problem. Stevie's doctor knew only about Stevie's medical problems, treating each new episode as though it were an isolated acute illness. He did not discuss, in any comprehensive sense, the overarching goals of Stevie's care.

If, instead, Stevie's doctor had approached Stevie's mother with the following questions, he might have better met the needs of the patient and family:

- What are you hoping we can accomplish with our medical care?
- Is there anything that you think is doing too much—anything that you would feel we would be doing *to* Stevie, rather than *for* him?
- Good and loving parents often worry about all of these things and more. Can we think through these decisions together?
- Over time, your answers may change as Stevie's condition changes. Should this occur, will you keep this conversation

going with me? I'd really like to do what is best for you and for Stevie, regardless of the circumstances of his illness.

An approach using such questions and statements enabled Stevie's mother to confidently make the transition from requesting no limitation of medical interventions to requesting no more than two days on a ventilator if his condition did not improve. With time, home visits, and interdisciplinary support, she later declined intensive care and after that refused even hospitalization, preferring that his care be conducted exclusively at home. Finally, she requested no intervention other than what was required to maximize his comfort at home—cough suppressants, antipyretics, music, and candlelight, with his family and friends bathing him in affection. Her concerns and doubts had been listened to along the way—at all times. Her love and dedication were affirmed and validated aloud. In the meantime, Stevie received regular medical visits and had effective amelioration of his symptoms and proactive treatment of his minor illnesses. His mother received support for her other roles, and volunteers allowed her the time and energy to attend to these other needs. She was never told she had to stop treatments for Stevie, nor were her values questioned. Her son's death was difficult for her, despite his long-standing illness, yet it was peaceful. Her family was intact at the time of Stevie's death, and each of the older children was succeeding in school.

Health care decision making for infants, children, and adolescents with life-threatening or life-limiting illnesses presents a wide range of challenges. One particular challenge is for young patients, their families, and the health care team to work together in making difficult decisions.

Imagine being asked whether you want to stop the provision of life support for your own child. For most parents, even momentary reflection on such a question will create an immediate sense of horror. Ill children and their families need all the support they can get when making such decisions. They require empathic communication, accurate information, a full explanation of the pros and cons of each potential course of action, and respect for their priorities and the choices they make. They also need to be respected and appreciated for their struggles, efforts, and pain, to share responsibility for medical decisions involving their child, and to feel that they will never be abandoned by clinicians.

Parent describing the need for collaborative decision making after her child's liver biopsy: "We needed a plan, we need to know where we are going, how long we are going, and what the game plan is." (Heller and Solomon 2003)

The aim of this chapter is to provide practical guidance to achieve collaborative decision making for children living with life-threatening conditions and their families. The material presented here has been developed in conjunction with an educational module, titled *Decision-Making in Pediatric Palliative Care,* for the University of Toronto's Ian Anderson Continuing Education Program in End-of-Life Care (McConnell and Frager 2003). The major challenges of such decision making, identification of the stakeholders involved, the process of discussing options and reaching consensus, and suggestions for conflict resolution within this process are discussed. Readers will be able to identify the participants in pediatric palliative care decision making and their respective roles; be more able to appreciate the need for ongoing, open, nonjudgmental communication to achieve the best decision-making collaboration possible; understand the legal and ethical issues that influence pediatric palliative care decision making; and have more tools for communication around pediatric palliative care decisions (see also chapters 2 and 5 in this volume).

What Are the Challenges?

DIVERSE AND UNUSUAL ILLNESSES

Life-threatening conditions in children are unusual and diverse, and few practitioners have a large experience with childhood terminal conditions. Each type of condition has a unique and frequently unpredictable time course, with its own treatment options and decision-making points (figs. 4.1 and 4.2). The duration, type, and intensity of care required varies tremendously across patients and for a single patient at different times. Pediatric patients have distinct physiological, pharmacokinetic, and developmental characteristics that influence the management of diseases and symptoms. The skill set required to manage this diversity may not be available in all locations, and families may be required to travel to distant tertiary care hospitals for care. Although most parents have no previous experience in making such difficult decisions, they often become more knowledgeable about their child's illness than the clinicians caring for them.

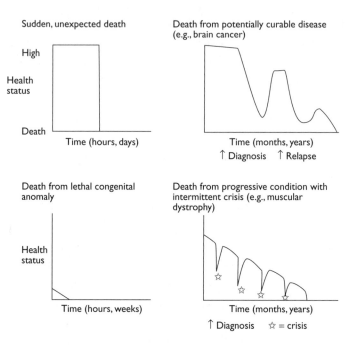

Figure 4.1. Trajectories of pediatric illness.

Source: Field and Behrman (2002). Reprinted with permission from National Academies Press.

Note: Other possible trajectories include that of a child who is seriously ill but later fully recovers.

UNCERTAIN PROGNOSIS

For many life-threatening childhood conditions, prognosis is uncertain. Improvements in medical and pharmacological therapy are helping more children live longer, but they are also making prediction more difficult. Children, families, and clinicians often have to make decisions in the absence of a clear vision of what the future might hold.

> *Parent lamenting the unwillingness of her physician to advise her on the best course of action: "She just gave us statistics and didn't really . . . she wouldn't even tell us, like, what she would do if it was her, because she doesn't know." (Heller and Solomon 2003)*

Children with life-threatening illnesses are living longer, but they do so with complex illnesses and therapy decisions, as well as enormous uncertainty

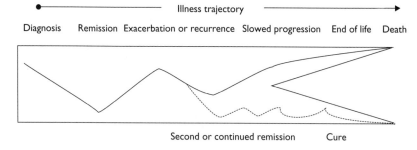

Figure 4.2. Decision points in the course of life-threatening pediatric illness.

about when, or whether, death will occur. These children and their families have an ongoing need for support, information, discussion of palliative care options, and open communication about death and the dying process—well before they find themselves facing it.

> *Mother describing informational needs after her daughter's sudden death from a prolonged cardiomyopathy: "I was frustrated a lot, but most of it was 'cause they didn't know. There was only one thing that I really wish that they had told me that they didn't. . . . They never said she was in danger of sudden death and that's really kind of what happened. I really wasn't prepared for that, for how she would die." (Heller and Solomon 2003)*

SURROGATE DECISION MAKING

Many children are unable to participate directly in decision making owing to developmental stage, medical condition, cognitive disability, or sedation. Surrogate decision makers, usually the child's parents, must therefore weigh the options and make decisions on the child's behalf.

> Faisal is a 14-year-old immigrant living with his older brother. He had a near drowning in an apartment complex pool and is now unable to breathe independently. He is receiving mechanical ventilation and is deeply comatose three days after the incident. His parents cannot get a visa to come to the United States.

Surrogate decision makers must try to understand and predict the child's responses to situations that they themselves have never personally faced. They

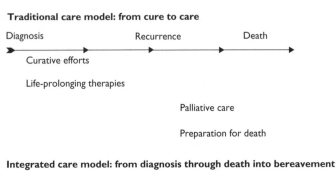

Traditional care model: from cure to care

Diagnosis   Recurrence   Death

Curative efforts

Life-prolonging therapies

Palliative care

Preparation for death

Integrated care model: from diagnosis through death into bereavement

Diagnosis   Death   Bereavement

Disease-modifying therapies

Symptom management

Communication, advance care planning, and death preparation

Family support

Figure 4.3. Traditional and integrated models of care in life-threatening pediatric illness.
Source: Field and Behrman (2002). Reprinted with permission from National Academies Press.

must make decisions despite personal anguish and distress, knowing that they will carry the burden of those decisions for the rest of their lives. Although clinicians cannot take on the full responsibility of decision making, they can use their knowledge, experience, and relatively lower level of emotional involvement with the patient to help the family weigh values, beliefs, and educated expectations to achieve the best outcome for the child (American Academy of Pediatrics 1995).

Decision making about acute or chronic life-threatening conditions requires ongoing discussion about the potential benefits, burdens, and risks of available management options. The timing and content of these discussions depend on the child's health and the urgency of the anticipated changes. The goals of palliative care should be introduced and discussed as early as possible in this process, even when the current goal of care is cure or prolongation of life and imminent death is not expected (see fig. 4.3) (American Academy of Pediatrics 2000).

The perceived benefits, burdens, and risks of palliative and other management options will vary with situations, with families, and, over time, with deterioration of the child's condition (American Academy of Pediatrics 2000). To respond appropriately to such variation and change, health care providers need to create an ongoing, evolving process of decision making rather than treating each decision as an isolated event (American Academy of Pediatrics 1994; Hinds, Oakes, and Furman 2001).

MAINTAINING HOPE

During all discussions with patients and families, clinicians must endeavor to provide accurate and realistic information without eroding hope. The maintenance of hope is essential to most families and patients coping with devastating disease and the possibility of death (American Academy of Pediatrics 2000; Contro et al. 2002). The focus of this hope may shift from hope for cure to hope for comfort or hope to get home, but its importance is not altered. For some children and their families, the hope for cure continues even unto death.

Parent describing the final hospitalization of her chronically ill child: "I guess down deep I thought he was really sick, but I went into this place thinking it definitely works miracles. . . . So I guess I didn't think he was going to die." (Heller and Solomon 2003)

Parent describing the communication with her health care team after her infant son was admitted to the hospital with an acute life threatening event and died thirty-two hours later: "Nobody told us the baby might die. . . . That was OK . . . because it let us have some time to hope and to be with him, spend those last hours with him." (Heller and Solomon 2003)

Society's Perception of Childhood Death

The death of a child is generally considered "unnatural" and one of the worst losses a family can suffer. Owing to an inherent need to do everything possible for an ill child, any technology or intervention tends to be considered simply because it is available if it holds even a small hope of prolonging life.

These decisions are sometimes made without reflection on the suffering imposed on the child or the impact on his or her quality of life. More appropriately child-centered decisions can potentially be facilitated by involving a clinician who is well known to the family and can provide continuity of care, by allowing sufficient time for detailed discussion and reflection about treatment options, and by developing balanced, evidence-based approaches to the use of technology and interventions with such children.

Health Care Providers' Grief

The experience of caring for dying children is highly stressful for clinicians and is accompanied by grief.

> *Physician describing the experience of caring for a child dying of cancer: "I manage to keep a certain distance, because I am deeply affected during the terminal period. I ought to say something to the parents but I am at a loss for words." (Papadatou et al. 2002, 348. Reprinted with permission of Jannetti Publications, Inc.)*

The training and work of clinicians is nearly wholly focused on "fixing" patients. Health care professionals can experience great role ambiguity and helplessness when they can no longer "fix" the problem and instead become bystanders to an irreversible disease process. The sadness clinicians experience when they find themselves unable to do the job for which they have been trained is significant and pervasive, and it may influence care decisions, leading to inappropriate attempts to continue to fix what cannot be repaired. Training in measures to support and comfort children and families can help clinicians feel more comfortable and competent when providing end-of-life care, leading to increased job satisfaction and decreased grief and distress.

Who Is Involved?

People who are commonly involved in decision making in pediatric palliative care are the ill child, parents, close family, and friends, extended family and community, and health care professionals (fig. 4.4). In the course of the child's illness, they interact not only with the child but also with one another.

THE ILL CHILD

Children usually know how ill they are and often find that talking about their hopes and fears is far more reassuring than silence. Children also are often aware of the wishes of authority figures, such as parents and physicians, and

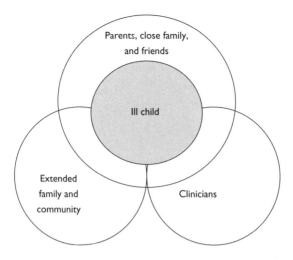

Figure 4.4. Interaction among the people commonly involved in pediatric palliative care decision making.

this may affect their ability to express their wishes and make coercion-free decisions (Leikin and Connell 1983). The life experiences of a chronically ill child can influence how they understand their illness, view their world, and evaluate treatment options.

> *An 11-year-old girl was offered the option of radiation therapy for pain control. She said: "I'm scared because I'm not so good at making decisions. My parents want me to have radiation, but a little voice in me tells me not to. . . . My mother always said that if I die, she wants me to die happy and at home. If I had radiation, I'd have to come into the hospital every day. And I don't know if radiation will really help, or if I would die anyway." (Sourkes 1995, 156. Reprinted by permission of University of Pittsburgh Press)*

There is evidence that children are both intellectually and emotionally capable of being involved in decision making about their own palliative care (American Academy of Pediatrics 1995, 2000). Children who suffer from life-threatening conditions need to be given as much information as they desire (presented in a way they can understand), to contribute to discussions, and

Exhibit 4.1. Play with stuffed toys

A 3-year-old boy played a game with a stuffed duck and a toy ambulance each time he was hospitalized. The duck would be sick and need to go to the hospital by ambulance. The boy would move the ambulance, making siren noises.

> *Therapist:* How is the duck?
> *Child:* Sick.
> *Therapist:* Where is he going?
> *Child:* To the hospital.
> *Therapist:* What are they going to do?
> *Child:* Make him better.
> *Therapist:* Is he going to get better?

During what turned out to be the boy's terminal admission, he played the same game with the duck. However, the ritual changed dramatically in its outcome:

> *Therapist:* How is the duck?
> *Child:* Sick.
> *Therapist:* Is he going to get better?
> *Child* [shaking his head slowly]: Ducky not get better. Ducky die.

Source: Sourkes (1995, 157–58). Reprinted by permission of University of Pittsburgh Press.

to be involved in decisions about their care, with due respect for their developmental level. They should be supported with the love and resources of their families. If the children themselves are unable to make decisions, they need to know that their families will do so for them. They need to be provided with health care that is appropriate to their condition and continuity of care throughout the course of their illness. Most young patients should be encouraged to ask questions and to express feelings and preferences concerning their care. During decision making, great weight should be given to any clearly expressed views. Some children can express themselves easily and clearly with words. Others respond better to a modified and creative approach, using art, music, writing poetry or prose, play acting, and storytelling (see exhibits 4.1 and 4.2). Such techniques can help the clinician assess the child's level of understanding, feelings, and perspectives, and may also decrease a child's fears and sense of isolation. There are valuable resources available and professionals, such as child-life specialists, who are experts in this area. The health care team should incorporate their expertise (IWK Children's Hospital 1991; Sourkes 1995; Stevens 2004b). Finally, children with life-threatening illness deserve

Exhibit 4.2. "If You Only Knew," poem by Barrie R. Pettipas, age 18

As I lie here in bed
So many thoughts go thru my head
Why have I not yet gone
Why must I continue on?
I've been chosen to survive
Even tho' it frustrates me to be alive
I've lost my sight and my taste
And my talent has gone to waste.
If you only knew what I'm going through
Then maybe you could see
Just how it's hurting me.
I just play games with my mind
I'll probably do this till the end of time
My body is so very weak
Even tho' it's sunny, the days are bleak
I'm in pain and so depressed
My whole life's a great big mess.
All the fears I have inside
The ones I cannot hide
Is it any wonder why
I break down and cry?
If you only knew what I'm going through
Then maybe you could see
Just how it's hurting me.

Source: With permission of and thanks to the family of Barrie Pettipas.

knowledgeable and respectful care that is considerate of their developmental stage, cultural, ethical, spiritual, and religious identities.

Adolescents with life-threatening conditions have special needs; in particular, they need help in balancing independence and autonomy with the requirements of their care as recognized by their parents and health professionals (exhibit 4.3). In addition to all the usual challenges of normal teens, they face complex and painful therapy, socially challenging changes in appearance, restrictions on normal teen activities, frequent absences from school and peer relationships, and increased dependence on family members. This can make it difficult for ill adolescents to establish a sense of autonomy and can lead to ambivalence and anger toward family members, particularly parents, and health care professionals (Woodgate 1998; Stevens 2004a).

Exhibit 4.3. Supporting adolescent decision making

Providing support:

- As much as possible, ensure privacy and confidentiality.
- Enable the adolescent to participate in his or her own care.
- In keeping with the adolescent's changing intellectual and emotional maturity and his or her expressed preferences, provide information concerning diagnosis, prognosis, and the benefits and risks of available treatment options.
- Encourage open discussion of treatment options and their likely outcomes, benefits, and burdens.
- Encourage expression of emotions, fears, and hopes.
- Answer all questions honestly and with empathy.
- Offer choices and opportunities for negotiation, even in small matters, whenever possible.

Promoting independence:

- Allow the adolescent to create an individualized space in the hospital—decorating as he or she wishes, allowing friends to stay overnight, and so forth.
- Enable interaction with other adolescents (ill and healthy) as much as possible.

Source: Data from Canadian Pediatrics Society (1994); Carr-Gregg et al. (1997); Stevens (2004a).

PARENTS AND CLOSE FAMILY

Families view themselves as "protectors" of their children, raising them to be healthy and free from danger, discomfort, and death.

A child's illness affects the entire family, testing their core values, relationships, and emotions to the limits.

It is the role of parents and close family members to solicit, assess, and respect the child's perspective on the decisions to be made about his or her care. If the child is unable or unwilling to make decisions, family members must act in the child's best interests and according to his or her values, to the degree that is applicable and reasonable.

Parents need information, provision of resources, and guidance in the decision-making process if they are to continue as "protectors" of their children during life-threatening illness. Family empowerment through decision making subsequently serves the parents in their bereavement (Todres, Earle, and Jellinek 1994; James and Johnson 1997).

Parent, talking about being involved in decision making for the child:
"[The health care professionals] treated me as an active member of the
treatment team. They would definitely listen. Before they made a deci-
sion they would always ask for my input. And they were honest about
not knowing how it was going to go, but they [assured me they] would
do everything they could to keep her within the comfort zone. That was
so important to me. And the fact that they acknowledged that this is
a situation that is not going to have a good outcome." (Contro et al.
2002, 15)

Parents and close family members must have access to basic needs, including food, privacy, sleep, and physical self-care, to maximize their own well-
being and their ability to participate in decision making. Their views should
be solicited respectfully and intensively and then listened to and understood
and incorporated into the plan of care. Their efforts and knowledge related
to the child's illness must be acknowledged by health care providers. They
need to know that they have the support of the health care team. Parents
and close family members need to have their obligations outside the health
care arena recognized and require assistance with obtaining access to community resources for the immediate family, especially siblings.

In the event they are unable or unwilling to decide for themselves the
course of their child's treatment and care, parents need to be confident that
substitute decision makers are available to act on behalf of their child. According to ethical principles, legislation, and hospital policy, there is a stepwise
chain of people (which varies between and within jurisdictions) who can be
designated as substitute decision makers for a pediatric patient judged incapable of making his or her own decisions (American Academy of Pediatrics
1994; Kluge 1995).

EXTENDED FAMILY AND COMMUNITY

Extended family members have often known and loved the child and the
family for many years. They will be the primary support for years after the
child's death. Thus, their role during the child's life is to support the child
and family and to provide wider perspectives and guidance during decision
making, as desired by and appropriate for the child and his or her family.

Extended family, however, also have needs of their own. They need to know
that their support and concern for the child and family is acknowledged,
respected, and valued. To the extent that the family relies on them for support

and guidance in making decisions about the child's care, they need to be provided with information and involved in discussions at the earliest possible stages. Their concerns, and doubts, if any, about the decisions made must be heard in a forum that does not add to the distress of the child or the child's family (Levetown 2002; Meyer et al. 2002).

HEALTH CARE PROFESSIONALS

Similarly skilled professionals differ in their recommendations about potentially life-sustaining interventions, based on attitudinal differences, country of origin, length of professional experience, religion, relationship to patient, and the number of intensive care unit beds in their health center (Webb, Wagner, and Wagner 1998; Randolph et al. 1999; Rebagliato et al. 2000; Carter and Bhatia 2001). They often share the societal value that "death is the enemy"; this can affect their professional interactions with seriously ill children and their families.

The role of health care professionals is complex. They must build a relationship of mutual respect and trust with the child and family, become familiar with the child's and the family's preferences regarding the degree of their involvement in decision making, and solicit their values and concerns. They will also be expected to help the child (as appropriate) and the family to understand the illness and available options, to evaluate those options and reach decisions, and to do so in a sensitive and respectful manner.

Health care professionals apply their knowledge, skills, and experience to ensure that the ill child receives care that is appropriate, desired (based on truly informed consent), and in his or her best interests (American Academy of Pediatrics 1994, 1995; Kluge 1995). They must be aware of the ethical and legal standards related to decision making in pediatric palliative care (American Academy of Pediatrics 1994, 2000). It is also their responsibility to ensure the effective and empathic communication of vital information to the child, his or her family, and their supporters.

Care should be taken that neither the child nor the family feels abandoned during, or overburdened by the responsibility for, decision making (Pinch and Spielman 1990; MacLean 1999; Street et al. 2000). Health care professionals must work collaboratively with other members of the interdisciplinary health care team and should enable or arrange for the provision of emotional and spiritual support for child and family. Finally, they are accountable for the care provided.

The needs of health care professionals are similarly complex. They must be allowed the time and private space to pursue continuing education in palliative care and access to knowledgeable and supportive colleagues. They must also have access to a process for reconciling disagreements and conflicts within the health care team. The importance and difficulty of their work needs to be individually acknowledged and their grieving process supported.

> *A clinician talks about the experience of caring for a dying child: "The most difficult aspect for me is when they all expect me to do something, yet I do not know what. In reality it's not dealing with death anxiety, but rather, with being there, unable to do anything and feeling medically and emotionally helpless and powerless." (Papadatou et al. 2002, 349. Reprinted with permission of Jannetti Publications, Inc.)*

What Decisions Need to Be Made?

A child's illness can follow many possible trajectories. At each stage, the goals of care may change and new decisions will have to be made. These goals can include cure, slowed progression of disease, remission, contribution to research, prolonged life span, achievement of life goals, maximizing normal life experience, maximizing periods of lucidity, comfort, maximizing family access, and care, and perhaps death, in a preferred location. These goals may or may not be achievable, depending on the patient's clinical status and the availability of treatments and resources. They are not necessarily mutually exclusive. Multiple goals may be identified and pursued at any one time, but often they must be prioritized to guide treatment decisions. Figure 4.2 illustrates one possible trajectory, and table 4.1 describes some aspects of decision making at various points along that trajectory.

PARTICIPATION IN CLINICAL TRIALS

A set of decisions faced by many patients and families, particularly when a child is afflicted with cancer, relates to participation in clinical trials and the pursuit of experiential treatments. At least 60 percent of children under the age of 15 who have cancer will enroll in clinical trials at some point in their illness (Levi et al. 2000). Such decisions require some understanding of complex information and risk concepts. Health care providers should strive to ensure complete understanding of such concepts, using graphic depictions

Table 4.1. Decisions during the trajectory of illness

Stage	Decision topics	Important factors	Approaches
Diagnosis Recurrence Exacerbation	• Attempting or forgoing treatments directed at cure or prolonging life • Participation in clinical trials or experimental treatments	• Existence and availability of treatments for amelioration or cure • Realistic chances for cure or improvement • Likelihood of benefit versus burden of treatment • Child's experience (including symptoms, isolation, being in unfamiliar surroundings, fatigue, quality of living) • Value of knowing that "everything possible was done" (may help family and clinicians during bereavement and prevent guilt, regret, and anger)[a]	• Find ways to incorporate the child's preferences • Find ways for clinicians to provide clarity about the options available and likely outcomes without destroying hope • Offer options within reasonable limits • Offer "time-limited trials" of therapy with defined goals and clear intervals for assessment
Remission	• Reintegration with school, peers • Degree of disclosure to child's peers, school officials	• Such decisions are not specific to any particular time point • Child's perception of burden versus benefit • Availability of health personnel to provide information before reintegration	Child's school and peers continue to be important, even during treatment

Slowed progression Approaching end of life	• Attempting or forgoing treatments aimed at prolonging life or relieving symptoms (including transplantation, mechanical ventilation, dialysis, vasoactive and other medications, chemotherapy, artificial nutrition and hydration) • Trials of experimental treatments • Location of care (home, community hospital, tertiary care hospital, or hospice)	• Family may need "permission" to change goals of care • Withdrawing and withholding treatment are legally and ethically equivalent but may feel different emotionally[b] • Decisions about each treatment must be made independently. However, no decision stands in isolation, and there should be frequent review and discussion of all current and planned interventions in the light of recent decisions[c]	• Ensure early discussions (before the imminent emergency) so that care is congruent with the long-held values and wishes of the patient and family, as determined during a nonurgent time • When a decision is equivocal, consider offering a time-limited trial • Evaluate the success of an intervention at defined intervals; discontinue if the risks and burdens outweigh the potential benefits • Provide ongoing support for the child and family • Tailor the location of care to the wishes of the child and family (visitors, privacy, decorations, rituals)

[a]Wyatt (1999).
[b]American Academy of Pediatrics (1994); Lantos et al. (1994); MacLean (1999); Wyatt (1999); Masri et al. (2000); Street et al. (2000).
[c]American Academy of Pediatrics (1994).

of probabilities, eliminating technical jargon from the discussion, and explicitly stating that neither the level nor the quality of care and support for the child and family will be adversely affected if the child does not enroll in the trial. The child should participate in the decision, as his or her perspective may differ significantly from the parents' (Nitschke et al. 1982). A researcher who is not clinically involved with the child's care may be of help in providing a noncoercive explanation.

Parents' desire to ensure that their child receives the most advanced treatments possible, and an altruistic desire to contribute to the care of other children, are factors that may contribute to decisions to participate in clinical trials. Therefore, an honest assessment of the likelihood of individual benefit must be disclosed, as well as benefits of not enrolling (including fewer lost opportunities and decreased pain and other discomfort) (Levi et al. 2000).

DO-NOT-RESUSCITATE DECISIONS

All too commonly, the consideration of palliative care options begins with a discussion about whether to resuscitate in the event of a crisis during a child's final hospitalization. This is unfortunate, for a number of reasons:

- Attempts at resuscitation of infants or children with life-threatening illnesses are rarely successful.
- Multiple discussions, over a lengthy period, are often required before families understand that a successful resuscitation is unlikely.
- Delaying discussion of do-not-resuscitate orders until death is imminent may not allow sufficient time for thorough consideration, leading to unnecessary guilt and regret that can extend far past the death of the child.
- The unnecessary exposure of health care workers to the provision of futile care can lead to job dissatisfaction and the loss of valuable and experienced workers (Mink and Pollack 1992; McCallum, Byrne, and Bruera 2000).

It may be helpful in the framing of discussions to refer to such orders as "do not attempt resuscitation" or "allow natural death" rather than the somewhat brusque "do not resuscitate."

ARTIFICIAL NUTRITION AND HYDRATION

Despite fundoplication and antireflux medications, Stevie was experiencing recurrent life-threatening reflux and aspiration. The option of forgoing artificial nutrition was discussed with his mother. She was concerned about Stevie's potential suffering and was guided to understand that he was unlikely to have discomfort because of his profound degree of neurological impairment. When asked specifically, she realized Stevie had never shown evidence of discomfort when efforts to feed him had failed. She was reassured that usual measures, such as keeping Stevie's mucous membranes moist and providing medications to ensure comfort if there were any behavioral indications that he had pain or other distress, would continue. She considered all the information provided and opted for continuation of artificial nutrition and hydration. With the next aspiration episode, she changed her mind, and these interventions were withdrawn.

Many clinicians and families find decisions about artificial nutrition and hydration (ANH) to be among the most difficult. Adults have an instinctual need to feed dependent children, and the prospect of withholding food and water can evoke strong emotions. These values and emotions should be acknowledged and discussed, but the following factors should also be clearly understood and considered:

- Decisions about ANH should involve evaluation of the benefits and burdens, primarily focusing on the child.
- Despite common perceptions, ANH does not appear to lengthen survival and often causes additional suffering.
- The provision of ANH by enteral or parenteral routes involves burdens of discomfort, bodily invasion, and decreased mobility and carries risks such as infection, obstruction, metabolic derangements, hepatic injury, and side effects.
- Patients may be more comfortable with complete withdrawal of nutrition rather than partial feedings.
- The simple intervention of moistening the oral mucosa, which families can do, can relieve any sensation of dryness accompanying limited fluid intake.
- Forgoing artificial nutrition and hydration in the final phase of life produces no discomfort; it is associated with increasing sedation and reduced choking, dyspnea, pain from edema, and skin breakdown (Nelson et al. 1995; Johnson and Mitchell 2000; Winter 2000).

INTERVENTIONS WITH ADVERSE SIDE EFFECTS

Treatments associated with adverse symptoms and discomfort are generally accepted when the treatment carries significant potential benefits, such as cure or prolongation of a good quality of life. However, a review of the goals of care is appropriate when the potential benefits are outweighed by the likely burdens, as perceived by the child and family. Factors to consider include the following:

- invasiveness and degree of discomfort associated with the intervention
- degree of symptom relief afforded by alternative, noninvasive measures
- location of care and other concomitant consequences of the intervention
- desire and capacity for retention of consciousness
- degree and duration of anticipated relief
- potential physical and emotional impact of the procedure
- proximity to death

MANAGEMENT OF SYMPTOMS IN ADVANCED ILLNESS

Sarah, a 14-year-old who had undergone treatment for a primitive neuroectodermal tumor of the brainstem and spine since the age of 8, was told that her pain might increase in the future and that it would most likely be controlled with medications that would not make her too drowsy or sedated. However, there was a small chance that the pain would not be completely controlled without her being asleep all the time. She was asked her opinion about what to do if that situation arose and clearly stated her preference for pain control even at the price of sedation if that were necessary. Her parents, who were present for the conversation, concurred. Though the need never arose, the child, family, and team knew what to do if it had.

In advanced illness, a generally realistic goal is optimization of physical and cognitive function with provision of adequate symptom relief through use of a combination of pharmacologic and nonpharmacologic measures (exhibit 4.4). On infrequent occasions, achieving both goals of comfort and function are not possible. Medications, including sedatives and analgesics, should be titrated to provide adequate relief from symptoms, even if this means that cognitive, respiratory, or cardiac function becomes compromised as a result (Fleischman et al. 1994; American Academy of Pediatrics 2000).

Exhibit 4.4. Guidelines for ethically grounded management of symptoms at the end of life

---

- The clinician consults with those having expertise in pain and symptom management at the end of life.
- The intention of the care is to provide relief of suffering with preservation of function, to the extent possible.
- The intention is not to cause or hasten the patient's death.
- Analgesic and sedating agents are given in response to pain or other distressing symptoms, such as breathlessness. Reasonable preemptive doses may be provided if distress is a likely consequence of an intervention, such as withdrawal of ventilatory support.
- The doses of analgesic and sedating medications are subsequently titrated, in a stepwise fashion, as needed to alleviate the patient's discomfort.
- If the patient is unable to communicate distress verbally, behavioral observations guide the use of analgesics and sedatives.
- The need for analgesics and sedatives, the doses given, and the patient's response are documented.

Source: Data from American Academy of Pediatrics (2000); Masri et al. (2000).

This practice is commonly referred to as *terminal sedation,* meaning sedation at the end of life, which can be easily misunderstood by patients, families, and clinicians as euthanasia or an active hastening of death (American Academy of Pediatrics 2000). Patients, families, and health care providers must clearly understand that these medications will be given only for the purpose of relieving symptoms and are not given to cause or hasten death. They may have a secondary, unintended, effect of shortening life by a few hours or days, though this is rarely the case.

CARE IN THE LAST DAYS OR HOURS OF LIFE

Once 18-year-old Juanita was allowed to participate in the discussion of her prognosis and preferences, she shared many hopes, fears, and dreams. She hoped that her mother, who was 54 and healthy and on whom she was dependent, would not predecease her. She also hoped that her mother, whom she loved dearly, would be able to cope without her. After receiving assurances about these concerns, she turned her hope to three events for the following weekend: to attend her cousin's high school graduation; to celebrate her nineteenth birthday at her favorite restaurant, twenty miles away; and to attend a memorial concert for her fallen idol. Juanita's dyspnea was difficult to control: she was receiving round-the-clock BiPAP and opioids routinely and was frequently sleepy. She clearly had very little time left. Given the temporal proximity of her goals, it was imperative to try to maintain consciousness while controlling dyspnea, allowing Juanita control over her degree of discomfort. She chose to sleep rather than attend the graduation, and at her birthday party she ate little, but with liquid oxygen, a backup generator, and a lot of excitement, she was completely alert and in no distress at the concert, for a full eight hours. She died comfortably two days later.

Proactive decision making about care during the last hours and days of life is made particularly difficult by our inability to predict the timing of specific symptoms and events. Planning for all the what-ifs and just-in-cases requires careful consideration of the patient's wishes, best interests, values, beliefs, and goals. It also requires a full understanding of the patient's medical situation and all the possible events or decision points that might arise before death.

Although they are unusual in pediatric care, advance directives and living wills are frequently used by adults to express their wishes concerning end-of-life care. They provide patients with some assurance that their wishes concerning end-of-life care will be considered even if they have lost the capacity to communicate those wishes at the time the decisions are implemented. Children can execute such documents. However, though ethically meaningful, these documents are not legally binding (Jefferson et al. 1991). Even in the absence of such a document or supporting legislation, families and clinicians have a moral obligation to attempt to honor the expressed views of the child patient (Browne and Sullivan 1999).

When? Getting the Timing Right

Finding the right time to introduce discussions concerning end-of-life care can be a challenge. Waiting for the "optimal" moment generally results in delaying discussions until the need for decisions is imminent. A better approach is to introduce the topic as soon as possible after diagnosis of any illness that could result in premature death.

The intensity of this introductory discussion should be guided by both the child's clinical situation and the child's and family's reaction to the introduction of the topic. For families facing an acute situation, such as a multiple trauma, the conversations need to be paced, but in short intervals.

Parent whose child died within forty-eight hours of admission following anaphylactic shock and cardiac arrest: "We wanted to be sure every possible chance was given to him, and sufficient time for his brain to heal and sufficient time to be sure this was irreversible. And we did." (Heller and Solomon 2003)

Some young patients and their families, especially those who have been living with a life-threatening condition for some time, have thought about these issues and may have talked about them among themselves. They may want to discuss their thoughts and wishes with a clinician but fear doing so because it might imply that they have given up hope for a cure or lost confidence in their health care team. Other patients and their families may not be ready to talk about these decisions in detail at first. For these families, early mention of palliative care can reduce the fear associated with such treatment options, allow time for thought, imply openness to alternative goals of care, and plant the seeds for decisions to be made over time (M. A. Mullen and M. Rattray, personal communication, July 16, 2002).

There remains a myth that the introduction of such topics can interfere with the patient's or the family's hope for cure or improvement. Most parents who recognize that their child is likely to die nevertheless maintain hope. At the same time, they are able to discuss their concerns and wishes about preparations for death and acknowledge that the lessening of suffering should be the primary goal of treatment (James and Johnson 1997; Wolfe et al. 2000). Thus the early discussion and integration of palliative care measures can be reassuring and lead to improved care and quality of life for seriously ill children (Pierucci, Kirby, and Leuthner 2001). Early discussions are also important because the child then has the opportunity to express his or her wishes concerning care options and may have enough time to achieve personal goals—take a meaningful trip, say good-bye to friends and family, prepare special mementos or legacies—while still physically and mentally capable.

Once such discussions are broached, periodic revisiting of the topic, initiated by the clinician or the family, may make later definitive discussions and decisions easier (Hinds, Oakes, and Furman 2001). This ongoing discussion allows patients and families to digest information concerning palliative care options, combine that information with their values, beliefs, and expectations, and build consensus.

How? The Cycle of Decision Making

Decision making in pediatric palliative care is cyclical in nature (fig. 4.5). The first step in effective decision making is to assess the patient's and family's styles of communication. This assessment may occur through observation or by explicit discussion of topics such as the following:

- How does the family currently communicate?
- Who is the primary decision maker?
- How much and in what format do the patient and family prefer to receive information?
- What information is shared with family members and with others?
- What information is shared with the patient? with siblings? with the extended family? How is the information shared?
- Are certain topics taboo?
- How does the patient communicate with his or her family?
- How are emotions and needs communicated? (Buckman 1993)

Additionally, disclosure of clinicians' culture, values, and attitudes toward confidentiality, truth telling, emotional involvement, uncertainty, the ethic of "do no harm," and futility, time constraints, and resource management—all of which are usually not known to patients and their families—is important to effective communication (Buckman 1993). Clearly stating the expectations and responsibilities of the clinician, the patient, and the patient's family is critical to effective decision making and high-quality care.

As in any health care relationship, it is essential to explore, acknowledge, and work with the cultural, spiritual, and ethnic beliefs and values of the family as a whole and the individuals within the family. Although certain ethnic and religious groups tend to have a shared sense of meaning and traditions surrounding death and dying, the variability among individuals may be greater than the variability among groups. Avoiding stereotypes and gently inquiring about the beliefs and values of each individual is the best approach (exhibit 4.5). The health care center's translation service (or the equivalent) can be an excellent source of information and advice in this area.

It is also important to explore, acknowledge, and work with the culture and values of the health care system and its individual professionals. These

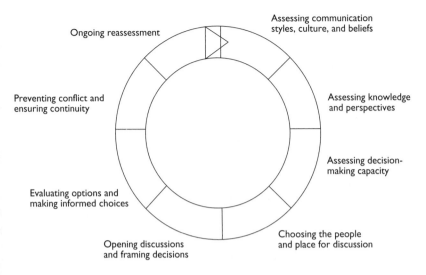

Figure 4.5. The cycle of pediatric palliative care decision making.

Exhibit 4.5. Culture and pediatric palliative care decision making

---

A family's cultural context can have a tremendous effect on their perceptions concerning such things as

- the child's role in decision making;
- who the key decision maker is (it may not be the same person as the primary caregiver);
- the degree of authority granted to the clinician in terms of decision making;
- the involvement of extended or geographically distant family members in decision making;
- the relative importance of quality-of-life concerns versus chances for cure or extension of life;
- the acceptability of options such as forgoing potentially life-sustaining interventions, including ventilation, and artificial nutrition and hydration;
- the use of analgesics and other interventions;
- the desire to have the child cared for in hospital or at home during the last period of life.

Source: Data from Hallenbeck (2001).

Exhibit 4.6. Approaches to discussing cultural issues with families

- Each time I meet a new family, it is helpful for me to understand how they make decisions. When do you want your child to be present for discussions? Who would you say is the person in your family whom everyone looks to for very important decisions? It would be useful to know these things when planning your child's care.
- Different people have different beliefs about medical treatments, such as pain medications like morphine and ventilator machines that help someone breathe. I would like to find out your thoughts on such things, just in case your child gets to the point where we start thinking about using them. It can be very helpful if we know about your beliefs ahead of time so that we can all work together.
- Some families need to consult with people in their community before making important decisions. It may be with a leader in their religious community, a respected elder, or someone who is a healer in their community. These consultations can be very helpful for some families. Is there anyone special whom you may want to talk with about these decisions?

factors help shape all health care decisions but are of particular importance when the decisions are related to dying (exhibit 4.6).

The next step is the assessment of the patient's and family's current understanding and perspectives concerning the illness, current care and priorities, and how they are coping. It is clear that this is rarely done. In fact children interviewed about their perception of their role in their care or the importance of their priorities indicate that they feel they are peripheral to the discussion (Young et al. 2003). The benefits of more directly involving children include greater adherence to the agreed-upon medical regimen, obtaining the critical input of information known only to the child-patient, developing and respecting the child's autonomy as an individual, and, in some jurisdictions, following the law. Exhibits 4.7 and 4.8 provide suggested questions for this type of assessment.

Finally, an assessment must be made concerning the child's capacity for health care decision making. The ethical principle of respect for autonomy supports the use of competence or capacity, rather than age or life experience, as the test when deciding whether an individual has the right to make his or her own health care decisions (American Academy of Pediatrics 1995; Kluge 1995; Sahler et al. 2000; Hinds, Oakes, and Furman 2001). A child or adolescent who has not yet reached the age of legal majority and is not considered an emancipated minor but is able to understand the proposed inter-

Exhibit 4.7. Suggested questions for the family

- Please tell me, in your own words, what you understand about your child's condition.
- Please tell me, in your own words, what you understand about the care being provided to your child at the moment.
- What things have you found particularly difficult to deal with during your child's illness? Who or what has helped you through them? What kinds of additional help do you need, if any?
- How have you been involved in decision making about your child's care up to this point? How have you felt about that involvement? How would you like to be involved?
- How have other members of your family (for example, your child's siblings or grandparents) been involved in discussions and decision making up to this point?
- What are your wishes about the care being provided to your child?
- If we were looking at a time when your child may not be able to get through the illness, can you tell me some of your wishes about that time? How would you like things to be?
- Do you have any particular worries about the time when your child may not be able to live through this illness?
- What are your fears or concerns about what your child is experiencing now? in the future?
- What are the most difficult things you are facing at this time? What do you think you might need to help you get through this time?
- What are your fears or concerns about what your child may experience if he or she is unable to live through this illness?
- Is there something that I could do, or avoid doing, to better help you and your family through this time?
- Is there something you can think of that would best help your child through this time?

ventions and their consequences is considered competent or capable of making his or her own health care decisions. In the United States, the child's decisions are not legally binding unless the child is an emancipated minor or of legal majority, but the principle of "mature minor" as described here mandates a moral obligation to honor the child's stated preferences, or at least consider them when formulating the plan of care.

Many children with life-threatening conditions have, through the course of the illness, achieved such a high level of maturity and understanding regarding the illness and its treatments that their decisions, even about life-and-death situations, are as valid as those of a competent adult. Capacity, however, can change with time, with the physical, cognitive, and emotional

Exhibit 4.8. Suggested questions for the child

- What do you think is happening to you? Why do you think it is happening? What do you hope will happen? What are you most afraid of?
- Please tell me about the medicines and other treatments you're getting today, this week, and at the moment.
- Why do you think you're getting these medicines and other treatments?
- How do these medicines or other treatments make you feel?
- When you first started getting these medicines or other treatments, did anybody talk to you about what you thought about them? What do you remember about that?
- What's been the most difficult thing you had to go through since you got sick? What helped you get through that?
- What's the most difficult thing you're thinking about right now? Who or what do you think could help you with that?
- What are the most important things you want to do in the next day, week, and month?
- If you had three wishes, what would you wish for? If you had three wishes and I could do magic to make them happen, what would you wish for? [The second wording is useful for stimulating the imagination of an older child or adolescent but should be avoided in a child who uses magical thinking to explain the illness.]

effects of illness on the child, and with the nature of the decision being made (American Academy of Pediatrics 1994). A 10-year-old boy with relapsing leukemia and pleural effusions, for example, may be considered able to clearly articulate the pros and cons of the therapeutic options and yet be considered incapable of making the decision to forgo life support owing to a perceived lack of appreciation of the permanence of death.

Within this clinical, ethical, and legal framework, clinicians have become responsible for evaluating every pediatric patient's capacity to make decisions and ensuring that the maximal input desired by the patient is accommodated (Canadian Pediatrics Society 1986; Nelson and Nelson 1992; American Academy of Pediatrics 1994; Kenny 1999). Exhibit 4.9 provides general guidelines for assessing capacity; health care professionals should refer to their own institutions for more specific guidelines or requirements. Such an assessment must be made at each decision point. Once made, the decision reached by a capable patient is durable and should be implemented subsequently even if the patient's capacity changes or the clinician disagrees with the decision made.

When the time arrives for definitive discussions and decisions, the setting and timing of conversations should be as conducive as possible. The best

Exhibit 4.9. General criteria for assessing capacity

To be considered capable of making decisions about his or her care, the patient must

- know that there is a decision to be made and be able to receive and appreciate information necessary for making that decision;
- be able to understand the potential consequences of each alternative;
- be willing to make a decision;
- be able to communicate the decision by some mode;
- be able to integrate the information in such a way as to produce the decision; and
- be able to weigh conflicting factors in a decision and reach a resolution by application of a stable set of values or priorities.

Source: Data from American Academy of Pediatrics (1994); Kenny (1999).

setting is one that is private and quiet. All the key people, as defined by the patient or designated decision makers and the health care team, are present. However, the clinician should be careful not to overwhelm the patient and family with a large number of health care professionals. Familiar personnel are most appreciated.

Parent, discussing the importance of talking with clinicians who are familiar to them: "The social worker who was there for four years with us and the oncologist . . . is the one who talked to us . . . and that, to me, was very important, because I didn't . . . want to hear it from anybody else except from her because she was more like personal, I think." (Heller and Solomon 2003)

Within the constraints of the clinical situation, as much time as possible should be set aside for these discussions. There is great variation in the amount of time required by physicians and families to agree on a course of action when the patient's illness is progressing toward death (Wall and Partridge 1997; McCallum, Byrne, and Bruera 2000).

Finding the words to begin a discussion of palliative care options can be difficult. Exhibit 4.10 provides some suggested language. However, the most important thing is to regard each family and patient as unique and to approach each discussion with an open mind. Often, simply starting with where the child is in a course of therapy, reviewing responses to treatments offered thus far, and asking how the child or family believes things are going

Exhibit 4.10. Suggestions for opening discussions

- I would like to take a few minutes to talk about some decisions about treatment for Maia that may come up in the future. As you know, it is possible that Maia's condition will get worse and that she may die. We are doing all we can to prevent that, but if that time comes, you and Maia may want to change the way she receives care. [Pause for response.] For instance, you may want to avoid a lot of procedures and time in the hospital, and you may choose to take her home and receive help to make her comfortable there. Maybe you are ready to talk about these kinds of things today, but it may take some time before you're ready. [Pause for response.] That's okay. I just want to let you know that I'm ready to talk about those kinds of things whenever you feel ready.
- Other families have told me that it can be very difficult to think and talk about decisions related to dying when they're still hoping for a cure. But the families whose children have died tell me that, when the time came, they were very glad they had considered and talked about those decisions beforehand.
- We can start talking now about the issues that may come up if your child's condition gets worse, but we don't have to make any of the decisions right now. You can think about it all, talk with your family, friends, spiritual adviser, family doctor, or whomever else you want. Then we can make the decisions bit by bit, as we go along.
- As we go along, it's really important that you ask whatever questions you have on your mind, even if you think they might be obvious or very difficult to ask. Just to give you an example, some parents who are thinking about taking their child home for care at the end of life want to know who they are supposed to call at the time of death. It's very difficult for them to ask about that but it's very important information for them to know. So whenever you have questions, about *anything*, please just ask. We will do our best to answer them.

will open the door for a more focused discussion. Being somewhat pointed in breaking the news that a disease's progression has not been altered by treatment may be necessary; parents often understand the gravity of an illness later than the professional health care team. But helping them to understand earlier may result in more thorough attention to palliative and comfort measures (Wolfe et al. 2000). As the discussion unfolds, incorporating or integrating palliative options for care into extant protocols or treatment regimens—provided that they remain appropriate and nonburdensome treatments—may ease the reality of needing to redirect the goals of care.

When framing decisions for families and patients, clinicians must sensitively present the available options within the reality of the disease process. Appropriate framing of the reasonable treatment options can make it easier for the child and family to understand the information presented, integrate

Exhibit 4.11. A suggestion for framing decisions when the options are limited

---

I wish we had more options than these. But there is no medicine, no surgery, and no amount of love, because you clearly love her very much, that will make your child better. You still have options and choices about where she receives care, whom you would like to be present, how her symptoms are managed, and things like that.

---

it into their view of the situation, feel supported, and face the necessary decisions. This may be important in preventing later doubts and guilt regarding the decisions taken.

The pattern and rapid progression of some diseases can make the success of certain intensive or invasive treatments extremely unlikely. Without appropriate framing of decisions, parents may pursue such treatments because they feel that not doing so would be equivalent to abandoning their child. If parents understand that because of the disease process or its trajectory certain treatment modalities will not work, they may be more confident in their decisions and may thereby avoid later misgivings concerning their choices. Exhibit 4.11 suggests one way of framing decisions at critical points in the trajectory of illness. It can also be helpful to provide reassurance that, whatever treatment is chosen, the parents will continue to be supported.

Special attention is warranted in the case of urgent decision making, when the family or the patient is not well known to the physician and decisions must be made quickly. Exhibit 4.12 provides some suggested language for starting such discussions. While extreme care must be taken to listen and speak with sensitivity and clarity, the same principles apply in this situation as in all others: attend to the needs of the family and encourage discussion of options as early as possible. It is important to use easily understood language, to repeat information, to give information in small and manageable chunks, and to check for understanding by asking the child and the family to repeat what they have heard in their own words.

It may be helpful to assign a member of the health care team to be the caregiver for the family. That person attends to the simple needs of the family—providing private space with a telephone, food, and other basic comforts—and can make an enormous difference in the family's capacity to absorb information and make decisions. The family caregiver can also be the primary source of updated information and the initiator of discussions concerning imminent or upcoming decision points.

Exhibit 4.12. Suggestions for framing urgent decisions

- We normally would not be asking you to make these decisions so quickly, and we recognize that it must be very difficult for you to face all of this at once. Is there someone who could help you sort through all of this information? Your family physician? Your pediatrician? Someone in your family? A friend? Your religious leader? Is there anyone you would like to be here to support you during this time?
- Many of the things that we're discussing are very difficult things to talk about. Some of them don't need to be decided right now, but I've found with other families in similar circumstances that it's useful to talk about these things well before we actually need to make the decision. If we don't and then the decision comes up very suddenly, we might not have enough time to talk it through properly.

Some families struggle to tell their child about his or her illness, treatment options, and possible death and do not know how to enable an older child or adolescent to obtain information about the illness and treatments or how to participate actively in decisions about their own care. Possible techniques and strategies in these situations are included in exhibit 4.13.

Patients and parents may also need suggestions for talking to family members and friends about the illness and treatment decisions (Hinds, Oakes, and Furman 2001). In general, the greater the number of family members and friends who understand the situation, the greater the support network available to the patient and parents. This may help prevent the common doubts and disagreements within the extended support network that can be devastating for parents, particularly after the child's death (Meyer et al. 2002). However, the burden of communicating with all of these people can be great. Useful techniques and strategies are included in exhibit 4.14.

Clinicians and parents often weigh available options differently, depending on their priorities, perspectives, and beliefs (exhibit 4.15). These differences in perspective, combined with ineffective communication, can make consensus building difficult and lead to disagreement or outright conflict between parents and clinicians (Abbott et al. 2001).

Once the realistic options have been presented, it is useful to have a structure for systematically discussing and evaluating each of them in turn. One such structure is a series of questions used to evaluate the likely benefits, burdens, and risks of each option (exhibit 4.16). Decision making through the weighing of pros and cons is a familiar process for many people. It is also the

Exhibit 4.13. Suggestions for helping families talk to a child with a life-threatening illness

- Suggest that the parents tell stories or read books that deal with the topics of illness and death in ways that are appropriate to the patient's level of development and disease progression (see the appendix for suggested readings).
- Ask questions about how the child usually communicates and likes to receive information. Does the child usually like to hear lots of detail or just the basics? Use this information to provide guidance to the family on conducting discussions with the child.
- Suggest age-appropriate language to use with the child when discussing illness and death.
- Provide guidance about the types of questions and reactions to expect from the child.
- Discuss creative methods of communicating, such as through play.
- Provide opportunities for the parents to talk to the parents of other children with similar illnesses.

Exhibit 4.14. Suggestions for helping parents talk to extended family and friends

- Convene a meeting with as many as possible of the family and friends present so that the health care providers can provide the same information to everyone and answer questions. When family and friends are at a distance, they can be included with the use of teleconferencing or by making an audiotape or videotape of the meeting that can be played for them later (Rylance 1992; Braner et al. 2000).
- Tell the patient or parents about easily accessible and accurate Internet sites to which they can refer family and friends for more detailed information (see the appendix for suggested websites).
- Provide the patient or parents with "info sheets" that contain concise but informative written descriptions of the illness, its prognosis and treatments, possible genetic implications, and so forth. These are useful to give to family and friends so that the patient and parents do not need to repeatedly communicate all of this information.

primary basis for ethical and legal decision making and should be applied to all decisions, even those that appear straightforward on the surface (Nelson and Nelson 1992; American Academy of Pediatrics 1994; Street et al. 2000; M. A. Mullen and M. Rattray, personal communication, July 16, 2002).

A process of this sort helps all the participants fully understand their own perspectives and those of the other participants on each of the available options. Such mutual understanding usually facilitates agreement; if disagreement

Exhibit 4.15. Factors influencing palliative care decisions

Physicians are most influenced by

- the family's or patient's expressed wishes;
- the probability of survival and predicted quality of life if the patient survives;
- the patient's current functional status;
- the availability of potentially effective treatments;
- information provided by other members of the health care team;
- the presence of unrelenting pain or other symptoms;
- fears of malpractice litigation.

Parents tend to be most influenced by

- recommendations and information received from health care professionals;
- the child's current quality of life, including pain and discomfort;
- the child's expressed wishes concerning continuing or not continuing treatment;
- the child's chance of improvement or survival;
- concerns about the adverse effects of treatment options.

Source: Data from Randolph et al. (1997); Wall and Partridge (1997); van der Heide et al. (1998); Street et al. (2000); Hinds, Oakes, and Furman (2001).

Exhibit 4.16. Evaluating treatment options

- How realistic is it that the intervention will cure the disease?
- If not able to cure the disease, will it prevent progression of the disease?
- Will the intervention improve the way the child feels?
- Could the intervention make the child feel worse? If so, for how long?
- What will it be like for this child to go through this treatment?
- What is likely to happen without the intervention?
- Will the intervention change the outcome for the child?
- What is the likely impact of this decision on the family?

Source: Data from Frager (1999).

exists, this process will clarify the exact nature of the disagreement and perhaps lead to a compromise or an agreement to disagree on that particular point but proceed on the basis of the consensus achieved in other areas (Nelson and Nelson 1992).

Informed choice during decision making about pediatric palliative care most often occurs as part of an ongoing process of discussion rather than a one-time event. The generally accepted components of an informed choice are outlined in exhibit 4.17.

Exhibit 4.17. Components of informed choice

Briefly, an informed choice is commonly considered to consist of four components:

- competency or capacity on the part of the decision maker
- disclosure of all appropriate information concerning the nature of the illness, the likelihood of benefit from reasonable treatment options, including pursuing no potentially curative or life-prolonging treatments, and the common serious and special risks and side effects of those treatments
- understanding of the provided information by the decision maker
- voluntary decision making, free of coercion or manipulation

---

Source: Data from American Academy of Pediatrics (1995).

Achieving this standard of informed decision making is an essential but difficult task for clinicians caring for critically ill children. It is also a process that can be easily and subtly manipulated by those involved, particularly by the physician.

Most parents want to play an active role in decision making about their child's care and to receive honest information about even the most difficult topics, and most are able to comprehend and work with complex medical information (Lesko et al. 1989; James and Johnson 1997; van der Heide et al. 1998; Levi et al. 2000). Uncommonly, parents feel overburdened by the responsibility of decision making and want clinicians to provide strong recommendations and effectively make the decisions for them (Lesko et al. 1989; Schlomann and Fister 1995; Levi et al. 2000). Exhibit 4.18 presents some suggested responses to parents who are uncomfortable being responsible for decisions about their child's health care. Disclosure and discussion of palliative care options should always proceed with sensitivity and compassion, regardless of the final decision. Decisions should be framed in such a way that the decision makers feel fully informed yet secure and trusting of the process.

During decision making, consensus building among the patient, parents or other surrogate decision makers, and the health care team is the best way to preempt conflict (American Academy of Pediatrics 1994). This is possible, in many cases, through appropriate framing of realistic options, effective and supportive communication, mutual understanding and respect, and the availability of sufficient time for discussion and evaluation of available options (Nelson and Nelson 1992; Randolph et al. 1997; Hinds, Oakes, and Furman 2001).

Exhibit 4.18. Suggested responses when a patient or family expresses discomfort with the responsibility of decision making

---

- When you think about this decision, what are your hopes? What thoughts have you had about it?
- I have heard you talk about a range of things that you would like for your child at this time. This gives us some guidance, and some of those things are possible. However, other outcomes are not going to be possible because. . . .
- The choice we have to make is really between options X and Y. Let's focus on just these realistic options. What do you think about them?
- We have talked about many different options for your child's treatment at this time. It can sometimes be very difficult for parents to make these kinds of decisions for their child. They feel that the responsibility is too much. Based on my relationship with you, knowing your values, and having helped many other families in this situation, I can recommend what I think is the best choice for your child, and you can tell me whether you agree or disagree. We will work together to find the best solution.

Exhibit 4.19. Sources of disagreement or conflict

The following factors or situations may increase the risk of disagreement and conflict:

- critical illness or an unexpected or severe event
- lack of prognostic certainty
- the involvement of a large number of primary and specialist health care providers
- previous experiences of others being cured or dying from the same or a similar illness
- insufficient or ineffective communication with health care providers
- the patient's or family's perceptions of unprofessional behavior by health care providers
- perceptions by health care providers about the patient's or family's "unrealistic" expectations for cure
- differences in religious perspectives, cultural beliefs, and values
- lack of a shared language or available translators
- lack of parental knowledge concerning the legal rights of adolescents and mature minors
- families with other ill members, internal conflict, geographical separation, parental separation or divorce

---

Source: Data from Nelson and Nelson (1992); American Academy of Pediatrics (1997); Browne and Sullivan (1999); Cutler et al. (1999); Abbott et al. (2001); Hallenbeck (2001); Contro et al. (2002); Stevens (2004a).

Exhibit 4.20. A general approach to managing conflicts during decision making

---

- Express genuine interest in resolving the conflict and a willingness to accept differences of opinion.
- Allow expression of the emotional components of the conflict and respond to them empathetically; then seek an agreement to focus on the discussions and decisions at hand rather than the emotions.
- Seek a detailed understanding and agreement concerning the root of a conflict, focusing on each party's understanding of the facts of the situation, the level of uncertainty involved, and the emotions, values, or beliefs that are shaping his or her perspective on the issue.
- If appropriate, seek agreement to a time-limited trial of the proposed treatment or change in care.
- Involve other professionals, such as ethics consultants, psychiatrists, social workers, spiritual advisers, trusted family advisers, and trained mediators, to help resolve disputes or facilitate a compromise.
- If the conflict cannot be resolved and no compromise decision can be reached, the treating physician has four options:
    - transfer care to another physician who will provide the care about which there is conflict or who may be able to reach a consensus with the patient or family
    - treat the patient according to the wishes of the patient or family but against the objections of the health care team
    - initiate legal proceedings to resolve the dispute
    - treat the patient according to the physician's understanding of what is best, against the wishes of the family, and place the burden on the patient or family to begin legal proceedings

---

Source: Data from Nelson and Nelson (1992); Buckman (1993); American Academy of Pediatrics (1995).

When disagreements occur, a systematic approach should be used to help all those involved understand one another's perspectives and rationale. The details of such approaches differ among authors, but the essential components are similar (exhibit 4.20). Chapter 2 in this volume addresses a number of these issues.

Seriously ill children are often cared for by a wide variety of general and specialist clinicians. Patients and their families often receive apparently conflicting information and advice from different clinicians, which can make decisions even more difficult. When the emphasis of care shifts toward preparing for death, the personnel involved in providing care are often different from those who facilitate decisions.

Maintaining continuity of care is obviously a difficult task, and patients and families are often left feeling abandoned, misunderstood, and unsupported

Exhibit 4.21. Suggested strategies for enhancing the continuity of care

---

- Involve one or more of the palliative care team members early in the trajectory of illness.
- Involve a community-based clinician who is well known to the family and can provide support throughout the trajectory of illness.
- Explain the health care team's methods of working and maintaining continuity (for example, the on-service and on-call schedules, timing of medical and family rounds, methods of communication between team members, and collective care arrangements).
- Where possible, designate one clinician as the key information source and arbitrator of care, especially when the prognosis is poor. When this is not possible, interdisciplinary meetings to achieve consensus on the prognosis and care plan, before discussions are held with the family, are essential to ensuring the consistency and continuity of information provided.
- Make explicit agreements about when to revisit or review the goals of care, progress of treatment, and alternative treatment options.
- Invite families to contribute to enhanced continuity of care (if they do not find it too burdensome) by
  - keeping a log book of symptoms, results, treatments, side effects, decisions taken, and so forth;
  - reminding clinicians about pending reports and consultations;
  - designating one family member to collect and coordinate information;
  - using e-mail and other means to maintain contact with distant clinicians;
  - tape recording meetings or important conversations for later clarification;
  - videotaping unusual or questionable symptoms or events that occur when a clinician is not present.
- Document all substantive discussions and decisions explicitly in the form of clear, specific, and detailed orders and explanatory progress notes. Orders for appropriate management of anticipated and ongoing pain and other symptoms should always be present in a patient's chart, including when a do-not-attempt-resuscitation or other order concerning potentially life-sustaining treatment is in effect.

Source: Data from American Academy of Pediatrics (1994); Todres, Earle, and Jellinek (1994); Abbott et al. (2001); Lister (2001); Contro et al. (2002).

at a time when the burden of uncertainty and emotional distress is at its peak (Altilio 2001; Lister 2001). Exhibit 4.21 outlines strategies to help lighten this burden.

Summary

The difficult process of making decisions for and with seriously ill children and their families can be improved by effective and empathic communication between and among health care providers and families, thorough medical knowledge, a willingness to admit uncertainty, and an exploration of values and concerns. The primary focus should remain on the child, but there are lifelong effects for surviving family members related to their decisions. Decision making should be viewed as a process, and a systematic approach to the process can lead to the best outcome for all involved.

Acknowledgments

Thank you to those who have encouraged and supported this work: the Advisory Committee and staff of the Ian Anderson Continuing Education Program in End-of-Life Care; many colleagues at the IWK Health Centre and from across Canada; Cancer Care Nova Scotia and Cancer Research and Education (CaRE); Bob Archuletta, M.D., chairman and medical director, Noah's Children, Richmond, Virginia; and Karen S. Heller and Mildred Z. Solomon, of the Initiative for Pediatric Palliative Care at Education Development Center, Inc., in Newton, Massachusetts.

References

Abbott, K. H., J. G. Sago, C. M. Breen, A. P. Abernethy, and J. A. Tulsky. 2001. Families looking back: one year after discussion of withdrawal or withholding of life-sustaining support. *Crit Care Med* 2:197–201.

Altilio, T. 2001. Learning from Liza. *J Pain Symptom Manage* 21:251–53.

American Academy of Pediatrics, Committee on Bioethics. 1994. Guidelines on forgoing life-sustaining medical treatment. *Pediatrics* 93:532–36.

———. 1995. Informed consent, parental permission, and assent in pediatric practice. *Pediatrics* 95:314–17.

———. 1997. Religious objections to medical care. *Pediatrics* 99:279–81.

American Academy of Pediatrics, Committee on Bioethics and Committee on Hospital Care. 2000. Palliative care for children. *Pediatrics* 106:351–57.

Braner, D. A. V., I. M. Laura, R. Hodo, L. Susanna, E. S. Miles, and B. Goldstein. 2000. Interactive web-based communication with referring physicians and families in the pediatric intensive care unit. *Crit Care Med* 28(Suppl. S):125.

Browne, A., and W. J. Sullivan. 1999. Advance directives: a third option. *Ann R Coll Phys Surg Can* 32:352–54. [Comments published in *Ann R Coll Phys Surg Can* 33:24–26.]

Buckman, R. 1993. Communication in palliative care: a practical guide. In *Oxford textbook of palliative medicine,* ed. D. Doyle, G. W. C. Hanks, and N. Macdonald, 47–60. Oxford, U.K.: Oxford University Press.

Canadian Pediatric Society, Adolescent Medicine Committee. 1994. Care of the chronically ill adolescent. *Can J Pediatr* 1:124–27.

Canadian Pediatric Society, Bioethics Committee. 1986. Treatment decisions for infants and children. *Can Med Assoc J* 135:447–48.

Carr-Gregg, M. R. C., S. M. Sawyer, C. F. Clarke, and G. Bowes. 1997. Caring for the terminally ill adolescent. *Med J Aust* 166:255–58.

Carter, B. S., and J. Bhatia. 2001. Comfort/palliative care guidelines for neonatal practice: development and implementation in an academic medical center. *J Perinatol* 21:272–78.

Carter, B. S., and S. R. Leuthner. 2003. The ethics of withholding/withdrawing nutrition in the newborn. *Sem Perinatol* 27:480–87.

Contro, N., J. Larson, S. Scofield, B. Sourkes, and H. Cohen. 2002. Family perspectives on the quality of pediatric palliative care. *Arch Pediatr Adolesc Med* 156:14–19.

Cutler, E. M., M. D. Bateman, P. C. Wollan, and P. S. Simmons. 1999. Parental knowledge and attitudes of Minnesota laws concerning adolescent medical care. *Pediatrics* 103:582–87.

Field, M. J., and R. E. Behrman, eds. 2002. *When children die: improving palliative care and end-of-life care for children and their families.* Committee on Palliative and End-of-Life Care for Children and Their Families, Board on Health Sciences Policy, Institute of Medicine. Washington, D.C.: National Academies Press.

Fleischman, A. R., K. Nolan, N. N. Dubler, M. F. Epstein, M. A. Gerben, M. S. Jellinek, I. F. Litt, M. S. Miles, S. Oppenheimer, A. Shaw, J. van Eys, and V. C. Vaughan III. 1994. Caring for gravely ill children. *Pediatrics* 94:433–39.

Frager, G. 1999. Pediatric palliative care. In *Palliative medicine secrets,* ed. S. K. Joishy, 157–73. Philadelphia: Hanley and Belfus.

Hallenbeck, J. L. 2001. Intercultural differences and communication at the end of life. *Prim Care* 28:401–13.

Heller, K. S., and M. Z. Solomon. 2003. The Initiative for Pediatric Palliative Care. Research data. Newton, Mass.: Education Development Center.

Hinds, P. S., L. Oakes, and W. Furman. 2001. End-of-life decision making in pediatric oncology. In *Textbook of palliative nursing,* ed. B. R. Ferrell and N. Coyle, 450–60. Oxford, U.K.: Oxford University Press.

IWK Children's Hospital. 1991. *Being here: writing by kids at the IWK Children's Hospital.* Halifax, N.S.: IWK Health Centre.

James, L., and B. Johnson. 1997. The needs of parents of pediatric oncology patients during the palliative care phase. *J Pediatr Oncol* 14:83–95.

Jefferson, L. S., B. C. White, P. T. Louis, B. A. Brody, D. D. King, and C. E. Roberts. 1991. Use of the Natural Death Act in pediatric patients. *Crit Care Med* 19:901–5.

Johnson, J., and C. Mitchell. 2000. Responding to parental requests to forgo pediatric nutrition and hydration. *J Clin Ethics* 11:128–35.

Kenny, N. P. 1999. Whose choice? therapeutic intervention. *Ann R Coll Phys Surg Can* 32(Suppl.):93–101.

Kluge, E. H. 1995. Informed consent by children: the new reality. *Can Med Assoc J* 152:1495–97.

Lantos, J. D., J. E. Tyson, A. Allen, J. Frader, M. Hack, S. Korones, G. Merenstein, N. Paneth, R. L. Poland, S. Saigal, D. Stevenson, R. D. Truog, and L. J. van Marter.

1994. Withholding and withdrawing life-sustaining treatment in neonatal intensive care: issues for the 1990s. *Arch Dis Child* 71:F218–23.

Leikin, S. L., and K. Connell. 1983. Therapeutic choices by children with cancer. *J Pediatr* 103:167.

Lesko, L. M., H. Dematis, D. Penman, and J. C. Holland. 1989. Patients', parents', and oncologists' perceptions of informed consent for bone marrow transplantation. *Med Pediatr Oncol* 17:181–87.

Levetown, M. 2002. Starting the quest to define optimal pediatric end-of-life care. *Crit Care Med* 30:263–65.

Levi, R. B., R. Marsick, D. Drotar, and E. D. Kodish. 2000. Diagnosis, disclosure, and informed consent: learning from parents of children with cancer. *J Pediatr Hematol Oncol* 22:3–12.

Lister, E. 2001. Liza's death: a personal recollection. *J Pain Symptom Manage* 21:243–49.

MacLean, B. 1999. Care of the dying child: withholding treatment. *Ann R Coll Phys Surg Can* (Suppl.):120–27.

Masri, C., C. A. Farrell, J. Lacroix, G. Rocker, and S. D. Shemie. 2000. Decision making and end-of-life care in critically ill children. *J Palliat Care* 16 (Suppl.):S45–52.

McCallum, D. E., P. Byrne, and E. Bruera. 2000. How children die in hospital. *J Pain Symptom Manage* 20:417–23.

McConnell, Y. J., and G. Frager. 2003. *Decision-making in pediatric palliative care.* Toronto: Ian Anderson Continuing Education Program in End-of-Life Care, University of Toronto.

Meyer, E. C., J. P. Burns, J. L. Griffith, and R. D. Truog. 2002. Parental perspectives on end-of-life care in the pediatric intensive care unit. *Crit Care Med* 30:226–31.

Mink, R. B., and M. M. Pollack. 1992. Resuscitation and withdrawal of therapy in pediatric intensive care. *Pediatrics* 89:961–63.

Nelson, L. J., and R. M. Nelson. 1992. Ethics and the provision of futile, harmful, or burdensome treatment to children. *Crit Care Med* 20:427–33.

Nelson, L. J., C. H. Rushton, R. E. Cranford, R. M. Nelson, J. J. Glover, and R. D. Truog. 1995. Forgoing medically provided nutrition and hydration in pediatric patients. *J Law Med Ethics* 23:33–46.

Nitschke, R., G. B. Humphrey, C. L. Saxauer, B. Catron, S. Wunder, and S. Jay. 1982. Therapeutic choices made by patients with end-stage cancer. *J Pediatr* 101: 471–76.

Papadatou, D., T. Bellali, I. Papazoglou, and D. Petraki. 2002. Greek nurse and physician grief as a result of caring for children dying of cancer. *Pediatr Nurs* 28:345–53.

Pierucci, R. L., R. S. Kirby, and S. R. Leuthner. 2001. End-of-life care for neonates and infants: the experience and effects of a palliative care consultation service. *Pediatrics* 108:653–60.

Pinch, W. J., and M. L. Spielman. 1990. The parents' perspective: ethical decision-making in neonatal intensive care. *J Adv Nurs* 15:712–19.

Randolph, A. G., M. B. Zollo, M. J. Egger, G. H. Guyatt, R. M. Nelson, and G. L. Stidham. 1999. Variability in physician opinion on limiting pediatric life support. *Pediatrics* 103:807–8.

Randolph, A. G., M. B. Zollo, R. S. Wigton, and T. S. Yeh. 1997. Factors explaining variability among caregivers in the intent to restrict life-support interventions in a pediatric intensive care unit. *Crit Care Med* 25:435–39.

Rebagliato, M., M. Cuttini, L. Broggin, I. Berbik, U. de Vonderweid, G. Hansen, M. Kaminski, L. A. A. Kollée, A. Kucinskas, S. Lenoir, A. Levin, J. Persson, M. Reid, and R. Saracci. 2000. Neonatal end-of-life decision making: physicians' attitudes and relationship with self-reported practices in ten European countries. *JAMA* 284:2451–59.

Rylance, G. 1992. Should audio recordings of outpatient consultations be presented to patients? *Arch Dis Child* 67:622–24.

Sahler, O. J. Z., G. Frager, M. Levetown, F. G. Cohen, and M. A. Lipson. 2000. Medical education about end-of-life care in the pediatric setting: principles, challenges, and opportunities. *Pediatrics* 105:575–84.

Sourkes, B. M. 1995. *Armfuls of time: the psychological experience of the child with a life-threatening illness.* Pittsburgh: University of Pittsburgh Press.

Stevens, M. M. 2004a. Care of the dying child and adolescent: family adjustment and support. In *Oxford textbook of palliative medicine,* ed. D. Doyle, G. W. C. Hanks, N. Cherny, and K. Calman, 806–22. 3d ed. Oxford, U.K.: Oxford University Press.

Stevens, M. M. 2004b. Psychological adaptation of the dying child. In *Oxford textbook of palliative medicine,* ed. D. Doyle, G. W. C. Hanks, N. Cherny, and K. Calman, 789–806. 3d ed. Oxford, U.K.: Oxford University Press.

Street, K., R. Ashcroft, J. Henderson, and A. V. Campbell. 2000. The decision-making process regarding the withdrawal or withholding of potential life-saving treatments in a children's hospital. *J Med Ethics* 26:346–52.

Todres, I. D., M. Earle, and M. S. Jellinek. 1994. Enhancing communication: the physician and family in the pediatric intensive care unit. *Pediatr Clin North Am* 41:1395–1404.

van der Heide, A., P. J. van der Maas, G. van der Wal, L. A. A. Kollee, R. de Leeuw, and R. A. Holl. 1998. The role of parents in end-of-life decisions in neonatalogy: physicians' views and practices. *Pediatrics* 101:413–18.

Wall, S. T., and J. C. Partridge. 1997. Death in the intensive care nursery: physician practice of withdrawing and withholding life support. *Pediatrics* 99:64–70.

Webb, S. A., M. T. Wagner, and C. L. Wagner. 1998. The effect of experience and profession on discussing end-of-life decisions with families in the neonatal intensive care unit. *Pediatrics* 102 (Suppl. 3):763–64.

Winter, S. M. 2000. Terminal nutrition: framing the debate for the withdrawal of nutritional support in terminally ill patients. *Am J Med* 109:723–26.

Wolfe, J., N. Klar, H. E. Grier, J. Duncan, S. Salem-Schatz, E. J. Emanuel, and J. C. Weeks. 2000. Understanding of prognosis among parents of children who died of cancer: impact on treatment goals and integration of palliative care. *JAMA* 284:2469–75.

Woodgate, R. L. 1998. Health professionals caring for chronically ill adolescents: adolescents' perspectives. *J Soc Pediatr Nurs* 3:57–68.

Wyatt, J. S. 1999. Neonatal care: withholding or withdrawal of treatment in the new-born infant. *Bailliere's Clin Obstet Gynaecol* 13:503–11.

Young, B., M. Dixon-Woods, K. C. Windgridge, and D. Heney. 2003. Managing communication with young people who have a potentially life-threatening chronic illness: qualitative study of patients and parents. *Br J Med* 326:305–10.

5

Communication at the End of Life

Ross M. Hays, M.D., Geraldine Haynes, R.N., B.S.N., J. Russell Geyer, M.D., and Chris Feudtner, M.D., Ph.D., M.P.H.

Compassion and love are precious things in life. They are not complicated. They are simple, but difficult to practice.

Dalai Lama (Dalai Lama and Borges 1996)

Quality at the end of life, and the possibility of meeting the expectations of both the patient and his or her family, is dramatically affected by the quality of communication with the patient's health care providers. When the patient is a child, he or she is often inextricably entwined with parents and family members throughout the exchange of information and the communication of treatment options and goals. However, most recent studies suggest that there continues to be room for improvement in patient-provider communication at the end of life (von Gunten, Ferris, and Emanuel 2000). Medical education in the United States has traditionally paid little attention to death, dying, and palliative care in general and to communication skills about these issues in particular.

With the advent of specialty and subspecialty medical practice, patterns of health care delivery have become increasingly fragmented. Care provided by multiple providers in different sites demands that communication between patient and family and providers, and among providers themselves, be the best possible. At the same time, such fragmentation of care or geographic dislocation makes optimal communication and documentation increasingly difficult. The convoluted arrangements for reimbursement also contribute to this disarray. In the United States, the medical reimbursement system does not compensate physicians as well for communicating as it does for performing procedures.

Toni was diagnosed with HIV disease as an infant. Her adoptive mother, Dawn, knew from her first meeting with Toni's physician that Toni had a life-limiting condition. Still, Toni lived for more than eight years. Her care was complicated—and sometimes confusing. During those eight years, Toni experienced chronic infections, recurrent pain, and deafness.

Toni was healthy and developed normally for the first years of her life, but when she was 5 years old, the available antiviral drugs lost their effectiveness. She developed acute pancreatitis and was hospitalized for the first of what would be more than forty hospitalizations. Hundreds of medical professionals were involved with Toni's care. Their communication with one another and with Dawn was inconsistent and led to confusion about care goals among the staff members and confusion between the staff and Dawn and Toni. Dawn was a nurse, and she maintained high expectations for good communication. She anticipated that her expertise and investment in Toni's care would be respected. She was prepared to accept her share of the responsibility in decision making and sought ways to ensure that the process served Toni's best interests.

The evolving theory and practice of palliative care suggests that improved quality of care at the end of life will be closely linked to four key areas:

- adoption of a patient-centered model of care
- quality of life in all areas of health care
- models of service delivery designed specifically to support patients at the end of life
- improvements in physicians' and other caregivers' communication skills

Educational initiatives and curriculums on communication skills needed by caregivers when confronted with death and dying have been developed and implemented by the American Medical Association, in their Education for Physicians on End-of-Life Care (EPEC) program and trainers' guide (American Medical Association and Robert Wood Johnson Foundation 1999). Furthermore, it is well recognized that among pediatric populations, communication needs to flow not only from provider to patient but also to (and through) the parent or guardian providing for the child. Such a triangle of care and communication is well described elsewhere (Levetown and Carter 1997). This chapter does not attempt to replace or duplicate those programs. Rather, it is designed to provide some of the theoretical background that supports improved patient-provider communication by exploring its ethical and developmental roots and to demonstrate how those origins have evolved into the creation of an innovative communication tool.

The Ethics of Communication

The ethical dimensions of communication are expressed in the relationships that health care providers develop with their patients, with society, and ultimately with themselves. Society expects that patients will be treated with honesty and, increasingly, with respect for their autonomy. For child patients who cannot speak for themselves, parental voices addressing the best interests of the child will be sought. Depending on the relevant cognitive development of the child, however, his or her understanding and voice will also be sought, whether it is to allow for information and education, to acquire individual assent, or to obtain real informed consent. All of these measures reflect the principle of respect for persons, generally characterized in the adult setting as respect for autonomy.

The satisfaction of patient, family, and provider may all be endangered when information is poorly delivered. The ethical dimensions of patient-provider communication represent the principles of beneficence, nonmaleficence, autonomy, justice, and utility. Their practical application is represented in the four domains of veracity, privacy, confidentiality, and fidelity.

VERACITY

Codes of medical ethics have traditionally ignored obligations and the virtues of veracity. The Hippocratic oath does not address veracity, nor does the Declaration of Geneva of the World Medical Association. As recently as 1980, the Code of Medical Ethics of the American Medical Association made no mention of veracity or truth-telling as either obligation or virtue, giving physicians unrestricted discretion about what to disclose to their patients. This changed in the 1997 edition of the code (American Medical Association 1997, 120, 125). The obligation to tell patients the truth has been advocated intermittently throughout the history of medicine. It was most clearly articulated in the seventeenth century by the French physician Samuel D. Sorbiere, who suggested that truthful disclosure might be a good idea but also strongly warned that telling patients the truth might seriously jeopardize medical practice (Gillon 1994).

The obligation to tell a patient the truth about his or her medical condition was characterized by ambivalence for the next four centuries. In the 1950s and 1960s, approximately 88 percent of U.S. physicians indicated that they preferred not to inform their patients of a cancer diagnosis (Oken 1961). The practice was so well accepted that there were even published methods for appropriate evasion or overt deceit. Physicians' attitudes began to change dramatically during the 1960s. By 1979, 98 percent of physicians surveyed reported that it was their policy to accurately disclose all diagnostic information to cancer patients (Novac 1979).

There are many reasons for the changes in attitude toward truth telling among physicians. Such reasons may include the availability of more treatment options for cancer, improved rates of survival from some forms of cancer, fear of malpractice suits, involvement of multiple team members in hospitals, altered societal attitudes about cancer, greater attention to patients rights, and increased recognition by physicians that communication is an effective means of enhancing patient understanding and compliance with health care.

Children require open yet flexible communication (Patient page: cancer and children 2002). One recently reported model for enhancing truth telling with respect to diagnoses of children includes the use of a model, or analogy. Jankovic and colleagues (1994) report the use of a flower garden analogy to enhance understanding, and alleviate stress, in conveying the diagnosis of leukemia to young children. Adolescent patients may require alternative approaches (Penson et al. 2002).

The obligation of veracity is based on the respect owed to others and is therefore rooted deeply in the principle of respect for patient autonomy (American Academy of Pediatrics 1995). This obligation is the primary justification and basis for rules of disclosure in informed consent. The obligation of veracity exists even when consent is not an issue and is the guiding precept of the duty of respect toward others. Veracity is closely related to the obligation of fidelity and promise keeping.

When any two parties communicate with each other, there is an implicit promise that both will speak truthfully and that they will not deceive each other. A patient encounters a contract or a covenant by entering into the relationship in therapy. Even though children may not legally be allowed to enter into formal contracts independent from their parents or guardians, the implied promise remains important. Such a contract includes the patient's right to have his or her wishes respected about receiving the truth regarding diagnosis, prognosis, and treatment procedures. Cultural beliefs may affect the patient's wishes, as might limitations on a family's desire for full disclosure and informed consent. Discerning the patient's and family's wishes can require experience, skill, listening, and time. In this truth-telling process (the contract), the health professional also expects to gain the right to truthful disclosures from the patient. Relationships between health care professionals and their patients ultimately depend on communication and trust. With respect to children, such dependence may, at times, be frustrated, as children, though generally more honest and forthright than adults, may act to protect their parents.

Christakis (1999) observes that professional norms in the United States at present generally support frankness, directness, and the sharing of information about diagnosis and therapeutic options, but they discourage bluntness in sharing prognostic information. There may be some concern, however, as to how rigorously this norm is adhered to (Larson and Tobin 2000). This attitude lends itself to cases of cautious disclosure of "bad news," whereby treatment possibilities are emphasized and the potential for a terminal prognosis is minimized. Cautious disclosure may use staged language, disclosing prognosis information in stages over time, providing the patient with only as much information as the physician believes is appropriate. "Benevolent deception," whether or not it is acknowledged, has long been a part of medical tradition. Its defenders suggest that disclosure of "bad news" (complete information), particularly the prognosis of death, sometimes violates the obligations of benevolence and nonmalevolence by causing patient anxiety and destroying the patient's hope. In the nineteenth century Samuel Johnson disagreed, saying, "I deny the lawfulness of telling a lie to a sick man for fear of alarming him. You have no business with consequences; you are to tell the truth. Besides, you are not sure what effects your telling him that he is in danger may have" (Donagan 1979).

Current thinking supports the notion that benevolent deception poses a threat to the special relationship of trust between physicians and patients and that it should not be practiced, even with very young patients (Surbone 1992). Another justification for nondisclosure is the reality that health care professionals can never know the whole truth. Physicians may say, "You can never tell what will happen," or "Each patient is unique." This approach, though technically honest, fails to respect the autonomy of the patient when it is used as a justification to provide vague or incomplete information. The ideal approach might be to formulate a standard of substantial completeness to provide each patient with the most appropriate and complete medical information comprehensible to and desired by him or her.

A third argument for nondisclosure, as implied above, is that some patients do not want to know the truth about their condition. At present, the majority of patients in the United States, regardless of age, want to know all relevant information about their diagnosis, prognosis, and future options and, in fact, regard access to this information as their entitlement in the health care relationship. The assumption by professionals that patients do not want to know is paternalistic and is most egregious when it wears the mask of respect for patient autonomy. Studies in the United States consistently find that patients want to hear the truth. Such views are not universally held. A study from Italy suggests that 50 percent of Italian women with breast cancer did not want to know their diagnosis (Mosconi 1991).

There are, then, certain culture-specific situations in which adult patients prefer not to have complete information about their diagnosis and prognosis conveyed to them. Whether these feeling hold true for children from these cultures has not been formally studied. Respect for autonomy suggests that cultural factors must be respected when considering disclosure to patients. Pellegrino (1992, 1735) warns against the use of assaultive truthfulness. He suggests that to "thrust the truth on a patient who expects to be buffered against news of impending death is a gratuitous and harmful misinterpretation of the moral foundations for respect for autonomy." A question for pediatric practitioners may be what to do when parents refuse to have the diagnosis revealed to their child without consulting, or considering, the preferences of the child. In such matters, practitioners may do well to assume the role of a trustworthy educator, informing the family of the fallacies and shortcomings of not openly discussing all of the information available to make sound decisions that truly respect the child patient.

A current challenge to veracity is the relationship between the provider, the patient (or, in the case of a child patient, the parents), and the institutions or agencies governing the financial resources necessary to pay for health care. Tension clearly exists between physicians' traditional understanding of their moral role as patient advocate and the new roles dictated by institutional structures that restrict both physician and patient choices about the use of financial resources. The understandable temptation toward deception in this system poses a threat to physician integrity and character as well as to the justice of the system. Nearly 50 percent of physicians surveyed by the Kaiser Family Foundation and the Harvard University School of Public Health (1999) admitted that they had sometimes exaggerated the severity of their patients' medical conditions to obtain payment for procedures that the physicians believed their patients needed. Another study conducted in the late 1990s suggests that 39 percent of physicians had exaggerated the severity of a patient's condition and altered a patient's diagnosis by reporting signs and symptoms that were necessary only for the purpose of justifying the patient's need to receive specific coverage. This tension can create serious conflicts of interest and represents a rapidly escalating dilemma in physician-patient fidelity.

PRIVACY

Respect for privacy received little attention in the law or in legal theory until the late nineteenth century. In the 1920s the U.S. Supreme Court employed an expansive "liberty" interest to protect family decision making about child rearing and education. The right to privacy is now said to protect liberty by demarcating a zone of private life that merits protection from state intrusion. The most dramatic example is the 1973 Supreme Court decision expanding the scope of privacy rights by overturning restrictive abortion laws. In their 1890 article "The Right to Privacy," Warren and Brandeis (1890) state that each individual has "the right to enjoy life and the right to be let alone" (cited in Halper 1996, 122). Privacy is a necessary condition for maintaining intimate relationships of trust and therefore pertains particularly to the patient-provider relationship.

The primary justification supporting this obligation is the principle of respect for autonomy. Health care providers respect persons by respecting their wishes not to be observed, not to be touched, and not to be intruded on. The right to privacy claims the right to prohibit unauthorized access and the right to authorize or to decline access. The principle of respect for autonomy therefore includes the right to decide as far as possible what will happen to one's person and body and to personal information about one's life, secrets, and health. In the provision of pediatric palliative care, the expectation of privacy in the patient-provider relationship may be tested in dealing with individual patient wishes, extended family or friends, schools, and the broader community. Parents and children together must set the tone for maintaining the proper degree of privacy balanced against potential competing interests.

CONFIDENTIALITY

Confidentiality is a branch or a subset of privacy in that it prevents re-disclosure of information originally disclosed within the confidential relationship. Under a pledge of confidentiality, a person to whom information is disclosed by another, whether verbally or by physical examination, agrees not to share that information with a third party without the confider's permission. Confidentiality can be justified in terms of autonomy and privacy rights: the argument from privacy views breaches of confidentiality primarily as violations of personal autonomy. There are also fidelity-based arguments, which posit the physician's obligation to live up to the patient's reasonable expectations of privacy and confidentiality as deriving from the general obligation of trust. Medical practice requires the patient to disclose private and sensitive information to the physician. When confidentiality is breached, a failure of fidelity corrupts the core of the patient-provider relationship. This may be most evident in dealing with sensitive adolescent issues.

Unlike veracity, rules of confidentiality have long been common in codes of medical ethics. Requirements of confidentiality appear as early as the Hippocratic oath and continue in the most recent version of the World Medical Association's Declaration of Geneva, which asserts an obligation of "absolute secrecy" and includes the following physician's pledge: "I will respect the secrets which are confided in me even after the patient has died" (cited in Beauchamp and Childress 1994, 419). The World Medical Association's international code of medical ethics states the most stringent requirement of all: "A doctor shall preserve absolute secrecy on all he knows about his patient because of the confidence entrusted to him" (cited in Beauchamp and Childress 1994, 419). At this time, such lofty admonitions are frequently ridiculed as little more than ritualistic formulas or convenient fictions publicly acknowledged by professionals but widely ignored and violated in practice. Siegler (1982, 1520) argues that confidentiality in medicine is a "decrepit concept." The concept that both physicians and patients have traditionally understood as medical confidentiality no longer exists in any meaningful way: it is systematically compromised in the course of routine medical care. Siegler's remark is based on his own experience: He admitted a patient to the hospital with the proviso that no one would have access to the patient's information other than those professionals directly involved in the patient's care. In retrospect, Siegler found that more than seventy-five people had had legitimate access to the confidential information regarding his patient (Siegler 1982, 1519).

It is clear that physicians can no longer protect their patients completely from breaches of confidentiality and that patients usually expect a more rigorous standard of confidentiality than actually exists. Given the interdisciplinary team model for palliative care provision, the traditional concept of confidentiality may need to be modified. Staff will require ongoing education on this issue.

FIDELITY

Fidelity, or trustworthiness, describes the faithfulness of one human being to another. The obligations of fidelity are best understood as norms that specify the moral principles of autonomy, justice, and utility. These principles justify the obligation to act in good faith to keep vows and promises, to discharge fiduciary responsibilities, to maintain relationships, and to fulfill agreements. Communication is the process by which this fidelity is expressed in the patient-provider relationship. Both law and medical tradition have traditionally distinguished the practice of medicine from business practices that rest on contracts and marketplace relationships. The patient-provider relationship is founded on trust and confidence. The provider is a trustee of the patient's medical welfare. Obligations of fidelity arise in this model whenever a physician establishes a relationship with a patient. The breach of fidelity is abandonment of that relationship.

Professional fidelity, or loyalty, has traditionally been conceived as the provider's holding the patient's best interests as the prevailing priority. It assumes that in the case of a conflict, a provider's self-interest will be subsumed to the patient's interests and that the physician provider will favor the patient's interests above those of all third parties. In practice, of course, this level of fidelity is rare; for example, physicians are not expected to care for patients completely free of charge. The pure concept of fidelity is also altered for the protection of the greater good of society; for example, public health issues such as immunization programs impose a small burden on the individual in order that society will benefit from decreased risk of disease. Fidelity is also sometimes modified in the interest of third parties, such as in maternal-fetal relationships. Institutional interests, such as requests for abortions in Catholic-sponsored care facilities, can sometimes override fidelity. Furthermore, in the pediatric context, providers must balance duties to the child patient with those directed toward parents, whose legal and socially recognized position of authority requires due consideration. These precepts of fidelity can affect communication and respect for an individual's wishes.

Perhaps no area of health care has greater conflicts regarding the obligations of fidelity than nursing. During the early evolution of nursing practice, nurses were discouraged from developing and acting on their own ethical judgments. The increasing importance of the hospital in health care eventually brought nursing under the dual command of physicians and hospital administrators. Codes of nursing ethics in the twentieth century clearly illustrate the sharply changing obligations and moral responsibilities of nurses. In 1950 the first code of the American Nurses Association stressed the nurse's obligation to carry out the physicians orders; the 1976 revision stresses the nurse's obligation to the client, including the obligation to safeguard both the client and the public from "incompetent, unethical, or illegal" practices of any person (Beauchamp and Childress 1983, 334).

More serious conflicts have weakened the traditional rules of fidelity in recent U.S. health care. Third-party payers and institutional providers increasingly impose constraints on medical decisions about diagnostic and therapeutic procedures. One result is that many physicians depend on these funding mechanisms essentially to set the standard for care. These mechanisms often function to limit and constrict the physician's fidelity to the patient through a mixture of incentives and disincentives. Conflicts of interest emerge in medicine when, in addition to the obligation to protect and promote their patients' interests, providers have personal, often financial interests that are at odds with fidelity or loyalty to their patients. The requirements of communication become diffused in these conflicts of interest, and providers are placed in the awkward position of having to determine whether to provide full disclosure to patients, to institutions, or to payers.

The ethical underpinnings of good communication continue to evolve in medicine in the twenty-first century. This evolution is guided by the expectations of society, the long tradition of ethical standards for health care practice, and the greater recognition of the individual's participation in his or her own decision making. Medical progress, particularly innovative approaches to end-of-life care, continue to create new challenges to patient-provider communication. A clear understanding of the ethical underpinnings of medical practice will help guide patients and providers in their continued attempts to speak plainly and truthfully about disease and to understand the choices available to each individual patient. While this is certainly true in conventional practice, it must be considered heavily with any anticipated uncontrolled, innovative therapies that may be pursued for children who are at risk of death.

Communication and the Child

Communicating medical information to children can be a formidable and complex task. The goal of communication is to clearly explain medical information, to improve their understanding of disease, to reduce their stress, to assist them in self-management, and to garner their compliance with medical advice and regimens (Masera et al. 1997; Spinetta et al. 2002). Accomplishing this with children of various ages can present a particular challenge. It requires considerable understanding of the language and cognitive skills of children at different ages. Considering the importance of explaining illness to children, surprisingly little research has been done on this subject. Existing research concerning children and medical communication has been dominated by a focus on children's conceptualization of illness and adults' estimation of children's understanding of illness. This research is based on the premise that knowing how children process and understand illness—that is, how they give answers about what causes their illness—can help adults in explaining diagnostic and prognostic information to them. Most descriptions of communication strategies for children are based on the cognitive-developmental or stage approach.

Bibace and Walsh (1980) suggest that children's conceptualization of illness corresponds to their cognitive development and maturation. They assert that a child's ability to understand illness and the explanation of prognostic information falls into developmental categories that can be loosely represented by the stages of cognitive development described by Piaget (1930): prelogical, concrete logical, and formal logical stages.

Prelogical explanations are observed in children from 2 to 6 years of age. Prelogical thought is characterized by children's incapacity to separate themselves from their social and physical environments. As a result, children in the prelogical phase of cognition offer explanations for cause-and-effect relationships by way of spatial and temporal perceptual experiences based on cues present in their own lives. The earliest developmental stage is described as phenomenism. Children who are functioning at this stage perceive illness as being caused by external concrete phenomena that may coincide with the illness but are inaccessible to them either spatially or temporally. In this stage, a child is incapable of explaining exactly how an illness occurs. When a child in this stage is asked to imagine a cause for illness, the most commonly offered explanation relates to contagion. Here, the cause of illness is found in people or entities that are close to but not particularly in contact with the individual child.

Children aged 7 to 10 use concrete logical explanations. At this stage, a child begins to differentiate between self and others and distinctly demarcates internal and external phenomena. Younger children in the concrete logical stage tend to continue believing that contamination is the primary reason for illness, but the child at this stage is often able to understand the difference between the cause of illness and the method of transmission. Sickness is often perceived as an action, an object, or a person separate from the child that is capable of damaging or injuring the child's body. The presumed method of contamination is often physical contact. As children mature, their explanations will begin to reflect internalization. In this stage, the agent of illness is external to the child's body, but the illness is understood to reside internally. This stage is the very beginning of the child's understanding about how different organs function.

At approximately 11 years of age, children begin to use formal logical thought and distinguish clearly between themselves and others. At this stage, children begin to demonstrate mature understandings of illness and classify causes of illness into physiological and psychological categories. A child at this stage can often differentiate thoughts and feelings and begin to understand the impact that thoughts and feelings have on the workings of their body. The physiological explanations usually describe the failure or malfunctioning of an internal physiologic process or organ. Children's explanations can be quite detailed and may involve a step-by-step internal sequence of events that culminates in an illness. Because the literature regarding explanation of illness to children relies heavily on Piagetian stage theory and its applications, most of the advice offered stresses categorized explanatory strategies for children at different cognitive levels.

Most researchers agree that the first step in good communication with children is understanding their point of view. Listening is critical to this understanding. The verbal development of children often does not enable a full description of their point of view. Tools other than words may be necessary to augment communication. It is helpful to learn each child's cultural, religious, intellectual, and experience level and personality type before attempting a difficult explanation. Understanding a child's current knowledge and understanding of her or his illness also facilitates communication. Dorn (1984) recommends asking children to describe what they believe is making them sick and, based on their responses, constructing an explanation that incorporates the child's understanding in an honest and truthful way. Asking a child to draw pictures to represent the nature of his or her illness can help a clinician gauge the individual child's level of understanding. Child-life specialists have specific training in this area.

The vocabulary for discussions with individual young children must be carefully chosen. The use of concrete operational terms can facilitate a child's understanding. It is important neither to underestimate nor overestimate a child's ability to understand complex information, and it is necessary to tailor vocabulary to the individual child's level of understanding. "Being concrete" includes avoiding health care jargon, technical terms, and euphemisms that have multiple meanings or lead to ambiguity. Examples include using the term *die* when talking with a child who has a terminal disease. Misconceptions can be formed by the thoughtless use of medical terminology. It is important to avoid the use of confusing terms such as "drawing" blood or "burning" sugar internally. A young child who is told that his knee is "inflamed" may be afraid that at some point his knee will actually catch fire.

Young children may lack the linguistic development, life exposure, medical experience, and attention span necessary to endure and understand long explanations. Moreover, their concrete level of functioning suggests the use of condensed, clear descriptions that lead children to form an accurate understanding about the outcomes and choices offered to them, whether the outcomes are positive or negative.

It is sometimes useful to incorporate figurative language, including the use of analogies, metaphors, or similes, when explaining an illness. The comparisons should be familiar to the child. Examples include describing the brain as a complicated computer or hemoglobin as a special boat designed to carry oxygen down the river of the bloodstream. Of course, these explanations would be useless to a child who is unfamiliar with computers or river navigation. In prospective controlled trials comparing the accuracy of children's understanding of illness, information provided with a figurative approach, using anecdotes and familiar metaphors, resulted in improved accuracy and longer retention as compared with straightforward descriptions of disease (Whaley 2000). These approaches can be successful with children who are at least 7 or 8 years old as understanding increases with age. When different figurative approaches were studied, it was found that younger children respond best to perceptual comparisons (comparisons based on shape, color, and texture), while older children respond better to functional comparisons (the heart as a pump or the kidney as a washing machine for the blood). The greatest liability in this approach is the tendency for providers to choose analogies and metaphors that are too advanced for individual children. Success is greatest when the figurative language is clearly reflected in patients' own descriptions of their experience with their disease.

Piaget's stage theory is limited, and research supporting it is relatively sparse. Two crucial factors need future investigation. First, a more clear understanding about what information children want to know is required. There is ample theory and research to ground discussion of children's ability to understand, but there is little to guide us to know how much children want to participate in the understanding of their illness. Second, communication requires the ability to understand what children need to know. It is important to understand the relationship between communication and understanding of disease, compliance, and clinical outcomes. Like adults, children appear to be more concerned with what their illness means to them in their everyday functioning and its effect on their daily life than on the physiology of the disease. Future research needs to consider children's experience with illness, rather than merely their cognitive developmental stages, as a starting place for the development of communication strategies.

When communicating with children, it is also necessary to recognize the crucial role of parents and to carefully incorporate parents into the information gathering and communication about disease, diagnosis, and prognosis. Rigid rules, such as explaining all information for children under age 7 and incorporating children in the discussion after age 7, ignore the capabilities, desires, and mores of individual children and their families. Flexibility is necessary, and a clear understanding of the wishes and desires of the child and the family is a prerequisite to good communication. Successful clinicians improve the efficacy of their communication by paying attention to both the content of the explanation of an illness and the process by which the communication is developed. They seek out creative approaches and use the resources of many members of the health care team, investing the necessary time to develop a genuine relationship with young patients and their families.

Improving Communication at the End of Life

Effective communication about palliative care continues to evolve in practice and theory, but there is clearly room for improvement. Shortcomings in communication are often manifested in a variety of disappointing clinical outcomes. Patients continue to die following unnecessarily prolonged hospitalizations, sometimes without adequate relief of pain and symptoms. Children may be at greater risk for prolonged hospitalization and disease-specific interventions as families and professionals attempt to maximally prolong a child's life. Too often, however, the child's preferences about such treatments are not adequately addressed, documented, or followed. Despite increasing awareness of the importance of communication, the need for major reform

Exhibit 5.1. The seven-step approach to communication

- Prepare for the discussion
- Establish what the patient and family know
- Determine how the information is to be handled
- Deliver the information
- Respond to emotions
- Establish goals of care and treatment priorities
- Establish a plan

---

remains. A study of physicians' communication patterns about advance directives has found that the average length of those discussions was 5.6 minutes and that physicians did 80 percent of the talking (Tulsky 1998).

One approach to improving competence in end-of-life communication is a six-stage protocol, originally promoted by Buckman (1992), for the communication of "bad news." The protocol has been adopted into the American Medical Association–sponsored Education for Physicians on End-of-Life Care (EPEC) program. Von Gunten, Ferris, and Emanuel (2000) expand Buckman's communication system to a seven-step method. The seven steps address communication, decision making, and the building of relationships (exhibit 5.1). The first three are used to prepare the patient, caregivers, and physician for discussion of important information. The last three are used to respond to patients' reaction and planning. The middle step is used to deliver information.

1. Prepare for the discussion by confirming medical facts, creating a supportive physical environment, ensuring that there is adequate time, and arranging for the appropriate people to attend—including, when possible, the child patient.

2. Establish what the patient and family know by using open-ended questions. Some parents may need to be counseled to be honest with their children.

3. Determine how the patient and family want the information to be delivered. This includes extent of information (in the United States, 90% of adult patients express a preference for full disclosure, regardless of the seriousness of the information) as well as methods of communication. It is important not to rely on assumptions about patient preferences based on the patient's chronological age and ethnic and cultural background. This step may be best

accomplished early in the patient-provider relationship, long before the need to discuss sensitive information is anticipated.

4. Deliver diagnostic and prognostic information. Use clear and unambiguous language, neither understating nor overstating the implications of the news. This conversation must be free of jargon and delivered in language the patient can understand, not in foreign medical terminology. Pace the delivery of information, giving many opportunities to ascertain the patient's reception of the information. Check for understanding.

5. Respond to emotions. Stop if the patient or family seems overwhelmed. The extent to which the provider is prepared to respond to any emotional reaction with respect and support will be repaid with a stronger patient-provider relationship. Having tissues handy is always a good plan.

6. Discuss the goals of care, a critical component of good communication. A clear understanding of the patient's goals, and the family's goals, will inform the future course of treatment. The use of open-ended questions encourages patients to formulate their values and preferences regarding the goals of treatment. This step is often revisited in subsequent meetings when the patient and caregivers have had the opportunity to absorb the medical information and when response to therapy becomes clearer. The first six steps logically lead to the final step, establishing a plan.

7. Establish a plan. In view of the considerations and interactions noted above, the mutually elaborated goals of care (step 6) should be used to make a plan for the patient's care that is consistent with family and patient values and goals. This may, at first, be a short-term plan with certain goals of gaining stability and comfort and measuring the patient's health and response to any provided treatments, interventions, or comfort measures. Reassessments need to be scheduled and incorporated into a more long-term plan for comprehensive management (von Gunten, Ferris, and Emanuel 2000).

Most commentators stress the value of using open-ended questions and extended listening when assessing a patient's preferences. Providers are often reluctant to use this approach because the patient's responses may be unpredictable. The open-ended question increases the provider's vulnerability by opening the door to uncomfortable emotional interactions, requests for services over which providers have no control, and the possibility of frustration, discouragement, and discomfort on the part of the provider. In these difficult situations, Lo and Quill (1999) suggest that providers keep several points in mind. First, although uncovering painful emotions may increase suffering in the short term, it may suggest a course of action that helps relieve greater suffering in the long term. Second, provider's emotional responses are often a good clue to the patient's and family's emotional state. When the physician feels discouraged or angry, there is a strong likelihood that the patient is also upset. Both patient and provider may enter into a more valuable and trusting relationship by honestly acknowledging their feelings. Third, providers become more effective and useful to the patient once he or she accepts the fact that their role is no longer to "fix" but is rather to come alongside the patient and share in his or her suffering. This rediscovery of compassion at the very heart of health care is long overdue. Finally, no provider should succumb to the temptation to accept sole responsibility for relieving the patient's suffering. The interdisciplinary team is no more valuable anywhere in medicine than in the care of patients at the end of life.

In discussions about the end-of-life phase, the child patient's and family's wishes and needs can be addressed in at least six different domains: patient goals; values of the family, caregiver, and patient; advance directives; do-not-attempt-resuscitation orders; plans for the relief of pain and symptoms; and attending to "unfinished business." These domains may need special consideration in the case of pediatric patients, for whom legal recognition of advance directives and processes whereby a do-not-attempt-resuscitation order can be obtained are special. Furthermore, children may require attention to particularly unique matters in addressing "unfinished business"—such as accomplishing unmet goals or leaving some kind of legacy. When the child patient, the parents, and the health care providers face the end of life together, these domains can be addressed in a logical and complete manner without resorting to uncomfortable, ill-timed, and artificial conversations. Improved communication will be accomplished by providing the patient and family with the freedom to clearly express their wishes to a health care provider and team who have the skills to listen.

A New Decision-Making Communication Tool

Improving communication at the end of life requires changes in knowledge, skills, and attitudes to incorporate the belief that shared decision making and strengthening of the patient-provider relationship will improve clinical outcomes. These attributes can be enhanced by the use of effective, tangible communication aids. Training in communication skills is included in most health care professional curriculums, but until now no standardized, consistent tools have been developed to document family-centered communication and decision making.

The Pediatric Palliative Care Consulting Service at Children's Hospital and Regional Medical Center in Seattle, Washington, has adapted a tool for ethical decision making to improve communication, clinical decision making, and care planning. This tool is a modification of the "four-box" method developed by Jonsen, Siegler, and Winslade (2001). The four-box approach was modified for use during patient care conferences to discuss the complex issues of pediatric palliative care. The original format, detailing medical indications, patient preferences, quality of life, and contextual issues and representing the ethical principles of beneficence, autonomy, utility, and justice, was designed to reduce the task of ethical case analysis to a practical and clinically relevant process. The original process was modified to be used as a patient-provider communication tool by including a fifth box, for discussion, and a sixth, for the plan of care. Discussants, date and length of conference, and patient history are noted, and a physician's signature on the plan of care validates orders noted in the plan.

In the typical first use of this model, the family and professional caregivers choose participants for the care conference. These participants may include the nuclear or extended family, primary and specialty care physicians, nurses, social workers, religious or cultural representatives, health plan case managers, teachers, home case managers, school counselors, physical and occupational therapists, child-life specialists, and others. A scribe, usually an experienced nurse or social worker, documents the conference on the decision-making tool form, separating out the items covered during the conference into their various "boxes" and suggesting areas for discussion that may not have been addressed. At the completion of the conference, the scribe reviews the form and the plan of care and modifies it as directed by the participants. The form is then transcribed to electronic format and sent to the family and ordering physician for review and signature. All conference participants and other designated caregivers (for example, specialists not present at the conference) receive a copy of the form, once it has been approved and signed.

The benefits of this process are both obvious and subtle and include but are not limited to the following:

- A common language and a reliable process for communicating and making decisions are developed.
- Medical indications, including risks and benefits, are clearly explained.
- A primary family representative may be identified.
- Preferences of patient and family regarding their options and choices are documented.
- Areas for conflict resolution (that is, decisions about treatment choices) are indicated.
- Resuscitation efforts may be discussed and noted.
- Factors felt by the patient to add to his or her quality of life are valued and noted.
- The context of the family's life, including the physical setting, intimate and wider circle of support (including family, friends, faith community, and the like), family experience, beliefs about the child's condition, and financial and health insurance concerns, are acknowledged and respected.
- The completed document is provided to the family for review and reflection. When the document is updated, reference to the earlier iterations of the plan can help provide the family and the professional care team with a view of the child's progress.
- Access to the document by the health plan case manager assists with verifying need for payment of chosen care modalities.

This process was evaluated in the pediatric palliative care demonstration project sponsored by the Promoting Excellence at the End-of-Life program of the Robert Wood Johnson Foundation at Children's Hospital and Regional Medical Center between 1998 and 2001. The use of the decision-making communication tool was found to have significantly improved both patient and provider satisfaction with the quality of communication. After several months in the project, families reported that the decision-making communication tool had been useful in building their confidence about their decisions for their child's care. Families also related that repeated use of the tool assisted their comprehension about the progress of their child's disease process.

In the beginning, generating these documents can be cumbersome, but with repetition the process becomes more intuitive and streamlined. In preparing to use the decision-making communication tool, consideration of questions that yield information in each of the areas is useful. The forms in exhibits 5.2 and 5.3 demonstrate some of these questions.

Exhibit 5.2. Decision-Making Communication Tool (Guidelines)

Patient Name:	Prepared by: Name of person recording the discussion
Date:	Present: Names of all participants, with titles, for future reference
Length of Visit:	

☒ First DMT
☐ Update

Physician of Record: Primary care or specialist
Care Coordinator: At clinic and/or at home

History of Present Illness

In this section, document the pertinent features of the child's illness to date. If the DMT is part of the standard medical record, then this is the location of the interval history section.

Medical Indications	Patient Preferences
In this quadrant document diagnoses, symptoms and treatments, including Risks and Benefits. The Benefits section may include expected cure rate and/or remission rate as well as expected length of remission when appropriate for the patient's diagnosis. The Risks section may include recurrence and complications rate.	In this quadrant document family and/or patient preferences/goals regarding:
	• Being informed
	• Being involved in decisions
	• Preferences for place of care
	• Expectations for this visit
	• Preferences regarding specific treatment options
	• Decisions about resuscitation

• Treatment(s) for Primary Condition:
    Benefit(s):
    Risk(s):
	If the patient is too young or unable to express preferences, the "best interest" standard is used and determined by the parents or legal guardians.

• Optional Treatment(s) for Primary Condition:
    Benefit(s):
    Risk(s):	

• Treatment(s) for Secondary and/or Temporary Condition(s):	
• Pain Management:	
• Nutrition:	

(continued)

Exhibit 5.2. *(continued)*

Quality of Life	Contextual Issues
The components of life that give value and meaning to the *patient* are documented in this quadrant. What does the child love to do? What gives the child comfort?	The physical, social and spiritual components of the daily life of the patient and family are documented in this quadrant.
<ul><li>Important activities</li><li>Important relationships</li><li>Personal identity</li><li>Emotional well being</li><li>Spiritual well being</li></ul>	<ul><li>Home environment</li><li>Who lives in the home?</li><li>Physical restrictions in the home</li><li>Who is the primary caregiver?</li><li>Extended family and friends</li><li>Cultural and spiritual issues</li><li>Financial/Insurance facts</li><li>Important family health history</li><li>Study protocols</li><li>Legal issues</li><li>Alternative health care options</li><li>Needs/opinions of professional caregivers</li><li>Members of the health care team:</li></ul> Insurance case manager Home Health Services case manager School personnel Social service agency case manager Other consultants

Patient Name: Date:

Discussion

This section documents the discussion between the health care team, the patient and family at enrollment. It details any discussion that supplements or enhances medical care goals and decisions for curative and palliative care, while giving balanced consideration for the elements identified in the quadrants above.

Plan

The plan of care is dynamic and is updated collaboratively in response to patient/family request, medical indications, and decisions reached by the care planning team. Each issue is noted separately. The provider signs the Decision-Making Communication Tool and each member of the team receives a copy.

Action: Who will do: By what date:

(continued)

Exhibit 5.2. (continued)

Action: Who will do: By what date:

Physician Signature _____   Date _____

Exhibit 5.3. Decision-Making Communication Tool (Example)

Following is an example of a completed DMT for a theoretical patient, Bill Smith. The form can be used for medical decision making in many settings. When used at the time of diagnosis, the form sets a pattern for sorting out choices that may be helpful to a patient and family throughout the course of an illness.

Patient Name: Bill Smith
Date: 5/31/00
Length of Visit: 1.0 hour
Physician of Record: Primary care/specialist
Care Coordinator: At clinic/at home

Prepared by: Name of scribe
Present: All participants with titles for future reference

☒ First DMT
☐ Update

History of Present Illness

14-year-old male, ALL Dx 1996. Relapse 1999. One year post BMT.

Medical Indications			Patient Preferences
Sx: Fatigue, bone pain, shortness of breath			Bill wants to participate in school play, April 2001. Wishes all Rx that will extend his life. State that his mother wants him to live as long as possible.
Options: No Rx	Benefits:	No intervention Able to remain at home	
	Risks:	Shortened life expectancy	
Palliative drugs (by name and dose)	Benefits:	Increased comfort/pain relief Sense of something being done	Bill prefers medicine that will allow him to function without sleepiness while having good pain relief.
	Risks:	Shortened life expectancy?	Bill reaffirms wish to live as long as possible.

(continued)

Exhibit 5.3. (*continued*)

Experimental protocol	Benefits:	Sleepiness vs. increased alertness Potential increase in life expectancy Contribution to medical knowledge	Bill prefers to use the experimental protocol, with the understanding that the use can be reviewed regularly. Bill is willing to endure more side effects if his life will be extended.
	Risks:	Dose-limiting toxicities Nausea/vomiting, hair loss, frequent lab draws	

Quality of Life	**Contextual Issues**
Bill loves • To spend time with his next-door neighbor/best friend/soccer teammate. • To act/perform in front of crowds and loves to act in every school play. • To spend mealtimes with his mother. These are special times.	• Is the only child in his family. • Lives with mother in an apartment on the third floor of a building near his school. • Father died of cancer when Bill was 2 years old. • No grandparents are living. • Insurance coverage for hourly care is limited to 8 hours per week. • Hospice coverage available. Physician has no experience with hospice care. • Further aggressive chemotherapy will require Bill and his mother to move to Seattle from their home in eastern Washington. • Bill's mother is concerned about losing her job, but wants to be near Bill.

Patient Name: Bill Smith   Date: 5/31/00

Discussion

Given the limited potential for cure and Bill's great wish to participate in the school play, his need to be at home with his mother and his wish to be close to his neighbor, simple chemotherapy was discussed as a probable first choice. The possibility of cure, even with the risks of aggressive chemotherapy, was the primary focus for Bill's mother. An extensive discussion of the risks and possible benefits of a trial of the new protocol gave Bill's mother hope and Bill is amenable to trying "one more time" if the treatment is ended in time for him to attend play practice and appear in the play. Bill says he knows more treatment is a "long shot" and that he wants to do some things with his mother and his friends while he can.

Plan

Action:	Who will do:	By what date:
1. Begin new protocol.	MD order	6/1/00
2. Mrs. Smith will take a two-week leave of absence from her job— remaining in Seattle through the first round of treatment.	Mrs. Smith	Immediately
3. Appropriate tests will follow the first round of treatment.	Team	7/16/00
4. Status meeting with Bill and Mrs. Smith.	Team	TBD
5. Bill will call his neighbor friend to make arrangements for e-mail contact/possible visit/telephone calls.	Bill	6/1/00

(continued)

Exhibit 5.3. *(continued)*

6. A referral will be made to the hematology/oncology social worker to assist Mrs. Smith with local housing.	Social Worker	6/1/00
7. If Bill needs assistance in walking, he and Mrs. Smith will consider moving to a ground-floor apartment.	Bill and Mrs. Smith	prn

Physician Signature_____   Date_____

References

American Academy of Pediatrics, Committee on Bioethics. 1995. Informed consent, parental permission, and assent in pediatric practice. *Pediatrics* 95:314–17.

American Medical Association, Council on Ethical and Judicial Affairs. 1997. Code of Medical Ethics: current opinions with annotations. Chicago: American Medical Association.

American Medical Association and the Robert Wood Johnson Foundation. 1999. Education for physicians on end-of-life care (EPEC Project): trainers' guide. Chicago: American Medical Association.

Beauchamp, T. L., and J. F. Childress. 1983. *Principles of biomedical ethics.* 2d ed. New York: Oxford University Press.

———. 1994. *Principles of biomedical ethics.* 4th ed. New York: Oxford University Press.

Bibace, R., and M. Walsh. 1980. Development of children's concepts of illness. *Pediatrics* 66:912–18.

Buckman, R. 1992. *How to break bad news: a guide for health care professionals.* Baltimore: Johns Hopkins University Press.

Christakis, N. 1999. *Death foretold: prophecy and prognosis in medical care.* Chicago: University of Chicago Press.

Dalai Lama and P. Borges. 1996. *Tibetan portrait.* New York: Rizzoli International.

Donagan, A. 1979. *The theory of morality.* Chicago: University of Chicago Press.

Dorn, L. 1984. Children's concept of illness: clinical applications. *Pediatr Nurs* 10: 325–27.

Gillon, R. 1994. Truth telling, lying, and the doctor-patient relationship. In *Principles of health care ethics,* 499–509. London: Wiley.

Halper, T. 1996. Privacy and autonomy: from Warren and Brandeis to *Roe and Cruzan. J Med Philos* 21:121–35.

Jankovic, M., N. B. Loiacono, J. J. Spinetta, L. Riva, V. Conter, and G. Masera. 1994. Telling young children with leukemia their diagnosis: the flower garden as analogy. *Pediatr Hematol Oncol* 11:75–81.

Jonsen, A., M. Siegler, and W. Winslade. 2001. *Clinical ethics.* 4th ed. New York: Macmillan.

Kaiser Family Foundation and Harvard University School of Public Health. 1999. Survey of physicians and nurses. Menlo Park, Calif.: Henry J. Kaiser Family Foundation. www.kff.org/kaiserpolls/loader.cfm?url=/commonspot/security/getfile.cfm& PageID=13233 (accessed February 19, 2004).

Larson, D., and D. Tobin. 2000. End-of-life conversations: evolving practice and theory. *JAMA* 284:1573–78.

Levetown, M., and M. A. Carter. 1997. Child-centered care in terminal illness: an ethical framework. In *Oxford textbook of palliative medicine,* ed. D. Doyle, N. MacDonald, and G. W. Hanks, 1106–17. 2d ed. Oxford, U.K.: Oxford Medical Publications.

Lo, B., and T. Quill. 1999. Discussing palliative care with patients. *Ann Int Med* 130:744–49.

Masera, G., M. A. Chesler, M. Jankovic, A. R. Ablin, M. W. Ben Arush, F. Breatnach, H. P. McDowell, T. Eden, C. Epelman, F. F. Bellani, D. M. Green, H. V. Kosmidis, M. E. Nesbit, C. Wandzura, J. R. Wilbur, and J. J. Spinetta. 1997. SIOP Working Committee on psychosocial issues in pediatric oncology: guidelines for communication of the diagnosis. *Med Pediatr Oncol* 28:382–85.

Mosconi, P. 1991. Disclosure of breast cancer diagnosis. *Ann Oncol* 2:273–80.

Novac, D. 1979. Changes in physician's attitudes toward telling the cancer patient. *JAMA* 241:897–900.

Oken, D. 1961. What to tell cancer patients: a study of medical attitudes. *JAMA* 175:1120–28.

Patient page: cancer and children. 2002. *JAMA* 287:1890.

Pelligrino, E. 1992. Is truth telling to the patient a cultural artifact? *JAMA* 268:1734–35.

Penson, R. T., P. K. Rauch, S. L. McAfee, B. J. Cashavelly, K. Clair-Hayes, C. Dahlin, K. M. Green, B. A. Chabner, and T. J. Lynch Jr. 2002. Between parent and child: negotiating cancer treatment in adolescents. *Oncologist* 7:154–62.

Piaget, J. 1930. *The child's conception of physical causality.* London: Kegan Paul.

Radovsky, S. 1985. Bearing the news. *N Engl J Med* 313:586–88.

Siegler, M. 1982. Confidentiality in medicine: a decrepit concept. *N Engl J Med* 307:1518–21.

Spinetta, J. J., G. Masera, T. Eden, D. Oppenheim, A. G. Martins, J. van Dongen-Melman, M. Siegler, C. Eiser, M. W. Ben Arush, H. V. Kosmidis, and M. Jankovic. 2002. Refusal, non-compliance, and abandonment of treatment in children and adolescents with cancer: a report of the SIOP Working Committee on Psychosocial Issues in Pediatric Oncology. *Med Pediatr Oncol* 38:114–17.

Surbone, A. 1992. Truth telling to the patient. *JAMA* 268:1661–62.

Tulsky, J. 1998. Opening the black box: how do physicians communicate about advance directives? *Ann Int Med* 129:441–49.

von Gunten, G. F., F. D. Ferris, and L. Emanuel. 2000. Ensuring competency in end-of-life care communication and relational skills. *JAMA* 284:3051–57.

Warren, S. D., and L. D. Brandeis. 1890. "The right to privacy." *Harvard Law Review* 4:193–220.

Whaley, B. 2000. Explaining illness to children. In *Explaining illness: research, theory and strategies,* ed. B. Whaley, 200–207. London: Lawrence Erlbaum.

Psychosocial and Spiritual Needs of the Child and Family

Stacy F. Orloff, Ed.D., L.C.S.W., Kathleen Quance, M.S., C.C.L.S.,
Sara Perszyk, R.N., B.S.N., W. Jeffrey Flowers, M.Div., and Erwin Veale Jr., M.Div.

> The day our child was diagnosed, the world changed. Nothing looked the same;
> even the colors of the sky and grass looked different. Our family was shaken in a
> way we did not know was possible. I didn't think we'd survive.
>
> *Parent of a child with a life-threatening disease*

Families with seriously ill children travel on an uncharted journey. There are
few road maps for this journey, and families often feel they are traveling alone.
Decisions must be made, often quickly. Families do not usually have much
time to "collect themselves" before beginning this journey. Given the pressure of time, families with a well-developed and cohesive support system have
a greater potential to use effective coping strategies; other families, perhaps
without a functional support system, may not develop effective coping strategies. The impact on the nuclear family, extended family, and community is
great.

The role of the health care team is to support the family and provide both
psychosocial and spiritual guidance as the family desires. As in all other
aspects of palliative care, the health care team supports family choice. It is
important that all health care providers be aware of common psychosocial
and spiritual care themes, with particular emphasis on family systems and
childhood development.

What do we mean by *family?* In today's society, there are many different
kinds of family. A common definition accepted by many family therapists is
that a *family* is "a group of individuals interrelated so that a change in any
one member affects other individuals and the group as a whole: this then
affects the first individual in a circular chain of influence" (Walsh 1982, 9).
Given this definition, it follows that the care team must be attentive to more
than the child's parents or guardians and siblings. Excellent palliative care

includes services to the child's larger family, including grandparents, other caregivers (including paid caregivers), and any other people identified by the child's parents or guardians as family members. Palliative care providers must be mindful that the child's family may define other community resources (for example, schools and service groups such as Boy Scouts and Girl Scouts) as part of their larger family system. Not all members of the extended family will live in the same city as the nuclear family. Palliative care teams must have systems to provide service to out-of-town family members.

Two families experiencing the same stressor will likely experience different outcomes—a fact denoted by the family therapy term, *equifinality.* Palliative care professionals must understand that each family is unique and that its need for psychosocial and spiritual care should be assessed individually. The best psychosocial and spiritual care assessments are ongoing, and they begin by asking families to share their concerns with the care team.

Particular attention must also be given to each family's cultural, religious, and spiritual needs. It is vital that palliative care providers have some working knowledge of different cultural norms and religious beliefs before assessing and providing psychosocial or spiritual care intervention. For example, most cultures have their own beliefs regarding sharing information about prognosis, funeral preplanning, and placing objects or pictures in the coffin. In many religions, there are certain rituals that must be performed before or after the death (Irish, Lundquist, and Nelson 1993). Any psychosocial or spiritual care assessment should include questions regarding religious, cultural, and spiritual beliefs.

Mark, a 16-year-old male, was diagnosed with Duchenne muscular dystrophy when he was five years old and in kindergarten. His mother told him his diagnosis at age 10, when he was in the fifth grade. Mark's mother had contacted the local hospice in her area for assistance in telling her son about his diagnosis. The palliative care counselor continued providing counseling to Mark and his family. By the time Mark was in seventh grade, he used a wheelchair full time. He had surgery that same year to lengthen his heel cord, in an attempt to preserve his ability to stand and walk a bit longer. By eighth grade, Mark was unable to bear weight at all.

Two years later, his neuromuscular scoliosis had progressed to the point where his parents elected to have Mark undergo a posterior spinal fusion. Mark was confined to bed postoperatively. He was admitted to the home health care program of the local hospice. From this point on, Mark experienced decline in function. He developed dysphagia and had subsequent weight loss. His total weight loss within a few months was more than 13 percent of his weight before the spinal fusion. Mark then had a percutaneous endoscopically placed gastrostomy tube (PEG) placement and began enteral feedings. One month later, he developed an upper respiratory illness and began choking on thick mucus. One choking episode resulted in a 911 call and a trip to the emergency room. Nebulizer and in-exsufflator treatments were begun, and a suction machine was ordered for the home.

Mark has a younger and an older sister living in the home. Both of his sisters have had many school problems. He is currently physically unable to attend school owing to his physical limitations and is home-bound. Previously, Mark had an episode in school in which he was left unattended in a restroom and was incontinent of urine and wet himself.

The family has many financial pressures. The parents frequently struggle to pay bills. Because of federal requirements regarding income eligibility, there have been a few months when the family is without Medicaid coverage. This lack of coverage creates severe economic hardship for the family. Mark's mother, a petite woman with back and neck problems, is limited in her ability to lift Mark. She also suffers from depression. The palliative care counselor has provided support to the entire family as well as individually to each family member. Mark's younger sister is a regular participant in the monthly sibling support group.

Diagnosis

The diagnosis of a life-threatening condition in a child is an earth-shattering event for any family. As the child and family move through the different phases of care—diagnosis, treatment, and cure, or death and subsequent bereavement—they require substantial support from an array of professionals. The sooner these resources are marshaled, the greater the likelihood that interventions will be successful in strengthening the family's and the child's coping abilities. The American Academy of Pediatrics, the International Work Group on Death, Dying, and Bereavement, and other organizations advocate an integrated model of palliative care for children living with life-threatening conditions. According to the model, palliative care begins at the time of diagnosis and continues throughout the course of the illness, whether the outcome is cure or death (American Academy of Pediatrics 2000; Davies 2000). Mark's case illustrates the challenges some families experience informing their child that he or she has a life-limiting disease. It took Mark's family five years to tell him.

The needs of the family during the diagnostic phase can differ to some extent, depending on how the diagnosis is made. Many times, the diagnosis is made after only a brief period of illness and abbreviated investigation or workup. Before diagnosis, the parents may have little warning that their baby or child has a problem. These parents most commonly express feelings of shock and disbelief. They often feel like they have been hit by a lightning bolt. A perfectly routine pregnancy may be interrupted by an abnormal ultrasound revealing a life-threatening in utero condition in the fetus. A baby may be born with a life-threatening condition after an uneventful pregnancy. A child may be playing T-ball one day and be abruptly diagnosed the next day with a life-threatening condition, such as cancer or an encephalopathy secondary to meningitis. When a diagnosis of a life-threatening condition is made in this fashion, many parents react with numbness, shock, and incredulity. Often, it is a physician they may have just met who informs them about the outcome of the diagnostic workup.

Uncertainty is almost always more difficult to cope with than any one particular diagnosis. If the family is presented with a differential diagnosis, the parents may focus on one or two diagnoses that they may be acquainted with, either through the media or from personal experience. In this information era, parents may take these several diagnoses and search the Internet to obtain as much information as they can. They may seek out experts and centers of excellence for their child's condition even before they have a firm diagnosis.

Cure-Oriented Treatment

Once a diagnosis is arrived at and curative treatment has begun, most families move past shock and disbelief into the treatment phase. They attempt to reestablish some measure of equilibrium and normalcy in their lives. Armed with information about the disorder and its treatment, they now cling to the hope of a cure (realistic or not) and endeavor to put their lives back in order. Their hopes and dreams are as vital to their continued daily functions as are eating and sleeping. Rather than shattering these perhaps unrealistic hopes, professional caregivers should assist the family to shift their hopes and dreams to outcomes they may be able to accomplish, such as to have the best family holidays ever or to enable their child to finish seventh grade.

Palliative Care

For many life-threatening conditions, a point is reached in the child's treatment when curative treatment is no longer possible or the side effects of the treatment become too onerous or too risky to justify continuing curative care. The family's period of relative tranquility is over. Regrettably, some families are told that there is nothing else that can be done for their child—at best a poor choice of words and at worst simply not true. There is *always* something that can be done for a child and family, even if it is only to be present for the family, to comfort them, to hold their hands, to let them know that others care. Often, much more than this can be done to ease the child's passage from this earth and to help the family cope with this devastating experience.

Ideally, palliative care services have been integrated into the child's care from the point of diagnosis, but in reality this is not often the case. At this transition phase, the concept of palliative care, or hospice care, is commonly introduced. For most families and professional caregivers, this is a difficult discussion. The ramifications of the transition for families may include giving up the team of health care providers they have come to trust and feel comfortable with for a new set of caregivers, such as the hospice team. The child's primary physician may continue to direct care if he or she is comfortable with providing palliative care. The child's other caregivers, including clinic, hospital, and home health nurses, social workers, child-life specialists, and various therapists, may or may not be involved in the child's care from this point on. The transition is so difficult that it often is delayed until it is evident that the child is actually dying. This delay in initiating palliative care can result in care that is crisis oriented, exacerbating the family's sense of vulnerability and helplessness. Establishing a framework for proactive decision making is made much more challenging with late palliative care referrals. In the case study, the hospice and palliative home care program was initiated early in Mark's diagnostic phase, making it much easier for the family to accept additional help as Mark's condition began to deteriorate.

In addition to the reservations that parents have about giving up their established team of caregivers, parents also resist the transition to hospice care because they equate hospice care with "giving up." Even if the parents recognize that the chances of cure are slim, they may still need to hang on to the slight hope for full recovery. A survey conducted by the Children's Hospice International (1998) indicates that one of the leading obstacles to providing hospice services to children is an association of the hospice concept with death rather than with life enhancement.

As it becomes evident that curative care may not be successful, many families seek out complementary or alternative therapies. These measures may also be sought as an adjunct to curative treatment from the start of care and may include herbal therapies, acupuncture, homeopathy, nutritional therapies, therapeutic touch or massage, prayer, and other modalities that may be culturally specific. Many families do not discuss these therapies with their traditional, or allopathic, physician. Some are afraid that their physician may not approve of what they are doing or might try to dissuade them from using complementary measures. Physicians and other health care professionals can keep the channels of communication open by listening without judgment and recognizing that the use of complementary therapies arises from the desire to leave no stone unturned. Most complementary therapies will not harm and may even benefit the child. Therapies that may have harmful effects on the child should be discussed with the family.

Incorporating the Child

Members of the palliative care team must have considerable knowledge about child development. Seriously ill children will often not talk with counselors and chaplains who seem uncomfortable with and uninformed about providing service to very ill children. Ill children frequently want to have some control over their illness and treatment and to participate in the planning and delivery of their health care. The primary care team must work with the ill child and his or her family to provide age-appropriate ways for the child to have a voice in the care-planning process. Issues of control will vary according to age. It may not be realistic for the younger child to decide whether or not to have chemotherapy, but the child could decide the location or time frame in which treatment is provided. Older children may have the cognitive ability to make decisions that affect treatment outcomes.

The palliative care team must address the following questions:

- When is it appropriate to ask the child what he or she wants?
- How will the family incorporate the needs and desires of the child in the decision-making process?

- How will the family and palliative care team address issues of informed consent?

The Palliative Care Foundation, in San Jose, Costa Rica, has published information on the rights of a child with a terminal illness, including the right to object to receiving treatment when cure is no longer possible and the right to have good pain control (National Hospice and Palliative Care Organization 2000). Family decisions may also depend on religious and cultural beliefs. The American Academy of Pediatrics has provided some guidance on the issues of parental permission, consent, child assent, and the consideration of religious beliefs in decision making for children (American Academy of Pediatrics 1995, 1997; Barnes et al. 2000).

Lack of understanding about the nature of the illness, disease progression, and prognosis can be the source of anxiety for the ill child. Health care providers must continually assess the child's level of understanding of the treatment process. Many children living with life-limiting conditions understand much more about their illness and health care in general than might be expected. Nonetheless, it is important to evaluate a child's specific level of understanding about diagnoses, tests, procedures, and treatments. Medical jargon and whispered or veiled communication can cause the ill child to become anxious. Ill children must be able to ask questions and obtain reasonable developmentally appropriate answers. Proper time must be given for children to ask questions. Frequently, children may have questions when their health care providers are not present. Not all children will feel comfortable asking questions of parents or other family members, and family members sometimes inadvertently give children the impression they are not comfortable discussing these "tough" topics.

For successful communication between children and their health care team, the team must provide effective interventions to enhance the child's ability to ask questions. One way the care team can be of assistance is by providing children with tape recorders to record their questions. The tapes can then be brought to the child's next appointment so the health care provider can listen to the tape with the child. Answers can be recorded on the same tape, enabling the child and his or her family to listen as often as necessary.

Ill children often feel isolated from their peers. Daily routines are often interrupted, and their illness can keep children from attending school for extended periods. It is important to find creative ways to encourage ongoing interactions with the child's peer group. Seriously ill children also often feel that they are the only ill children their age. Children with life-limiting conditions need opportunities to socialize with other ill children. Increased socialization is especially important during treatment, as it increases opportunities for children to talk about issues that concern them. How does a child, a concrete thinker with a limited concept of time, understand and express things such as hope, cure, and remission? Children frequently worry about symptoms and prognosis. Peers are often better able to encourage hope, as they have actually gone through similar experiences. Self-esteem and self-image can be enhanced through these socialization events. Support through informal group meetings is also important.

Ill children also need a sense of normalcy. As much as possible, the family should provide ongoing normal activities for the child. Leisure activity can be helpful. Many communities offer camplike retreats for ill children. It is also advisable, if feasible, to consider sending the ill child back to school, youth group activities, and other outside activities. If the child is unable to return to the classroom or youth group activities, care providers and families should consider creative ways to bring peers and their activities into the child's home. Mark's condition deteriorated to the point where he was not able to attend school. The psychosocial counselor understood that Mark still desired to socialize with peers and arranged for hospice teen volunteers to visit with him at home.

Parents

The family experiences many stresses during the time of the child's illness. Parents are confronted with the unimaginable situation that their child may precede them in death. Anticipatory grief issues begin immediately at the time of diagnosis. Parents have lost a part of their future. No longer may they assume without question that their child will provide a family legacy into the future. Important anticipatory grief issues to address include the following:

- assisting the family to stay connected with the child
- assisting with communication issues both within the family and with health care providers
- providing support to the family with any funeral preplanning they may wish to do
- assisting family members in creating lasting memories that will comfort them after the child dies (National Hospice and Palliative Care Organization 2000)

Parents may question previously held religious and spiritual views. Anger with a Supreme Being is not unusual. Parents may feel in some way responsible for their child's illness. An important role of parents is to be the child's protector, and the parents of an ill child no longer feel that they can protect their children. Treatment may include painful procedures, and long-term pain and symptom management issues are a reality. Parents of children born with genetic or metabolic disorders may blame themselves, or each other, for the illness. It is important that issues of anticipatory grief be addressed from the time the child is diagnosed with a potentially life-limiting disease.

For many parents, this time period puts much stress on the marital relationship. Husbands and wives frequently express emotions differently. Although the couple may understand that there is no right or wrong way to express feelings, it is not unusual for one spouse to be more verbally expressive than the other. This may well create a situation in which one spouse may feel the other is not as emotionally affected by the diagnosis or illness. Sexual intimacy may also be affected during this time period. For some couples, sexual intimacy may be a way to affirm life and support their need to be close to each other. Others may experience a lack of sexual desire. Many couples fear that their marriage may break up because of these stresses. Research in this area has yielded evidence demonstrating support both for and against the disintegration of the marital relationship when a child has a life-threatening illness (Armstrong-Dailey and Zarbock 2001). Recognizing that parents are also a marital unit is important. Frequently, psychosocial professionals' focus on the adults only as the child's parents negates the impact of the illness on the parents both as individuals and as marriage partners. Group support can affirm the stresses on the marital unit by providing opportunities for the adults to get to know other couples who have ill children. Ongoing support groups are most helpful.

Siblings

The bond between siblings is strong and is marked by much intensity. Within the family unit, it is siblings who will spend the greatest proportion of their lives together. Cicerelli (1995) defines sibling relationships as "the total of the interactions (physical, verbal, and nonverbal communication) of two or more individuals who share knowledge, perceptions, attitudes, beliefs, and feelings regarding each other, from the time that one sibling becomes aware of the other" (Cicerelli 1995).

Siblings must share their parents' time, attention, and affection. During the diagnosis and treatment process, parental attention will focus predominately on the ill child, often leaving healthy siblings feeling left out. For families living in rural areas, children's hospitals may be far from home, and healthy children must therefore be left at home with caregivers while the parents stay with the hospitalized child. Hospital visitation protocols still vary around the country and may make it difficult for families to be together when the ill child requires hospitalization. Technological interventions such as video hookups through computers, e-mail, and conference calls can assist family members to stay connected with one another.

Psychosocial concerns are similar for all children. How these concerns are acted out behaviorally and psychologically varies according to the age of the sibling. Although magical thinking is often associated with younger children, the palliative care counselor must address this issue with all siblings. Magical thinking can result if the child is not given age-appropriate information regarding the illness, its symptoms, and the possible causes of the disease. Siblings frequently argue with one another, and in the course of an argument it is not uncommon for one child to say to another, "I hate you and wish you were dead." Magical thinking might allow such a child, particularly a young one, to feel responsible for the illness of a sibling. Older children may worry about "catching" the illness. Mark's younger sister, Jane, had a difficult time as Mark's condition deteriorated. She benefited from attending the monthly meeting of the sibling support group sponsored by the local hospice provider. At this group, Jane was able to meet other children with ill siblings. It was the first time, she said, she felt that someone other than her counselor understood what she was going through. Good assessment and accurate information will help to ease most of these concerns.

Siblings may also feel anger toward the ill child and their parents. Healthy siblings frequently feel that the ill child is getting an overabundance of attention—attention that could be given to them. Siblings frequently express anger that they are no longer able to participate in many outside activities or, if they do participate in other activities, that their family is rarely there to watch. Even if a parent is physically present, emotionally he or she may seem distant to the child. Children do not often understand why their parents act differently and frequently interpret the parents' emotional distance as a reaction to something the child may have done to upset the parent. Many palliative care programs provide specially trained volunteers to serve as mentors to siblings. Although the volunteers cannot take the place of the child's parents, they can provide a consistent adult presence in the life of a child with a life-threatening illness.

Some siblings also describe feeling ashamed or embarrassed. Children with a neurologically impaired brother or sister may feel uncomfortable being out in public with a sibling who looks and acts different. Many of these children do not know anyone who has a sibling with a similar illness. Introducing children who have siblings with similar diagnoses helps them cope with these feelings. Sibling support groups also provide opportunities for children to talk about their neurologically impaired siblings without feeling ashamed or embarrassed.

Families

When a family is faced with the reality of caring for a child with a life-threatening condition, the foundation of that family is shaken. Some families crumble under the strain of caring for a sick child, some plod on barely surviving, while other families not only remain standing but also find inner resources they did not know they had. Families in the midst of the twenty-four-hour-a-day turmoil of caring for a child with a life-threatening condition need some means of stepping away from these pressures. Caring for a child with a life-threatening disease is a taxing responsibility that can often overwhelm the family's resources (Diehl, Moffitt, and Wade 1991). The everyday tasks of chauffeuring a healthy sibling to soccer practice, walking the dog, and doing the dishes, or going on a family vacation, can be challenging, if not impossible, for a family with a seriously ill child. Parents' days can be filled with trips to various specialists' offices, hospital stays, ordering supplies and equipment, coordinating with home nursing agencies, dealing with insurance or Medicaid care managers. A division of labor frequently occurs in two-parent families, one parent, usually the mother, serving as the ill child's primary caregiver. The primary caregiver must stay home with the ill child while the other parent attends to the family's business. This makes it difficult for a family to be a family. Parents often serve, by default or of their own choosing, as their child's nurse, home health aide, social worker, mental health counselor, spiritual counselor, case manager, and health care system advocate. Support programs for families of children with life-threatening conditions have not kept pace with these other trends, and, as a result, such families are under more pressure than ever.

These circumstances frequently place families under financial stress. Given the amount of time required to care for an ill child, parents may find it difficult to maintain employment. One or both parents may lose a job, which increases secondary losses such as insurance and other employee benefits. The impact from financial strain on the family can be immense, and palliative care professionals must be prepared to provide guidance to families experiencing financial stress.

Respite Care

Respite care is designed to give families a break from intense caregiving obligations. Respite care is defined as the provision of care for the ill child by alternative care providers, enabling parents to take time off from the exhausting care these children require. Some families are able to marshal their own resources, coordinating a cadre of caregivers including extended family and friends, to provide their own respite care. In fact, as much as 90 percent of respite care may be provided informally by families (Shantz 1995). This usage pattern may be a matter of necessity rather than choice, as the availability of respite services varies considerably from one community to another. Children with life-threatening illnesses often have complex care requirements, requiring the respite care provider to have specific training regarding that child's care.

The families with the greatest need for respite care are those who fall through the cracks of the existing programs. Their child's care may be too complex for a lay caregiver program but not complex enough to be granted around-the-clock nursing care. Thus the burden of their child's care falls almost entirely on the parents' shoulders. Without adequate respite, these families can crumble under the chronic stress of this caregiving obligation. Respite care is consistently identified by families as a priority need (Cohen and Warren 1985). For many families, "respite care becomes a vital service— a necessity, not a luxury" (National Information Center for Children and Youth with Disabilities 1996, 3). It is intended to prevent parent burnout and to allow the child with a life-threatening condition to remain at home. The provision of such services by tertiary care children's hospitals and community hospitals with pediatric units, reimbursed through state-sponsored support programs, may be an area for improvement in the next few years.[1]

Coordinating Care

Children living with life-threatening conditions are cared for by a variety of caregivers and in many settings, including the home, community hospitals, pediatric or specialty hospitals, nursing homes, medical day care centers, foster homes, and hospice homes. The dilemma many families face is coordinating all these services.

Primary care physicians, such as pediatricians and family doctors, home health nurses, school nurses and teachers, hospice personnel, Medicaid and insurance case managers, and often a multiplicity of pediatric subspecialists, are frequently involved in the care of such a child. For a child whose illness requires technological support, as many as seven people may be designated as case managers.

Often, depending on the treatment regimen or acuity of the child's illness, the child moves from one care setting to another with regularity and frequency. In these diverse settings the child's treatment goals can vary substantially. This can be disturbing and stressful for the child and family, as the following example illustrates.

> Shawn, a child with a terminal condition cared for by a hospice team, is on limited gastrostomy feedings because he is not able to tolerate full feedings. His parents are not ready to discontinue all feedings because they do not want him to "starve to death" and feel he still has some "quality time" left. Shawn requires hospitalization at a local children's hospital for a brief "tune-up" for relief of symptoms. On his admission to the hospital, the admitting pediatric resident reviews Shawn's weight and total twenty-four-hour fluids and promptly "scolds" the parents for not feeding their son enough. The resident failed to ask about or even consider the parents' goals for their child.

Parents of children with life-threatening conditions are often obliged to serve as coordinators of care between the various physicians caring for their child. Each physician may care for a different organ system or manage one of the child's medical problems, but the child is rarely viewed as a whole person. Frequently, these specialists disagree about the child's diagnosis or treatment regimen. This can be stressful for parents. Someone must consider the child as a whole. It is essential that at least one individual take into account the family as a unit, as well. In many instances, the pediatrician or family physician will serve this role. Regrettably, not all pediatricians and family doctors have the desire, training, or even the time to function in this role.

Parents may also find it necessary to provide supervision of their child's outpatient caregivers, including home health aides; in-home shift nurses; physical, occupational, and speech therapists; medical day care personnel; and school nurses and teachers. Parents often directly observe the care rendered by these caregivers and can be best positioned to make judgments about its quality. They frequently find this an undesirable responsibility to assume, fearing that any negative feedback they provide about a particular care provider may place their relationship with him or her in peril. The parents are apprehensive that the care provider may retaliate against their child in some way. On the other hand, if the parents do not promote high-quality care for their child, the child will, in some measurable way, suffer from second-rate care.

It is a rare parent who is suited to "wear all these hats"—advocate, coordinator, and supervisor. Infrequently, parents will relish their role as their child's health care system key worker. Most parents, however, find it to be a demanding and draining experience. Innovative programs are being developed to provide such a key worker for families with severely ill children; such programs could serve simultaneously to reduce the family's stress level and to improve outcomes for children with life-threatening conditions.

Spiritual Dimensions of Pediatric Palliative Care

Any conversation on health care that seeks to be inclusive of the total person must include a discussion of the spiritual dynamics associated with illness, loss, and bereavement. Benson (1999) describes health care as a three-legged stool, the legs being surgical and therapeutic interventions, pharmaceutical and medicinal treatments, and self-care. Spiritual care is at the forefront of self-care. An examination of the word *spirituality* reveals a much deeper and all-encompassing concept, one that is within all of us. Spirit is a natural dimension of every person (VandeCreek and Burton 2001), and even decisions made in everyday transactions have a spiritual component. The spiritualist John Mane (1987) describes it as follows:

> The spiritual life is not a specialized part of daily life. Everything you do in the day from washing to eating breakfast, having meetings, driving to work, solving problems, making more problems for yourself once you have solved them, watching television or deciding instead to read, going to a

restaurant or movie or going to church, everything you do is your spiritual life. It is only a matter of how consciously you do these ordinary things, how attentive you are to the opportunities they offer for growth, for enjoyment, and how mindfully, how selflessly, how compassionately you perform them. Yet to live spiritually all the time, everyone needs to take specific times to focus on the spiritual dimension before everything else.

Rather than overt religious acts, spirituality has much to do with how we choose to live and be a part of society.

Perhaps nothing affects these types of decision as much as the illness of a child. A child's struggle with severe illness is troubling even to people who do not have any relationship with that child. Hospitals experience no shortage of people volunteering their time to assist children. A common spiritual value is that children are innocent and pure and should be exempted from the most difficult elements in life, such as pain, suffering, illness, and death. The illness of a child undermines a sense that life is fair and predictable. Often with the illness and death of a child, the adults touched by that child experience continuing losses. In addition to the immediate suffering of the child, dreams of a "normal" life crash and are replaced by harsh realities of adjustment to the new definition of *normal.* Things did not happen according to the natural plan. The death of a child strikes a chord of injustice. The loss of a child is devastating to the family unit, as much of a family's life centers around the children. In the years ahead, as other children pass milestones, the bereaved family will feel the loss again. The first day of school, birthdays, and graduations are all events that re-create the sense of loss and remind the family of the death. Health care professionals must come to an understanding of how spiritual issues are dealt with in the confines of a health care system and how they themselves might become more sensitive to the spiritual dimension.

All children and families have the right to spiritual care. "Healthcare organizations are obligated to respond to spiritual needs because patients have a right to such services" (VandeCreek and Burton 2001). The role of a trusted pastor, priest, rabbi, or shaman can be crucial. A trained chaplain should be a vital member of the health care team to ensure that spiritual care issues are addressed. Palliative care programs must be able to provide spiritual care support.

Spirit implies energy and power. "The word spirituality goes even further and describes an awareness of relationship with all creation, an appreciation of presence and purpose that includes a sense of meaning" (VandeCreek and Burton 2001). From its root meaning, it is often translated in sacred literature as "wind." When a person is confronted with the crisis of illness, particularly illness in a child, spiritual energy and strength are pushed to their limits and tested for their ability to provide comfort and hope even in the face of despairing odds. It is incumbent on any health care provider to develop the ability to inquire about spiritual resources within the family unit and to take note of how these resources might help the family in crisis.

While health care providers may feel comfortable asking a patient or parent about such things as bowel habits, they avoid a question as simple as "Do you participate in any particular faith group?" Studies, however, indicate that seriously ill children and their parents would like their health care providers to ask these questions. According to one such study, as many as 70 percent of patients are aware of one or more spiritual needs related to their illness (VandeCreek and Burton 2001). Studies of patients in acute care hospitals indicate that between one-third and two-thirds of all patients want to receive spiritual care (VandeCreek and Burton 2001). The Joint Commission on the Accreditation of Healthcare Organizations addresses the need for spiritual support by specifically noting patients' fundamental right to considerate care that safeguards their personal dignity and respects their cultural, psychosocial, and spiritual values (VandeCreek and Burton 2001).

Given that spiritual issues must be addressed with the pediatric patient and family, the question is how to define such a broad topic in a manner that gives personal attention to individual wishes. A question as simple as "Do you have a particular faith?" may elicit a myriad of responses. The word *faith* has a range of interpretations, from a particular religious organization to a challenging of the laws of nature and a desire for a miracle. For some evangelicals, for example, the question of faith asks whether a person has enough belief or trust in a higher power to reverse the realities of the given situation. Others hear this inquiry as asking whether one has specific practices that enhance one's life, such as meditation, fasting, reading sacred texts, or attending fellowships. The absence of religious language is not an indication of a lack of spirituality. Religion and spirituality are not one and the same.

It is a mistake to assume that only adults understand spiritual issues and possess spiritual resources. Children appear to understand these issues as well, if in a simpler and more honest way. Natural curiosity leads the child to ask direct questions and to accept direct answers. Children often accept the existence of spiritual beings and the continuation of life on another plane. They have yet to complicate life with specific questions of how. When asked to believe or trust, this is a natural response. It is important that children be included in these discussions at whatever level of comprehension is appropriate and that specific attention be given to their wishes. Many health care providers who work with terminally ill children in health care settings have heard young children speak of having conversations with God, seeing angels, or wondering aloud how all that we call our world came to be.

There are many different ways to assess spirituality in seriously ill children. Health care providers must become more aware of the many different formal and informal assessment tools available. One such example is the spiritual history inventory (Matthews 1998), which assesses four dimensions of spirituality: faith, influence, community, address (abbreviated as FICA). The first step addresses the role of religious faith or spirituality in the child or family's life. The next inquires into the way the individual views himself or herself religiously or spiritually. The care team may then offer many different interventions, such as the reading of sacred writings, the playing or singing of sacred music, or other rituals that bring comfort to the patient and family. A thorough assessment includes questions regarding family religious or spiritual rituals.

The Children's Project on Palliative/Hospice Services, under the auspices of the National Hospice and Palliative Care Organization, has developed guidelines for assessing spirituality in ill children and their families. The guidelines have distinct questions that can be used with the ill child, siblings, parents, and grandparents. There is also a section for the family that does not have a particular religious belief system (Davies 2000; Davies et al. 2002).

Assessing the family's use of rituals is important. Prayer, defined as talking to God, is an important part of the spiritual lives of many people. Members of the health care team should encourage children and their parents to be open and honest in their prayers. Prayer involves not only talking to God or one's Higher Power but also listening inside one's head, heart, soul, and being.

What is wanted or expected from prayers? Literal healing, getting well and out of the bed, is perhaps the thing that people most want. Prayer may sustain hope even when medical evidence does not support cure. And hope can be a healing balm even to the last breath.

Prayers of acceptance are also important. They can be of great comfort to the child and the family, as well. Sometimes children linger if they sense that the family is still holding on. Giving them permission to rest and stop the fight, in conversation and in prayers, can be one of the most loving things anyone can give to dying children. The option of having prayers said aloud should be given. Prayer during pastoral visits may be greatly appreciated. Prayers offered spontaneously from the heart and traditional written prayers all have their place. It is most important to question what the child and family may want regarding the ritual of prayer.

Baptism is another important ministry ritual. In an emergency situation, any person can baptize. Receiving Communion and baptism may be the two most frequently requested, and performed, rituals. These rituals may be administered in any location in the hospital or home. Babies have been baptized in the operating room. Anointing with oil is another important ritual in some religious traditions. Such acts must not be perceived to be magical. They do not guarantee miraculous healing. These powerful rituals should be understood and acknowledged as part of the mystery of faith. The most important thing is that the patient and his or her family receive whatever ritualistic ministry is significant to them.

Dietary and cleansing rituals may be important issues for the child and family. Kirkwood (1993) provides information regarding rituals for persons entrusted to the care of the palliative care team. Such reference material should be made available to the health care team, as they may not be knowledgeable about the beliefs of all their patients. A child of the Muslim faith, for example, may want to sit or lie facing Mecca; something as simple as moving the bed will be greatly appreciated by the family. Family members may want to read sections of the Koran, and members of the Sikh faith may receive comfort from hearing readings of the Guru Garantha Sahab when dying (Kirkwood 1993).

Making confession, being given absolution, and receiving the last rites are all important to some as death approaches. Others are indifferent about such formalities; and for still others, these rituals are not part of their spiritual or faith tradition. Some people prefer to have their privacy respected and may genuinely desire solitude. Children may be especially shy and are likely to be much more so when critically ill. Conversation should be brief during this time. Physical space while trying to offer spiritual support should be respected. Commonsense rules for interacting with children, such as not sitting on the bed and touching only as appropriate, are essential for establishing and maintaining trust. In some cases, being sure that the child is not left alone is a preferred practice. Chaplains in the hospital, hospice, or palliative care setting can and do perform these rituals for patients and their families. The child and family may prefer that their own rabbi, priest, or shaman be contacted. The family should be asked what they are praying, hoping, or longing for on their faith journeys. When they ask for ritualistic ministry, sacramental ministry, and prayer, what are they expecting to happen? Having faith does not guarantee that one will get exactly what one wishes for in life. Tragically, there are persons who view prayer and particular passages from the Bible as magical remedies to all ills. There must be awareness of the great chasm between sincere and genuine faith and magical thinking.

Early intervention by the chaplain may help with these issues. At the least, a chaplain or other religious counselor can serve as a liaison between a child, his or her family, and their spiritual or faith community. Relationship is a key word here. The rabbi, priest, shaman, or pastor may indeed already have a loving and solid relationship with the persons involved.

Absent Faith?

What about children and families who have little or no professed faith? What about those who do not "believe" at all? In addressing the needs of these people, their belief and the dignity of their spiritual position, or lack thereof, deserves equal respect. Perhaps the illness of their child has damaged or forever cast aside what was once a strong faith. This can happen when cliché theology is offered by well-meaning friends or family members, such as "God needed a new angel" or "Another flower has been plucked for heaven's garden." Is it any wonder that children and their family members get angry with God when such theology is sent their way? Who can dare to tell dying children or their parents how to feel or what to believe? The novelist Flannery O'Connor (1979) once wrote, "Let me tell you this: faith comes and goes. It rises and falls like the tides of an invisible ocean. If it is presumptuous to think that faith will stay with you forever, it is just as presumptuous to think that unbelief will."

In Mark 9:24 the father of an ill child prayed, "Lord, I believe. Help thou my unbelief." When death is imminent, people of faith may fear that their faith is inadequate. Many people suffer with painful guilt and believe that God is punishing them for some sin or because their faith has not been strong enough. They may conclude that because their faith is weak, their prayers have also been weak. Thus healing as they had hoped for will not come. Again, people cannot be made to believe and have faith. One can extend love to them. One can strive to offer hope. Daring to simply be there with a dying child speaks volumes. In itself, it proves that love for that child and family is real. One must not worry about what to say.

Not all issues can be discovered early in a spiritual assessment. The tremendous weight of guilt and a sense of isolation may lie undetected beneath the surface for many people and can alienate them from the help they so desperately need.

Conclusion

Children living with life-limiting conditions and their families have the right to expect the highest quality of care from their palliative care providers. This care includes staff who are competent to guide families as they embark on this difficult journey through the curative health care system. As guides, palliative care staff must be capable and skilled in turning their knowledge of the emotional, psychosocial, and spiritual needs of family into specific professional tasks to assist each family member. The information presented in this chapter is just the beginning. All palliative care professionals must commit to continued learning about the psychosocial and spiritual care needs of the child and his or her family.

The assertion has often been made, "I am not afraid of death. I am afraid of dying." While we do what we can to alleviate physical pain, we must also do all that is within our collective power to ease spiritual pain wherever we find it as the dying process is happening in our presence. Finding hope, comfort, and peace in the face of death is the right of every suffering soul. Father Henri Nouwen (1984) may have provided the best perspective:

> When we honestly ask ourselves which persons in our lives mean the most to us, we often find that it is the person who instead of giving advice, solutions, or cures, [has] chosen . . . to share our pain and touch our wounds with a gentle and tender hand. The friend who can be silent with us in a moment of despair or confusion, who can be silent with us in our hour of grief and bereavement, who can tolerate not knowing, not curing, not healing, and face with us the reality of our powerlessness, this is the friend who cares.

Note

1. On March 28, two bills were heard before the Massachusetts Joint Health Care Committee. *An Act to Provide Pediatric Palliative Care to Children with Life Limit-*

ing Illnesses in the Commonwealth (S565/H1759) was presented by members of a coalition that developed the bill, including Joanne Wolf, M.D., Dana Farber Cancer Institute; Paul Thayer, PediCare Franciscan; Maureen McGrath, R.N., Hospice of the North Shore; Rigney Cunningham, Hospice and Palliative Care Federation of Massachusetts; and Mrs. Sandie Aiello, parent of 3-year-old Kayla, a three-year hospice patient who died in the care of Health Care Dimensions. Mrs. Aiello's compelling testimony anchored the panel and clearly moved the legislators present. If passed, and subject to appropriation, the bill would have established a pediatric palliative care program at the Massachusetts Department of Public Health to provide direct care services to children with life-limiting illnesses (ages infant to 18) and their families. Services would complement, not compete with, existing care provided by other professional caregivers. These services, depending on the unique needs of the child, could include consultation for pain and symptom management, social services, spiritual care, counseling and bereavement services, volunteer support, and up to forty-eight hours of respite care each year. On referral by a professional caregiver such as a physician, hospital, or visiting nurse association, these services would be provided on a fee-for-service basis by a limited number of licensed hospices selected by Department of Public Health on the basis of demonstrated expertise and capability in pediatric palliative care. Unfortunately, the bill did not pass (Joanne Wolf, M.D., Dana Farber Cancer Institute, personal communication, January 16, 2002).

References

American Academy of Pediatrics, Committee on Bioethics. 1995. Informed consent, parental permission, and assent in pediatric practice. *Pediatrics* 95:314–17.

———, Committee on Bioethics. 1997. Religious objections to medical care. *Pediatrics* 99:279–81.

———, Committee on Bioethics, Committee on Hospital Care. 2000. Palliative care for children. *Pediatrics* 106:351–57.

Armstrong-Dailey, A., and S. Zarbock, eds. 2001. *Hospice care for children.* 2d ed. New York: Oxford University Press.

Barnes, L. L., G. A. Plotnikoff, K. Fox, and S. Pendleton. 2000. Spirituality, religion, and pediatrics: intersecting worlds of healing. *Pediatrics* 106:899–908.

Benson, H. 1999. Health, illness, and the use of conventional and unconventional medicine and mind/body healing. Paper presented to the Spirituality and Healing Conference. Boston, December 11.

Children's Hospice International. 1998. Survey: hospice care for children: Executive Summary Report. Alexandria, Va.: CHI.

Cicerelli, V. G. 1995. *Sibling relationships across the lifespan.* New York: Plenum.

Cohen, S., and R. D. Warren. 1985. *Respite care: principles, programs and policies.* Austin, Texas: Pro-Ed.

Davies, B. 1999. *Shadows in the sun.* Philadelphia: Brunner/Mazel.

————. 2000. International Work Group on Death, Dying, and Bereavement. Alexandria, Va.: National Hospice and Palliative Care Organization.

Davies, B., P. Brenner, S. Orloff, L. Sumner, and W. Worden. 2002. Addressing spirituality in pediatric hospice and palliative care. *J Palliat Care* 18:59–67.

Diehl, S., K. Moffitt, and S. Wade. 1991. Focus group interview with parents of children with medically complex needs: an intimate look at their perceptions and feelings. *Children's Health Care* 20:170–78.

Irish, D. P., K. F. Lundquist, and V. J. Nelson, eds. 1993. *Ethnic variations in dying, death, and grief.* Washington, D.C.: Taylor and Francis.

Kirkwood, N. A. 1993. *A handbook on multiculturalism and religion.* Harrisburg, Pa.: Morehouse.

Mane, J. 1987. *The inner Christ: a combined volume of word into silence, moment of Christ, the present Christ.* New York: Darton, Longman, and Todd.

Matthews, D. 1998. *The faith factor: proof of the healing power of prayer.* New York: Penguin Putnam.

National Hospice and Palliative Care Organization. 2000. *Compendium of pediatric palliative care.* Alexandria, Va.

National Information Center for Children and Youth with Disabilities. 1996. Respite care. *NICHCY News Digest,* June, 1–8.

Nouwen, H. 1984. *Out of solitude.* Notre Dame, Ind.: Ave Maria.

O'Connor, F. 1979. *The habit of being.* New York: Farrar, Straus and Giroux.

Shantz, M. 1995. Effects of respite care: a literature review. *Perspectives* 10:11–15.

VandeCreek, L., and L. Burton, eds. 2001. A white paper: professional chaplaincy: its role and importance in healthcare. *J Pastoral Care* 55:81–97.

Walsh, F., ed. 1982. *Normal family processes.* New York: Guilford.

7

Holistic Management of Symptoms

Richard Hain, M.B.B.S., M.D., M.Sc., M.R.C.P., F.R.C.P.C.H., Sharon Weinstein, M.D.,
James Oleske, M.D., M.P.H., Stacy F. Orloff, Ed.D., L.C.S.W.,
and Susan Cohen, M.A., A.D.T.R., C.C.L.S.

Palliative care for children is distinguished from conventional medical management by basing care goals and means of achieving them on holism, derived from the Greek word for "everything." One interpretation of this word in medical situations views the child in the context of the family.

In fact, although important, this is just one aspect of holism. In its wider sense, holism (also known as a biopsychosocial model) embodies the observation that, in the same way that physical objects possess height, breadth, and depth, all human experience occurs simultaneously in three dimensions, conventionally labeled the physical, the psychosocial, and the spiritual. Physical issues are self-explanatory; psychosocial concerns involve the effects of an experience or illness on how an individual person feels about himself or herself and interacts with others. Spiritual (or, perhaps better, existential) issues refer to how an individual understands the meaning of an experience. This often invokes an overtly religious framework of belief, but issues of paradigm shift, guilt, belief, and doubt are common existential experiences, irrespective of formal religious conviction.

The World Health Organization's (1998) definition of palliative care emphasizes the physical, emotional, and spiritual care of the patient and his or her family. A common error is to imagine that each symptom falls into one category or another. For example, we may imagine pain to be a physical symptom and guilt to be an existential one. A systematic approach may demand that we examine the three dimensions separately, but a process of reintegration is then necessary in our application of the principles to patient care.

Every symptom, like all human experiences, occurs simultaneously in all three dimensions.

The first principle underlying good symptom control in pediatric palliative care, then, is that the approach is holistic. The second is that a rational and analytical approach is applied nonetheless. Good evidence and sound scientific principle should govern care. That a child is unlikely to survive does not reduce the importance of considering the pathophysiology of symptoms and adopting a rigorous approach to history taking and examination. The third principle should underpin all medical practice: no medical intervention should be considered, either for investigation or for treatment, unless the benefit of the intervention is judged to outweigh the burden to the patient. For example, the burden of an isotope bone scan that may require an injection and will certainly necessitate a hospital visit is clearly justified at the initial diagnosis of cancer or when relapse is first suspected. However, the procedure's value is much less when metastatic disease is already recognized and a child has an established history of localized bone pain. Under these circumstances, the diagnosis is already so clear that a bone scan may be judged superfluous.

In summary, care of the child for whom there is no prospect of cure should be rigorously rational, caring, and compassionate. When appropriate weight is given to all the dimensions of a child's symptom experience, a rational approach to care, one that balances burdens and benefits to the child, will result.

Complementary Therapies

In recent decades, there has been increasing public use of complementary and alternative medicine (CAM). The incorporation of CAM into routine allopathic medical care has become known as integrative medicine. The National Center for Complementary and Alternative Medicine of the U.S. National Institutes of Health defines complementary and alternative medicine as a broad range of activities and interventions that are outside standard allopathic medicine. They have become increasingly popular, and consumers are spending large amounts of personal money on CAM. Neuhouser et al. (2001) note that 66 percent of children with cancer use some form of CAM. Complementary and alternative medicine includes self-care practices such as relaxation, which can be performed by an individual without assistance, and

Exhibit 7.1. An approach to considering complementary and alternative medicines in pediatric palliative care

---

- Consider each practice separately, based on the specific situation.
- Gather data on safety.
- Gather data on efficacy.
- Elicit beliefs and preferences of the patient and his or her family.
- Present appropriate recommendations to patient and family.
  - If there is sufficient evidence of unacceptable risk and efficacy data are lacking, advise against the practice.
  - If risk is uncertain and efficacy data are lacking, advise accordingly (that is, that a medical recommendation cannot be made).
  - If efficacy data are sufficient, balance risk information in the usual risk-benefit analysis and advise accordingly.

---

acupuncture or other interventions that are generally performed by a licensed practitioner who has met credentialing requirements. Many "therapies" and dietary supplements (including herbal remedies) are unregulated. The degree of scientific evidence supporting some of these practices is extensive; for others, however, it is entirely absent. Factors influencing individuals' choices of CAM interventions are poorly understood. Specific cultural practices and the belief systems upon which they are based should therefore be fully appreciated by the professional health care team, especially in the pediatric setting. Health care professionals are further advised to approach patients and families in a respectful and organized way when discussing CAM interventions (exhibit 7.1). Tolerance of harmless CAM practices, encouragement of helpful practices, and knowledge of harmful practices or therapies is critical to effective patient-centered care.

Management of Pain and General Symptoms

Data on the prevalence of symptoms among dying children are gradually becoming available (Hunt 1990; Hain et al. 1995; Mallinson and Jones 2000; Wolfe et al. 2000; Hain and Hughes 2001). Patients present with symptom complexes related to diagnosis and stage of disease as well as to therapeutic interventions. Symptoms change over time and in response to primary and palliative treatments, necessitating frequent reevaluation for symptom control.

The diagnosis of pain in children can be difficult. Some children can clearly detect and describe their pain. For others, particularly those who are non-verbal or preverbal, a change in behavior is the only clue. Health care professionals must respect the knowledge of usual caregivers, particularly the family. A therapeutic trial of analgesia may be the only way to distinguish pain from other causes of distress. Assessing and measuring children's pain is also difficult. Many scales are available, but most are more suitable for research than for clinical applications. There is a need for tools that assess more global aspects of quality of life, particularly for children who are terminally ill.

Diagnosis of Pain. A number of misperceptions have traditionally been attributed to the child's experience of pain, illustrating the pitfalls of considering pain as a single, objective, physiological phenomenon. For much of the twentieth century, it was thought that children suffered pain less intensely than adults. The difference between a baby's and an adult's response to a painful stimulus was assumed to derive from a difference in perception of pain rather than response. One early study even concluded that "the neonate's experience of pain is equivalent to that of a deeply anesthetized adult" (McGraw 1941).

A second observation was that the nervous system of a neonate also differs from the adult. The relative lack of myelination in a neonate's nervous system similarly led to the fallacious but understandable inference that the demyelinated fibers transmit pain less intensely than fully mature, myelinated ones.

Recognition that pain is a subjective phenomenon (World Health Organization 1998) has led researchers to find ways to uncover the child's own experience of pain rather than rely on adult interpretation. It now appears that children in fact experience pain as intensely as adults. New hypotheses to explain this unanticipated phenomenon have included the idea that many of the fibers that are unmyelinated in the neonatal period are those that inhibit pain. Thus the pain experience of neonates may be even more intense than that of adults (Craig and Grunau 1993). Furthermore, early experiences of pain affect subsequent perception (Fitzgerald, Millard, and MacIntosh 1988; Porter, Grunau, and Anand 1999; Anand 2000a, 2000b).

Nevertheless, there is still a tendency on the part of adults, and particularly health care professionals, to underestimate a child's experience of pain. Despite the availability of safe and effective anesthesia, painful procedures such as circumcision and bone marrow biopsy are still performed on conscious children without even local anesthetics or postprocedure analgesics (Hain and Campbell 2001). Adults often judge that for children, pain is relatively trivial and that adequate analgesia is an unnecessary—perhaps even dangerous—treatment. Insurers seem to agree, creating further disincentives to providing procedural pain management for children, at least in the United States.

Pain in Pediatric Palliative Care. In adult palliative medicine, the study of pain control is, thus far, essentially the study of cancer pain. Children with cancer probably account for fewer than half the referrals to pediatric palliative care (Hain and Hughes 2001); the remainder have a wide range of nonmalignant conditions, often complex neurodegenerative disorders. Many of the principles of good pain control developed for adults can safely be extrapolated, but pain in children presents some unique challenges. Baker and Wong (1987) present one commonsense approach, summarized by the acronym QUEST:

- Question the child.
- Use rating tools.
- Evaluate behavior.
- Sensitize parents (and staff).
- Take action!

There are many different ways of classifying pain. Table 7.1 lists four such classifications, of which the most helpful at diagnosis is perhaps the causative. Once a management plan has been instituted, a more empirical classification based on responsiveness to opioids becomes helpful. Clearly, the classification systems are linked; for example, neuropathic pain is more likely than soft tissue pain to be only partially opioid responsive. A diagnostic classification based on responsiveness to therapy emphasizes that, irrespective of the underlying cause, opioids will usually provide the most effective relief (Cherny 2000).

Table 7.1. Classifications of pain

Classification	Category of pain	Description
Pathophysiological	Nociceptive Physiological (somatic and visceral) Pathological (somatic and visceral) Neuropathic Compression (somatic and visceral) Injury (peripheral, somatic, and visceral) Central Sympathetic-mediated	Useful classification for understanding pathophysiology; in this way, clinicians can suggest interventions most likely to be effective. Limitation is that although it appears comprehensive, it in fact encompasses only the physical aspects of pain and excludes behavioral components.
Causative	Soft tissue pain Bone pain (osteopenia and infiltration) Nerve pain Central pain Muscle spasm Colic "Total pain" (emotional, spiritual, and interpersonal)	Simple, empiric clinical classification. Useful as it clearly links cause for pain with interventions likely to be effective. Not all types of pain fit into this classification, and there is a risk of too closely associating cause with specific intervention.
Temporal	Acute Chronic Recurrent Continuous	Important to make the distinction, as cause, assessment, and management are all different. Particularly important in assessment of pain in children, whose acute response to pain may be short lived.
Responsiveness to opioids	Opioid responsive Partially opioid responsive Opioid resistant	Helpful pragmatic classification. Emphasizes that opioids are the first line of treatment for most pain in palliative care, irrespective of underlying cause.

Source: Adapted from Twycross (1997, 18–24).

Diagnosing Pain in Nonverbal or Preverbal Children. Recognizing that a child is in pain is not always easy for the health care professional. If, as has been said, the normal child is always either sleeping or playing, behavior can give a valuable clue that a child is in pain, even in the absence of verbalization. It is important always to consider pain in the differential diagnosis of altered behavior patterns, such as a child who becomes distressed when being moved. Behavioral changes that indicate pain may, however, be subtle. A child may be able to avoid pain but only at the expense of normal social interaction, giving the child an affect resembling depression (Gauvain-Piquard et al. 1999). It is not always possible to reliably exclude the presence of pain in a child; a therapeutic trial of analgesia may therefore be justified. It is important that appropriate doses of the right analgesia are used.

The longer the observation of behavior patterns in an individual child, the more reliable the assessment of pain. Thus the child's family and primary nurses or other consistent caregivers are more likely to accurately identify pain-related behaviors than physicians and others with more limited contact. The pediatrician should respect the assessment of those who know the child best.

In assessing whether a child is likely to experience pain as a result of an intervention, it is not sufficient simply to ask, "Under the same circumstances, would I be in pain?" Irrespective of whether a child is capable of verbalizing pain, if pain is likely, adequate analgesia and even anesthesia should be provided.

Assessment of Pain. Once pain is diagnosed, it should be measured to provide an indication of how effective treatment has been, and the child should be engaged to provide insights into his or her perception of it. Although the numerous pain scales for children have been recently reviewed (Hain 1997; Franck, Greenberg, and Stevens 2000), it is still relatively unusual for a pain assessment tool to be available in an acute pediatric unit, owing to weaknesses in the concept or practicality of many of the tools or possibly the continued low priority given to pain management in many busy acute care units.

Quality of Life. Pain scales play a number of important roles in assessing the effectiveness of a new approach to analgesia. For example, it is important to know that an analgesic relieves pain rather than anxiety. In evaluating the effectiveness of pediatric palliative care, however, it may be that simply measuring pain is of little value. The ultimate intention of palliative care is to improve a child's quality of life. Good pain management is an important part of this, but there is a need for reliable tools to measure more global aspects of the quality of life. Such tools have been developed for some subgroups of children (see, for example, Colver and Jessen 2000; Gee et al. 2000).

Treatment of Pain. The World Health Organization's pain ladder (World Health Organization 1984, 1998; Ventafridda et al. 1987) is familiar to many clinicians around the world, though perhaps not widely used in the United States (fig. 7.1). For mild pain, management starts with simple analgesics such as acetaminophen on an as-needed basis. For more severe pain, the ladder suggests that a fixed-dose combination opioid, such as codeine plus aceta-minophen, be tried. In practice, the main benefit of this step is probably simply to give the family time to adjust to the need for major opioids, the final step of the ladder, such as morphine, diamorphine (not available in the United States), oxycodone, hydromorphone, and fentanyl.

A number of general principles are associated with this simple approach:

- Medication should generally be given orally. A number of alternative routes are available, including intravenous, subcutaneous, trans-cutaneous, transmucosal, rectal, nasal, epidural, and intrathecal. Nevertheless, the enteral route (oral or through gastronomy tube) is preferred for most children most of the time.
- The use of appropriate adjuvants should be considered at all levels of pain. Adjuvants are medications that are not usually prescribed for pain relief but offer analgesia in certain situations, including some anticonvulsants and antidepressants for neuropathic type pain, nonsteroidal anti-inflammatory drugs for musculoskeletal pain, anticholinergics for colic, and muscle relaxants for pain caused by muscle spasm. Although each of these may be effective for a partic-ular sort of pain, opioids are usually more effective than any of them for moderate to severe pain, irrespective of the cause (Cherny 2000).
- Opioids should always be given regularly (around the clock) to treat moderate and severe pain, with additional doses prescribed to be used as necessary for breakthrough pain.

There are three phases in initiating analgesia for pediatric patients: select-ing a starting dose, titrating the dose, and maintenance. The starting dose of a major opioid can be selected in one of two ways. If the child is already

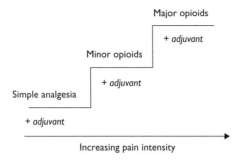

Figure 7.1. World Health Organization Pain Ladder.
Source: Adapted from World Health Organization (1998).
Note: Some authors avoid the terms *major* and *minor* opioids, preferring instead *opioids for moderate to severe pain* and *opioids for mild to moderate pain* to acknowledge that some opioids are intermediate. A large dose of a minor opioid is pharmacologically identical to a small dose of a major opioid; it can be argued that in children the middle step is redundant.

taking a minor opioid (such as codeine), conversion can be made to the equivalent dose of oral morphine (table 7.2). Alternatively, an empiric, starting dose of one milligram per kilogram of body weight a day can be selected (Hull 1999).

The total daily dose should be given as six doses at regular four-hour intervals. The intention of this regular dose is to keep the child from experiencing pain, and it should be given even when the child's pain is under good control. Inevitably, there will be some episodes of breakthrough pain; an additional dose of analgesia, equivalent to the regular four-hourly dose (that is, one-sixth of the total daily dose), should be prescribed and available on a one- to four-hour basis. The half-life of morphine is variable; frequency of breakthrough dosing must be tailored to the individual.

Most children will become drowsy in the first twenty-four to forty-eight hours of commencing or increasing morphine therapy. This usually resolves spontaneously, with no need to adjust the dose. Explaining this to both the child and the family in advance of its occurrence provides reassurance and decreases anxiety.

The purpose of titrating the dose is to establish the individual child's optimal opioid dose for effective relief. Good pain relief is indicated by the need for only one or two breakthrough doses a day. If more frequent breakthrough

Table 7.2. Relative potencies of some "major" and "minor" opioids, extrapolating from adult data

Opioid	Route	Potency relative to oral morphine (24 hours)
Codeine	Oral	0.10
Dihydrocodeine	Oral	0.10
Tramadol	Oral	0.20
Morphine	Oral	1.00
Morphine (sustained release)	Oral	1.00
Morphine	Subcutaneous infusion	2.00
Morphine	Continuous subcutaneous infusion	2.00
Diamorphine	Subcutaneous infusion	3.00
Diamorphine	Continuous subcutaneous infusion	3.00
Fentanyl	Patch	150.00
Fentanyl	Continuous subcutaneous infusion	150.00
Alfentanil	Continuous subcutaneous infusion	30.00
Hydromorphone	Oral	6.0–7.5
Hydromorphone (sustained release)	Oral	3.75–7.5

Source: Adapted from Back (2001, 207–9).

medications are needed, it is necessary to increase the regular dose by simply adding the additional doses to the total daily dose and prescribing it, again, as six equal doses given at four-hour intervals. The breakthrough dose should increase proportionally, remaining a sixth of the total daily dose.

Once the child's opioid requirements have been established, the doses can be given in a more convenient form. For many children, slow release formulations of morphine will be appropriate. As the child's condition progresses, other approaches, such as intravenous or subcutaneous infusions or transcutaneous formulations, may be indicated. Whatever form regular dosing takes, it should always be accompanied by access to appropriate doses of breakthrough medications, generally using the same medication for around-the-clock and breakthrough pain. However, it is not unusual for a child to have regular opioid therapy using a fentanyl transdermal patch, with oral morphine syrup for breakthrough pain, because no oral formulation of fentanyl is available.

Adverse Effects of Opioids. Constipation is almost universal among children taking major opioids. The problem is frequently exacerbated by relative dehydration and inactivity. Any prescription of major opioids in children should therefore be accompanied by prophylactic stimulant and softening laxatives. Bulking agents are inappropriate in this setting.

Opioid-related side effects have different frequencies in the adult and pediatric populations; nausea and vomiting occurring less frequently, and urinary retention and pruritus more often, in children than adults. Pruritis generally responds to antihistamines. There is some evidence that ondansetron and oral naloxone can help (Nelson et al. 1988; Sanger and Twycross 1996; Pal, Cortiella, and Herndon 1997). If dose escalation results in intolerable adverse effects, an alternative opioid should be considered.

Special Considerations When Using Opioids in Children. Relatively little research has been published on the use of opioids in pediatric palliative care. It appears that children may clear morphine more quickly than adults and that the half-life is therefore somewhat shorter in children (Hain et al. 1995; Hunt et al. 1999). However, there is wide interpatient variability of morphine half-life. Scaling the adult dose of morphine down per unit weight for children does result in a similar serum concentration. Clinical experience indicates that the principles for use of opioids developed in adult palliative medicine can be extrapolated safely to children, though this premise has not been subjected to rigorous study. If anything, children appear to be rather resistant to both the toxic and the beneficial effects of opioids, compared with their adult counterparts. Respiratory depression, a much-feared complication, has been reported rarely in children (Gill et al. 1996) but not in a palliative setting.

There is some research on the pediatric use of morphine and diamorphine, fentanyl, hydromorphone, and meperidine (pethidine). Of these, the incidence of seizures probably makes meperidine too toxic for use in pediatric pain relief now that experience with alternatives has grown. Oxycodone and tramadol have yet to prove any role for themselves in pediatric palliative care. Methadone is particularly useful for neuropathic pain (Carpenter, Chapman, and Dickenson 2000; Sang 2000; Stringer et al. 2000; McDonnell, Sloan, and Hamann 2001), but experience in children is limited to case series (Shir et al. 1998). Diamorphine (heroin) is a highly effective opioid that is highly soluble and therefore ideal for continuous infusion, but unfortunately it is not available in North America. Hydromorphone, which is five to ten times as potent as morphine but otherwise similar, is particularly useful in the setting of fluid restrictions and need for high-dose opioids.

ANXIETY AND FEAR

Though we have all been children, for most adults the memory is so far removed from our daily lives that it is difficult to draw on the experience. Furthermore, pediatricians are rarely experienced in recognizing and managing psychological symptoms. Comprehensive care for a child with a life-threatening condition thus requires the advice and support of psychiatrists, psychologists, counselors, and other professionals outside of medicine.

A child's anxiety, like that of an adult, is based on prior experience and understanding. The child who undergoes a bone marrow aspirate while conscious will forever afterward find even coming into the pediatric oncology department stressful and frightening. Those working with children acknowledge the close and complex relationship between the attitude of the child and that of his or her parents. It is not enough simply to explore the fears of the child; a complicated web of perception and understanding must be uncovered to reassure the whole family and help reestablish a normal family dynamic.

The mainstay of pharmacological therapy for anxiolysis in children is the benzodiazepine class; however, some young children and some with brain injuries respond paradoxically to this class of medication. Benzodiazepines range from ultra-short-acting ones, such as midazolam, through those with intermediate half-life, such as lorazepam, to longer-acting ones, such as diazepam. Midazolam is a particularly useful drug, especially for procedure-related anxiety. It can be administered subcutaneously, by injection or infusion, intranasally, and even orally (Bentley et al. 2002). In intervening to prevent a panic spiral, with children and parents mutually exacerbating each other's anxiety, it is clearly important to select a route with rapid onset of action.

Although benzodiazepines cause sedation as well as anxiolysis, it is important to remember that not all sedatives relieve anxiety. Chloral hydrate, for example, does little to alleviate anxiety. Nozinan (levomepromazine) is an effective sedative (Chater et al. 1998) but has an unproven role in the relief of anxiety. The distinction between sedation and anxiolysis should also be borne in mind when advocating the use of other medications prescribed wholly or in part for their sedative effect, such as phenobarbital.

DEPRESSION

Depression in children is probably underrecognized. Particularly in adolescents, the syndrome closely resembles that of adults and may respond to commonly prescribed medications, such as the serotonin reuptake inhibitors. Tricyclic antidepressants, such as amitriptyline and nortriptyline, may have a role. An advantage of these medications is that they may also alleviate other symptoms. For example, they are powerful adjuvants in neuropathic pain, and their anticholinergic effects may provide useful antiemesis as well as act as soporifics.

AGITATION

Agitation is a difficult symptom to manage in children, as in adults. It is typically multifactorial, caused by environmental factors as much as those specific to the individual child. Multiple medications are a common cause, although children are probably more resilient than adults to the plethora of pharmaceuticals that are typically coprescribed in the terminal phase. This underlines the need to review medications frequently, reducing the number wherever possible. It is also important to exclude organic causes, such as infection (particularly sepsis of the respiratory or urinary tract) and undiagnosed pain, that can cause or mimic agitation in children unable to articulate their experience. This is a particular challenge in children with learning difficulties.

Where an organic cause cannot be found, neuroleptics such as haloperidol may have a role. Haloperidol is relatively nonsedating and is also a powerful antiemetic that can be combined with other medications in a single syringe (Vermeire and Remon 1999). Benzodiazepines once again have a role. Levomepromazine, which is both neuroleptic and sedative, is often a particularly helpful medication in the terminal stages.

Phenobarbital (phenobarbitone) has been reported by clinicians to be a useful drug in the management of agitation caused by cerebral irritation, which frequently complicates acute anoxic or septic insult to a child's brain and may be a feature of some neurodegenerative conditions. Phenobarbital can be given by mouth or by infusion. Phenobarbital is familiar to pediatricians and is an anticonvulsant, important because seizures commonly complicate cerebral irritation.

DISORDERED SLEEP

Disordered sleep patterns are common in pediatric palliative care, particularly in brain-injured patients. Sleep disorder, like most other symptoms, is multifactorial. There is accordingly no single agreed-upon approach, but the following recommendations may be effective:

- *Rationalize medications:* Children with disordered sleep are typically on many different medications throughout the day. Many of these are potentially sedative. As a first step, medications should be reordered so that all sedative ones are given at night.
- *Emphasize the distinction between day and night, including the distinction between time for sleeping and time for being awake:* During the day, the child is encouraged to be active within the constraints of his or her condition. The curtains are open and, weather permitting, so are the windows. At night, activity and interruptions are kept to a minimum, and the room is kept dark and quiet.
- *Introduce new medications:* A number of medications can be useful in trying to regulate the sleep-wake cycle. Melatonin is a rational choice at night because it mimics the normal circadian rhythm (Jan 2000). Benzodiazepines can be useful if the child is not already receiving them. The half-life of diazepam is about eight hours, allowing the child to sleep through the night. Midazolam infusion overnight is more controllable because the drug is rapidly cleared once the infusion is discontinued in the morning. Chloral hydrate is an effective sedative but relatively irritating to the stomach. Furthermore, it is difficult to take in the volumes required for older children, and long-term use is dangerous.

FEEDING

The need to nurture and feed a child is a fundamental part of a parent's identity. At the first sign of flagging appetite, parents will often ask for medication to restore the child to normal food intake. However, few interventions can actually achieve this. Reluctance to eat can, of course, be related to other gastrointestinal symptoms, some of which are reversible. Where the cause is early satiety caused by gastric compression, metoclopramide, with or without steroids, may be effective. Other important organic conditions to consider and treat are oral thrush, the side effects of chemotherapy—vincristine can cause metallic or other altered taste—xerostomia from radiotherapy, and untreated nausea. Steroids can produce a transient stimulation of appetite, and there may be an occasional role for a short course, but prolonged use leads to disproportionate adverse effects. There is usually little to be gained from considering other pharmacological approaches.

In fact, poor appetite is usually more of a concern to the family and professionals than it is to the child. To be forced against one's will to eat can be as unpleasant as being denied food when hungry. With this in mind, the first goal is to explore issues of feeding and appetite with the family and the child, in particular, to establish what giving or withholding nourishment means to them. This process can uncover profound differences between the family's values and understandings and those of the professional team about the child's condition and prognosis.

Even without pharmacological intervention, food can be made more attractive and palatable. A child may be more comfortable eating many small meals a day rather than a few large ones. Favorite meals, attractively presented on small plates or saucers, can often tempt the child to eat. It is important to remember that mealtimes are a favorite battleground for children, even in the absence of life-limiting conditions; it is best to avoid allowing food to become an issue, if at all possible.

Technical advances mean that it is now possible to be artificially fed through nasogastric or, increasingly, gastrostomy tubes. It is rarely in the dying child's best interests for life to be artificially and unnecessarily prolonged in this way (Royal College of Paediatrics and Child Health 1997; British Medical Association 1999). Anorexia is part of the natural progression of disease, and artificial nutrition may add to the patient's symptom burden—for example, by worsening respiratory secretions.

GASTROINTESTINAL SYMPTOMS

Pain and dysfunction of the gastrointestinal tract are common in pediatric palliative care, related either to the disease process or to side effects of treatment. Assessment includes eliciting symptom intensity and symptom distress for each gastrointestinal symptom. Strategies for symptom relief depend on the presence or absence of mechanical obstruction and potential for reversibility, if present. Inflammatory processes associated with infection may be reversed. Noninfectious, treatment-related inflammation of the gastrointestinal tract usually responds to medical therapies. Treatment of central nervous system etiologies of nausea and vomiting involve correction of the underlying process (for example, raised intracranial pressure). If obstruction is present and reversible, all attempts to promote proper motility should be undertaken. If obstruction is present and irreversible, symptoms of pain, dysphagia, nausea, vomiting, abdominal distention, and constipation must be treated. Opioids and other analgesics given to treat pain are likely to cause persistent bowel slowing; therefore, constipation should be anticipated and prevented.

Nausea and Vomiting. Antiemetic agents should be selected on the basis of their mechanism of action and an understanding of the etiology of nausea and vomiting. Centrally acting drugs can cause sedation, confusion, and extrapyramidal side effects. Newer agents that produce selective 5HT3 blockade may be more effective for chemotherapy-related nausea and vomiting. Prokinetic agents are selected when there is motility disturbance and when constipation is a concurrent problem.

Constipation. Constipation may be relieved with dietary measures and increased fluid intake. If medications are needed, a combination of gentle stimulant laxative and stool softener is generally effective. Osmotic agents and stronger laxatives may be required. In some cases, enemas may be required to evacuate the colon and rectum before initiating an effective laxative program. Careful dosing of an oral opioid antagonist (for example, naloxone) can help relieve otherwise refractory opioid-induced constipation (Meissner et al. 2000). It must be dosed cautiously to avoid reversing the desired analgesic effects of opioids.

Irreversible Intestinal Obstruction. When intestinal obstruction is irreversible and severe nausea and vomiting accompany dysmotility of the gastrointestinal tract, pharmacologic bowel paralysis is warranted. Octreotide, a long-acting analogue of somatostatin that reduces secretions, has been used to treat high-output vomiting associated with bowel obstruction in adults.

Diarrhea. Uncontrolled diarrhea may threaten the integrity of a patient's skin, leading to painful breakdown and increased risk of sepsis. Opioid derivatives can be effective in reducing diarrhea. Octreotide is helpful for high-output diarrhea (Mercadante 1994).

Oral Hygiene. Simple measures such as use of ice chips, wet sponges, or glycerin swabs can maintain a comfortably moist oral mucosa in the final stages of life, when general dehydration naturally occurs. Pineapple chunks or ascorbic acid dissolved on the tongue can help keep the mouth feeling fresh. However, care must be taken in children whose swallowing is impaired and those with oral or esophageal ulcerations.

Mucosal bleeding from the mouth and nose are particularly common in the setting of advanced hematopoietic malignancy. Bleeding from the nose may originate from a single source, in which case it can be arrested by application of a pressure dressing or by cautery. Fibrinolytic agents, such as tranexamic acid, can be effective applied topically (Avvisati et al. 1989) or systemically (Dean and Tuffin 1997). Oral agents to promote platelet aggregation may also be effective.

RESPIRATORY SYMPTOMS

Symptoms of respiratory distress (dyspnea, cough, and difficulty with secretions) are common. Clinical evaluation is directed to identify mechanical interference with breathing and structural lesions causing cough or airway irritation. Whenever possible, physical interventions to relieve mechanical interference should be considered. Simple measures such as repositioning the patient, improving airflow in the room (for example, by opening a window), and providing a less physically crowded environment may relieve air hunger. Oxygen supplementation may relieve dyspnea in the setting of hypoxia, but most patients find facemasks uncomfortable, as they contribute to the feeling of suffocation. Nebulized air, bronchodilators, and chest physiotherapy may be helpful. Where accumulation of cellular debris is the cause (for example, in cystic fibrosis), inhaled mucolytics such as n-acetyl cysteine can help loosen thick secretions and make them easier to clear.

Systemic benzodiazepines and opioids are very effective for dyspnea and cough. Hiccup may be caused by gastric distention and is a common reversible side effect of corticosteroids. Phenothiazines may be useful for hiccup. At end of life, noisy breathing with wet secretions (the death rattle) may be distressing to family members. Discontinuation of exogenous fluids (intravenous, subcutaneously, by gastrostomy tube, and so on) as well as agents to dry secretions, such as anticholinergics (glycopyrronium and hyoscine), may be effective in this setting. Some anticholinergics are available in a transdermal patch, making them ideal for use in children.

URINARY SYMPTOMS

Reduction of urine volume may be associated with the natural progression of disease. Renal failure may be part of the terminal progression and usually results in a relatively painless death. For urinary symptom control, clinical evaluation is indicated, to identify mechanical interference with micturition and neurogenic urinary dysfunction. Urinary retention is a common side effect of opioid and anticholinergic medications. It also may result from extreme constipation. Urinary incontinence may be secondary to retention (overflow). Painful bladder spasms may be related to mechanical irritation or neurogenic dysfunction. If strategies directed at improving urinary flow are unsuccessful, intermittent or indwelling catheterization should be considered. Pain resulting from renal or ureteral obstruction is effectively managed with diversion techniques. Pain should otherwise be treated symptomatically with analgesics and antispasmodics.

SKIN PROBLEMS

Pruritus. Medications known to cause itching should be discontinued, if possible, and rashes treated with emollients, humidified air, or topical and systemic medications, as needed. Less conventionally, ondansetron and oral naloxone have been tried for opioid-induced pruritus. However, when opioids are the cause, it is more appropriate to first consider conversion to an alternative agent. Fentanyl may cause less pruritus than other available agents.

Pressure Sores. Pressure sores (decubitus ulcers) are generally preventable. The bedridden patient should be assessed for risk of pressure sores and predisposing factors reversed whenever possible. Excellent bed care includes skin hygiene, frequent position changes, and avoidance of hard surfaces and shearing forces on body parts. Once a bedsore is established, care is directed to promote healing of tissues and may include local dressings, debridement, and antibiotic therapy.

Malodorous Tumors. Even with excellent nursing care, tumors may erupt through the skin, becoming necrotic, malodorous, and distressing to the patient and family. Good room ventilation and frequent change of room deodorizers may help. Specific charcoal or algae-containing dressings, as well as topical and systemic antibiotics, will minimize odor and anaerobic infection.

OTHER SUPPORTIVE CARE CONSIDERATIONS

Family caregivers may be instructed to regularly inspect indwelling catheters for proper positioning, functioning, and signs of infection. They may also assist with catheter care and administration of medications and nutritional supplements, which may increase their personal satisfaction with caring for their child.

The patient with impaired mobility should be assisted to be out of bed as much as is desired. Again, family members may be instructed by occupational or physical therapists in such techniques and may participate as they feel comfortable. Change of rooms and even brief trips out of doors can be beneficial, providing relief from boredom and feelings of entrapment for both patient and family.

EMERGENCIES

Raised Intracranial Pressure. Raised intracranial pressure is characterized by headaches, nausea, and vomiting that are typically made worse by lying down and are at their most severe first thing in the morning. Acutely raised intracranial pressure is relatively rare, except in association with some brain tumors. A short-term solution is to give high dose steroids parenterally, conventionally dexamethasone. Radiotherapy or surgical placement of a ventricular shunt may be needed, bearing in mind the discomfort that raised intracranial pressure can cause.

Spinal Cord Compression. Compression of the spinal cord is relatively rare in children compared with adults. It can complicate the management of cancer, in particular, neuroblastoma. Even in the palliative phase, spinal cord compression is treated as an emergency. Initial treatment is high-dose parenteral dexamethasone, followed by radiotherapy as the definitive treatment. Surgery may be needed if, on balance, the potential benefit to the child outweighs the burden of a possibly prolonged and painful hospital admission.

Obstruction of the Superior Vena Cava. Obstruction of the superior vena cava presents with a feeling of fullness in the head and headaches that are worse when lying down or when the pressure is increased by Valsalva maneuvers (for example, sneezing or coughing). Symptoms include facial fullness and plethora, as well as dilated superficial veins over the upper thorax. The jugular vein is typically distended and nonpulsatile. Symptoms of obstruction of the superior vena cava include discomfort, dyspnea, and panic. Superior vena cava syndrome is a common complication of mediastinal lymphoma but can also be caused by thrombosis (for example, following long-term total parenteral nutrition through a central line). Management of the underlying cause relieves the obstruction. For tumors, treatment consists of high-dose steroids followed by radiotherapy; for clot, thrombolysis followed by anti-coagulation may be indicated.

Intractable Seizures. Children with brain injuries, malformations, and neurodegenerative diseases often suffer from seizures, which increase in frequency and severity as they reach the terminal phase. Often, these children are taking numerous anticonvulsants, but paradoxically, this profusion of medications may become epileptogenic, worsening rather than abating the seizure disorder; the solution is often to simplify the regimen to one or two anticonvulsants. Seizure control can be secured rapidly and effectively with the use of syringe drivers of phenobarbital or midazolam (or both). Breakthrough seizures can be managed with rectal diazepam (or, outside of the United States, paraldehyde). If the child is at home, these formulations allow the parents to administer the drugs rapidly as soon as the seizure begins. Other benzodiazepines such as clobazam (limited availability) may be effective and should be offered on the advice of the local pediatric neurologist.

It is likely that seizures are more distressing for the family than for the child who experiences them. As death draws nearer, it may not be appropriate to treat minor seizures or those of short duration. It is important to be sure that the burden of the interventions offered to the child—which will be both inconvenient and sedating—are offset by a positive impact on his or her quality of life. It is often reassuring to parents and caregivers to be informed that seizures lasting only five or ten minutes will do little harm to the child. It is always important, however, to acknowledge that seizures, however harmless, may be very frightening to watch.

Hemorrhage. Although sudden catastrophic hemorrhage is greatly feared by many parents, in practice it is rather rare; patients at highest risk are children dying from lymphoproliferative disorders that create dysfunction in or reduction in the number of platelets. Some leukemias are associated with coagulopathies. These risk factors can be exacerbated by the indiscriminate use of nonsteroidal anti-inflammatory drugs, which can interfere with platelet aggregation. Once again, it is often more helpful to talk through the issue than simply to offer pharmacological solutions.

The fear of acute hemorrhage may be based on a series of much smaller bleeds, typically from the oral mucosa or from the nose. It is often possible to identify a localized bleeding point, which can be cauterized. Tranexamic acid and ethamsylate, administered topically or systemically, may both have a role here. Tranexamic acid is an antifibrinolytic agent that inhibits the breakdown of clots. Ethamsylate works by increasing platelet aggregation, and its effect will therefore depend on the presence of normal numbers of circulating platelets.

Where severe hemorrhage is considered a likely terminal event, it may be helpful to ensure that there are green, black, or red towels available at the patient's bedside. A small volume of blood can look frighteningly large when it has come from your own child, and these towels serve to reduce the visual impact of a hemorrhage. If hemorrhage occurs in a conscious child, sedation may be helpful; midazolam, which is both quick acting and of short duration, is most commonly recommended.

Adjunctive Therapies

CHILD-LIFE THERAPY

Play has been said to be a child's work and a way for the child to make sense of the world. "The event of hospitalization seriously threatens the quality of play and the extent to which the child may engage in it. Because play is so important to the growth of the child, to impede play is to discourage normal development" (Thompson and Standford 1981). Having opportunities to play can help a child work through a stressful situation by gaining mastery and expressing fears and anxieties.

Child-life specialists receive classroom and supervised clinical training in the use of guided play to facilitate a child's understanding of and comfort with medical procedures. All child-life specialists are trained in anatomy and medical terminology and have both practicum and internship experience in children's hospitals.

Parents often ask for assistance in discussing diagnosis, treatment, and prognosis with their ill child. It is important that parents be offered the opportunity to meet with a child-life specialist so that their concerns can be addressed, as child-life specialists are trained to communicate medical information to children in developmentally appropriate terms and can either do so directly or coach parents in how to do it themselves. Child-life specialists can also help the parents understand the ramifications in the family system of withholding information from children, and they can play a significant role as advocate for hospitalized children and their families by communicating any concerns or miscommunications to the other members of the care team.

During an early hospitalization, Emily, a 3-year-old child with cancer, confided to the child-life specialist that she was scared to have any lab work done while she was in her bed. The child-life specialist communicated this to other team members, and blood samples were thereafter taken in the treatment room.

Child-life specialists use distraction techniques with children, such as blowing bubbles or reading a "push the button book," to reduce procedure-related anxiety, giving even very young children an important sense of control and encouraging focus during uncomfortable times. An important function of child-life therapists is to provide the needed creative opportunities for ill and medically compromised children to express feelings and concerns (Rubin 1992).

Procedure-Related Discomfort. The child-life specialist is never in a position to implement a procedure that inflicts pain, and he or she is thus a safe haven. As an example, a child-life specialist would never participate in restraining a child for a procedure; however, it would be appropriate for her to explain the importance of being still during the procedure and to practice coping mechanisms with the child, such as deep breathing or guided imagery exercises. Child-life specialists can ensure that the team provides parents with appropriate choices for participation in their child's procedures; parents usually prefer to remain in the supportive role of hand-holding, storytelling, and comforting immediately after the procedure.

Family-Centered Care.

Emily lived with her mother, father, and 10-year-old brother, Andrew. Communication difficulties were frequent, and each family member used different styles of coping with Emily's illness and prognosis.

"Normal" limits and boundaries were not enforced for Emily; however, Andrew was treated normally in terms of expectations in school and participation in home-based activities. This lack of consistency in parenting was difficult for Andrew to understand and created resentment toward his parents.

Child-life specialists assist families in developing and maintaining their own healthy sense of balance in the face of crisis and abnormality. Normalcy and consistency are comforting to children, especially during times of stress and uncertainty. During the active treatment phase the family focus is primarily on the ill child, and a sense of normalcy can be difficult to maintain. A child-life specialist can serve a pivotal role in encouraging families to practice self-care and regain a sense of balance in the family unit. Healthy siblings need opportunities to partake in everyday occurrences such as birthday parties, soccer games, and faith-based events. Attending to the needs of the parents, including their own well-being, is an important part of providing good care to the ill child (Leff-Tanner, Chan, and Walizer 1991).

Adjustment to Illness. For children with chronic conditions, treatment may be protracted. Children who must maintain a particular medical regime often find it hard to do so for long periods of time. Parents may grow weary from the battle of "forcing" a child to comply with medical treatment. Child-life specialists can assist during this difficult family time by using behavior modification techniques and positive reinforcement systems. The child-life specialist can also help by empowering the ill child with appropriate involvement in his or her own self-care.

CREATIVE ARTS THERAPY

The creative arts offer unique and novel ways to assist dying children during a time of ultimate separation and departure. Whether the modality is art therapy, dance and movement therapy, or music therapy, creative arts therapists help children make the transition from the familiar into a world that is unknown. Dying is a process that, even in the company of others, concludes with aloneness. It is a time when sensory and bodily experiences diminish and children turn inward toward a deep sense of ultimate quiet and stillness.

Establishing a Spiritual Foundation for the Work of Creative Arts Therapy. Creative arts therapists adopt a palliative model integrating curing and compassionate healing throughout the course of care; these concepts and practices change emphasis over time. Careful observation and attention to maintaining continuity during transitions can facilitate important awareness and potential acceptance during the dying process. Mindfulness about subtle shifts within therapeutic sessions provides an arena for children to creatively express and solidify otherwise less identifiable feelings and concerns; the creative process itself brings to life ideas that may not be readily verbalized.

The creative process permits opportunities to address one's wholeness with a deep and sacred understanding of meaningful elements. Creative rituals expressed through art, dance, and music supersede verbal communication and interaction, approaching themes with heightened attention and intention. Fear, sadness, and confusion, for example, may be manifest in a simple gesture, song, or magazine image; children thereby find new groundwork for relating inner content. Activities pertaining to dynamics, color, tone, and form give rise to fresh ways of experiencing and sharing important issues. Within creative arts therapy sessions, rituals provide a means by which to integrate body, mind, and spirit while moving beyond the limitations of verbal communication. Concerns related to illness, treatment, and death are expressed through symbols and metaphor. Imaginative storytelling, dance, and fantasy depict significant ideas and feelings that may otherwise remain hidden and unavailable to child, family, and medical caregiver. When medical caregivers and family members become involved in the creative process and interaction, the creative arts therapy experience reduces isolation within the hospital environment as well as at home. Usual ways of relating to one another are expanded. Typical roles and boundaries relax, and interactions may express a sense of playfulness and spontaneity that is therapeutic for all. Creative rituals facilitate the expression of important developmental tasks and promote essential feelings of trust.

Creative Arts Therapy in the Dying Process. In working with dying children, the creative arts therapist attends to nuances of eye contact, body posture, images, energy level, interactive style, and verbal references, each of which may provide entry points for exploring relevant therapeutic issues. As with all caregivers, the creative arts therapist must be attuned to the family's religious and cultural beliefs so that he or she may join those ideas rather than impose their own practices and beliefs. Through creative arts therapy, there is an acknowledgment of the completeness of the child's life, however brief. The child is empowered and reassured about potentially experiencing a wide range of emotional responses. Children, especially those who are severely ill, need to explore their unspoken inner experiences, and the creative arts therapist can provide a mechanism for this important exploration.

The Specific Modalities of Creative Arts Therapy. Dance and movement therapy focuses on body movement as a manifestation of thoughts and feelings.

Dance and movement are each viewed in their broadest context to encompass elements of traditional dance forms, patterns of movements, gestures, postures, and more subtle aspects of nonverbal communication. A fundamental premise is that psychological characteristics and processes, such as affect and cognition, are expressed consistently through nonverbal means. The uniqueness of dance and movement therapy is that psychological and body-oriented constructs are intimately interrelated: one necessarily implies the other, and it is merely the perspective or "point of entry" that differentiates them. Therapeutic modification of any of these elements, therefore, leads to changes in the others (Cohen and Walco 1999).

Dance and movement therapy offers opportunities to experience the body in more positive and pleasurable ways, even when physiological systems are shutting down. Mirroring breathing patterns, facilitating small gestures, using touch, and developing a sense of wholeness are all part of the dance and movement therapy experience. The dance and movement therapist observes and understands how a child's personality traits, interactive style, and mode of communication are conveyed nonverbally and can then promote understanding and awareness on those levels. As the dance and movement therapist develops a sense of empathy by kinesthetically mirroring the body movement qualities of the child and his or her family, a powerful sense of acceptance ensues. The therapist witnesses the child's movement behaviors in his or her own body, reflects them sensitively, and provides the groundwork for developing new insights. The body "speaks" to dance and movement therapists, and it is the therapist's task to decipher what the body is trying to communicate in order to help children deal with the emotional toll of illness, treatment, and dying processes. Through body movement, contact with others, communication, and expression are all encouraged (Mendelsohn 1999). Children can gain an increased sense of confidence in their bodies and learn ways to relax. Movement can provide a playful way to release tension. Emotional issues can be addressed symbolically.

Art therapy can also be used as an assessment tool to provide further information about the child's response to illness, treatment, and dying. Through art therapy, children can express their feelings by creating a visual image of their fears, anger, frustrations, and fantasies; the art therapist can then communicate these feelings to the child's family and medical team. Art therapy provides tactile stimulation, distraction from pain, an opportunity for choice, and a means to achieve mastery. Art is a familiar language for all children.

What they cannot say in words can often be expressed through images. Figure 7.2 presents a drawing by Sharon, a 15-year-old suffering from acute myeloid leukemia.

Sensitively improvised music therapy can help a frightened child feel less threatened and can initiate the establishment of trust and rapport. Music therapy can reduce a child's isolation by including family members or medical staff in sessions, increasing opportunities for positive interactions. Improvisational music therapy is used to engage, empower, and focus children undergoing painful medical procedures and can be a useful tool for processing their experiences afterward. Active songwriting and improvisation can be used to encourage children to relate their experiences and explore their feelings within a creative structure. Various tones, musical dynamics, and rhythm are utilized to decrease pain, stress, and anxiety by promoting distraction, release, soothing, or comfort.

The progression of disease processes may engender a sense of lack of control. Within the experience of creative arts therapy, children can regain a sense of involvement with their own care.

Applying Creative Arts Therapy within a Developmental Perspective of Dying. The application of creative arts therapy varies according to the age and developmental level of the child. Each stage affects subsequent stages in a multifaceted manner, however, and thus rigid conceptualization by age and developmental milestone is not helpful. General guidelines are, however, appropriate.

- *Birth to three years old:* Concerns such as separation anxiety and primary caregiver attachment in very young children are chiefly expressed through crying (Faulkner 2001). The need for close and continuous physical contact is paramount. Empathic contact and stimulation can provide the basis for a secure sense of boundaries for young children when their routines are continually changing and they are exposed to aversive sensations. The dance and movement therapist may use voice, breath, touch, and movement to help a young child experience various regions of the body by developing a sense of bodily organization and awareness. Use of touch and light stroking can develop a feeling of being contained within a rather undefined environment. It is important that stimulation across various channels (voice, breath, touch, and movement) be integrated

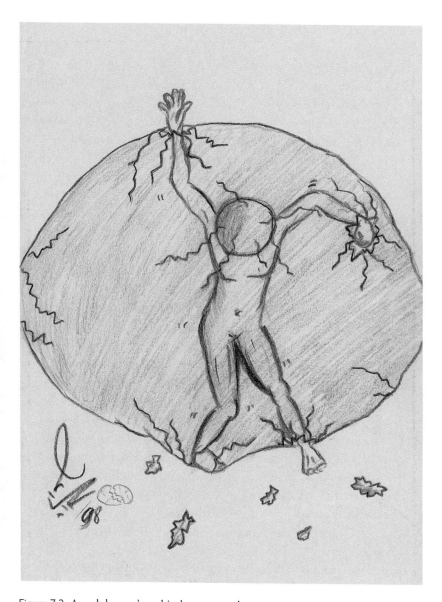

Figure 7.2. An adolescent's ambivalence toward autonomy.
Source: Drawn by Sharon, 15 years old. Provided by Dr. Miryam ben Arush and art therapist Analia Magen, Haifa, Israel.

and synchronous, facilitating greater assimilation for the young child.

Music therapy can also provide a "holding atmosphere," offering familiar songs and lullabies to the child. Family members and medical staff can join together in music, working toward a common goal of comforting and soothing a child approaching the end of his or her life. This can have a powerfully positive impact on family members. Sometimes health care staff or hospice workers choose to be involved with these activities. Siblings may participate as well, allowing them to be a part of this important transition, joining in the musical activities and gently touching their dying sibling's body. A deep sense of ritual and intimacy arises from this act for all participants.

- *Three to six years old:* General therapeutic goals include helping the young child modulate emotions and adapt to the demands of a given moment (Cohen and Walco 1999). Dying children in this age group may have anxiety about going to sleep, separation, and immobility. To allay some of these fears, the creative arts therapist begins where "the child is" and provides contact, reassurance, and gentle instruction in addressing the child's fears. Body movement activities provide the basis for exploring a range of feelings. The dance and movement therapist may first invite the child to explore extremes in movement (for example, strong and light, big and small, quick and slow) and then facilitate a sense of modulation and control by exploring the gradients between the extremes. Physical contact and reassurance, along with verbal comments that offer support and acceptance, may provide a sense of integration on a body level. Through art therapy, children can create symbols through their drawings, depicting relevant themes and images pertaining to their experience. Their stories can be discussed and developed through the art-making process. This can enhance the child's understanding of the dying process in a less threatening manner. Creating meaningful family images and objects builds common themes and helps the whole family begin to attain a sense of closure.

    The music therapist sings familiar childhood songs while inserting different "feeling" words that may describe the child's situation, creating in the child a sense of validation and support. Furthermore, improvisational music-making gives children the chance to play instruments, expressing various emotional and behavioral qualities through rhythm and melody. A musical progression may begin quite chaotically but develop into something more organized and melodic with the assistance and guidance of the music therapist. When this happens, the child may perceive mastery and regain a sense of control.

- *Six to twelve years old:* Vulnerability regarding peer rejection owing to changes in physical appearance from illness and treatment may cause isolation and withdrawal in children six to twelve years old. In contrast, the ability to be problem solvers and to utilize logical thought can provide essential coping skills for children in this age group. As children begin to assimilate relational issues of isolation and separation, themes of body integrity and loss become increasingly important. Children in this phase need to have their bodies treated with careful respect, to be offered specific factual information, and to have as much control over their situation as possible.

Exploring feelings related to the dying process, both nonverbally and verbally, opens new ways of understanding challenging concerns. The creative arts therapist can offer a range of choices (for example, choosing instruments, movement props, art materials) to facilitate a sense of control and discovery in the child. Acknowledging the child's pace and style of expression is crucial as the therapist begins to integrate the child's thought, behavior, and emotion. Through the arts, children begin to interrelate various components of death and can integrate difficult emotional elements such as fear, anxiety, and alienation. Rituals bring in sacred elements as children attempt to attain a sense of peace when saying good-bye to loved ones.

- *Twelve years and older:* Socially and emotionally, healthy adolescents are moving toward more independence and autonomy, though still dependent upon parents and family members for reassurance at times. A chronically or terminally ill child is challenged in achieving these normal transitions and milestones. Personal beliefs are investigated and may be influenced by symbolism in art forms and religion.

Adolescents facing the end of life are capable of speculating about the comprehensive implications and ramifications of death. They have an adultlike understanding about the end of their own lives, as well as the impact it has on other people and on society as a whole.

Facing death may invoke anger, fear, and sorrow. Balancing a range of needs becomes a delicate proposition. Hospital staff and family members negotiate the teenager's need for privacy, closeness, and independence in just the right doses. Because their peer group is so significant, adolescents need opportunities to interact with friends in an effort to obtain closure and may also have a strong drive to document their lives in a global context.

Facing the reality of premature death can be expressed in nonverbal forms that potentially facilitate greater acceptance. Observation of the teen's body movement dynamics (gestures, postures, interactive style) can help others understand some of the issues that are otherwise difficult to communicate.

Creative arts therapy provides adolescents with an important avenue by which to identify emotional material that may be difficult to access by verbal language alone. Art images and symbols, key themes in recorded music, musical improvisation, and songwriting provide teenagers with alternative, less threatening mechanisms with which to explore the dying process. The creation of videotapes, art objects, murals, and dances enable adolescents to say good-bye and leave a legacy.

The Value of Creative Arts Therapy for Children with Terminal Illness. Across the developmental continuum, play, imagination, and creativity provide natural outlets for expression. The unique interests, concerns, and fascinations of each child can be conveyed through the heroes, stories, and themes that become manifest in the creative process. When children want others to understand their inner experience, nonverbal communication vehicles may be essential tools.

Confronting terminal illness and the end of life requires the identification of feelings and the development of mechanisms that allow these feelings to be safely shared with others. Creative arts therapy brings a richness and potency to that expression. Resolving conflicts, decreasing isolation, and maximizing comfort are essential in attempting to gain ultimate peace and acceptance. For caregivers, there are unique opportunities to participate in an intimate experience as children and their families face final separation. In the words of Saint-Exupéry's (2000) Little Prince, "One runs the risk of weeping a little, if one lets himself be tamed."

References

Anand, K. J. 2000a. Effects of perinatal pain and stress. *Prog Brain Res* 122:117–29.

―――. 2000b. Pain, plasticity, and premature birth: a prescription for permanent suffering? *Nat Med* 6:971–73.

Avvisati, G., J. W. ten Cate, H. R. Buller, and F. Mandelli. 1989. Tranexamic acid for control of haemorrhage in acute promyelocytic leukaemia. *Lancet* 2:122–24.

Back, I. N. 2001. *Palliative medicine handbook.* 3d ed. Cardiff, Wales: BPM Books.

Baker, C. M., and D. L. Wong. 1987. QUEST: a process of pain assessment in children. *Orthop Nurs* 6:11–21.

Bentley, R., J. Cope, M. Jenney, and R. D. W. Hain. 2002. Use of intranasal/oral mida-zolam in paediatric palliative care. *Arch Dis Child* 86 (Suppl. 1):A76.

British Medical Association. 1999. *Withholding and withdrawing life-prolonging medical treatment: guidance for decision making.* London: BMJ Books.

Carpenter, K. J., V. Chapman, and A. H. Dickenson. 2000. Neuronal inhibitory effects of methadone are predominantly opioid receptor mediated in the rat spinal cord *in vivo. Eur J Pain* 4:19–26.

Chater, S., R. Viola, J. Paterson, and V. Jarvis. 1998. Sedation for intractable distress in the dying: a survey of experts. *Palliat Med* 12:255–69.

Cherny, N. I. 2000. The management of cancer pain. *CA Cancer J Clin* 50:70–120.

Cohen, S. O., and G. A. Walco. 1999. Dance/movement therapy for children and adolescents with cancer. *Cancer Practice* 7:34–42.

Colver, A., and C. Jessen. 2000. Measurement of health status and quality of life in neonatal follow-up studies. *Semin Neonatol* 5:149–57.

Craig, K. D., and R. V. E. Grunau. 1993. Neonatal pain perception and behavioral measurement. In *Pain in neonates,* ed. K. S. J. Anand and P. J. McGrath, 67–105. Vancouver: Elsevier Science.

Dean, A., and P. Tuffin. 1997. Fibrinolytic inhibitors for cancer-associated bleeding problems. *J Pain Symptom Manage* 13:20–24.

Faulkner, K. W. 2001. Children's understanding of death. In *Hospice care for children,* ed. A. Armstrong-Dailey and S. Zarbock, 9–22. 2d ed. New York: Oxford University Press.

Fitzgerald, M., C. Millard, and N. MacIntosh. 1988. Hyperalgesia in premature infants. *Lancet* 1:292.

Franck, L. S., C. S. Greenberg, and B. Stevens. 2000. Pain assessment in infants and children. *Pediatr Clin North Am* 47:487–512.

Gauvain-Piquard, A., C. Rodary, A. Rezvani, and S. Serbouti. 1999. The development of the DEGR(R): a scale to assess pain in young children with cancer. *Eur J Pain* 3:165–76.

Gee, L., J. Abbott, S. P. Conway, C. Etherington, and A. K. Webb. 2000. Development of a disease specific health related quality of life measure for adults and adolescents with cystic fibrosis. *Thorax* 55:946–54.

Gill, A. M., A. Cousins, A. J. Nunn, and I. A. Choonara. 1996. Opiate-induced respiratory depression in pediatric patients. *Ann Pharmacother* 30:125–29.

Hain, R. D. 1997. Pain scales in children: A review. *Palliat Med* 11:341–50.

Hain, R. D., and C. Campbell. 2001. Invasive procedures carried out in conscious children: contrast between North American and European paediatric oncology centres. *Arch Dis Child* 85:12–15.

Hain, R. D., and E. Hughes. 2001. Children referred for specialist palliative care: first 25 patients. Paper presented at the spring meeting of the Royal College of Paediatrics and Child Health. York, U.K., April 5.

Hain, R. D., N. Patel, S. Crabtree, and R. Pinkerton. 1995. Respiratory symptoms in children dying from malignant disease. *Palliat Med* 9:201–6.

Hull, D., ed. 1999. *Medicines for children.* London: Royal College of Paediatrics and Child Health.

Hunt, A. M. 1990. A survey of signs, symptoms and symptom control in 30 terminally ill children. *Dev Med Child Neurol* 32:341–46.

Hunt, A., S. Joel, G. Dick, and A. Goldman. 1999. Population pharmacokinetics of oral morphine and its glucuronides in children receiving morphine as immediate-release liquid or sustained-release tablets for cancer pain. *J Pediatr* 135:47–55.

Jan, M. M. 2000. Melatonin for the treatment of handicapped children with severe sleep disorders. *Pediatr Neurol* 23:229–32.

Leff-Tanner, P., J. M. Chan, and E. M. Walizer. 1991. Self-understanding and reaching out to sick children and their families: an ongoing professional challenge. *Children's Health Care* 20:230–39.

Mallinson, J., and P. D. Jones. 2000. A 7-year review of deaths on the general paediatric wards at John Hunter Children's Hospital, 1991–97. *J Paediatr Child Health* 36:252–55.

McDonnell, F. J., J. W. Sloan, and S. R. Hamann. 2001. Advances in cancer pain management. *Curr Pain Headache Rep* 5:265–71.

McGraw, M. B. 1941. Neural maturation as exemplified in the changing reactions of the infant to pin prick. *Child Dev* 12:31–42.

Meissner, W., U. Schmidt, M. Hartmann, R. Kath, and K. Reinhart. 2000. Oral naloxone reverses opioid-induced constipation. *Pain* 84:105–9.

Mendelsohn, J. 1999. Dance/movement therapy with hospitalized children. *Am J Dance Ther* 21:65–80.

Mercadante, S. 1994. The role of octreotide in palliative care. *J Pain Symptom Manage* 9:406–11.

Nelson, T. W., J. K. Lilly 3d, J. D. Baker 3d, and J. A. Ackerly. 1988. Treatment of pruritus secondary to epidural morphine: prophylactic v. PRN naloxone. *W V Med J* 84:183–85.

Neuhouser, M. L., R. E. Patterson, S. M. Schwartz, M. M. Hedderson, D. J. Bowen, and L. J. Standish. 2001. Use of alternative medicine by children with cancer in Washington state. *Prev Med* 33:347–54.

Pal, S. K., J. Cortiella, and D. Herndon. 1997. Adjunctive methods of pain control in burns. *Burns* 23:404–12.

Porter, F. L., R. E. Grunau, and K. J. Anand. 1999. Long-term effects of pain in infants. *J Dev Behav Pediatr* 20:253–61.

Royal College of Paediatrics and Child Health, Ethics Advisory Committee. 1997. *Withholding or withdrawing life saving treatment in children: a framework for practice.* London: Royal College of Paediatrics and Child Health.

Rubin, S. 1992. What's in a name? child life and the play lady legacy. *Children's Healthcare* 21:4.

Saint-Exupéry, A. de 2000. *The little prince.* Orlando, Fla.: Harcourt.

Sang, C. N. 2000. NMDA-receptor antagonists in neuropathic pain: experimental methods to clinical trials. *J Pain Symptom Manage* 19 (Suppl. 1):S21–25.

Sanger, G. J., and R. Twycross. 1996. Making sense of emesis, pruritus 5HT- and 5HT3- receptor antagonists. *Prog Palliat Care* 4:7–8.

Shir, Y., Z. Shenkman, V. Shavelson, E. M. Davidson, and G. Rosen. 1998. Oral methadone for the treatment of severe pain in hospitalized children: a report of five cases. *Clin J Pain* 14:350–53.

Stringer, M., M. K. Makin, J. Miles, and J. S. Morley. 2000. D-morphine, but not l-morphine, has low micromolar affinity for the non-competitive N-methyl-D-aspartate site in rat forebrain: possible clinical implications for the management of neuropathic pain. *Neurosci Lett* 295:21–24.

Thompson, R. H., and G. Standford. 1981. *Child life in hospitals: theory and practice.* Springfield, Ill.: Charles C. Thomas.

Twycross, R. 1997. *Symptom management in advanced cancer,* ed. R. Twycross and A. Wilcock. 3d ed. Oxford, U.K.: Radcliffe Medical.

Ventafridda, V., M. Tamburini, A. Caraceni, F. De Conno, and F. Naldi. 1987. A validation study of the WHO method for cancer pain relief. *Cancer* 59:850–56.

Vermeire, A., and J. P. Remon. 1999. Compatibility and stability of ternary admixtures of morphine with haloperidol or midazolam and dexamethasone or methylprednisolone. *Int J Pharm* 177:53–67.

Wolfe, J., H. E. Grier, N. Klar, S. B. Levin, J. M. Ellenbogen, S. Salem-Schatz, E. J. Emanuel, and J. C. Weeks. 2000. Symptoms and suffering at the end of life in children with cancer. *N Engl J Med* 342:326–33.

World Health Organization. 1984. *Cancer as a global problem.* Geneva: World Health Organization.

———. 1998. Guidelines for analgesic drug therapy. In *Cancer pain relief and palliative care in children,* 24–28. Geneva: World Health Organization–International Association for the Study of Pain.

8

Bereavement

Betty Davies, R.N., Ph.D., J. William Worden, M.Ed., Ph.D.,
Stacy F. Orloff, Ed.D., L.C.S.W., Maria Gudmundsdottir, R.N., Ph.D.,
Suzanne Toce, M.D., and Lizabeth Sumner, R.N., B.S.N.

Inherent in pediatric palliative care is the understanding that the child will die. The death of one's child is possibly the most difficult loss to grieve. This is especially true when the child is young and depends on the parent for life-sustaining activities. For this reason, the care that is provided does not stop at the moment of death; the care must continue for family members as they struggle with their loss and try to relearn their world (Attig 1996). Parents, siblings, grandparents, and all those others who were a part of the child's life need the informed support of health care professionals as they grieve.

Family Grief

For families, the death of a child symbolizes the loss of a future—the dream that this child will continue the family's legacy into the future. A child's death reverberates through the family in untold ways. Heartfelt grief is also noted by the larger community that surrounded the child, such as the child's peers and classmates, teachers, members of the family's faith community, and the health care professionals involved in the child's care. This deep-rooted grief may be experienced for many years (Rando 1993). The family unit and individual family members are forever changed by the experience.

Providing effective grief interventions in anticipation of a child's death will increase the family's ability to negotiate the difficult bereavement journey after the child's death. The parents should be provided with literature on bereavement and access to support groups. The hospital staff should not neglect the care of the extended family, especially siblings but also grandparents and others. If at all possible, caregivers should recognize the death by attending the visitation or memorial service, phoning the family, or sending a card. If an autopsy is performed, the physician should meet with the family when the results are available, discuss implications for subsequent pregnancies, and review the bereavement process. Support needs to be continuing. The infant or child may be especially missed at special times, such as birthdays, the anniversary of the death, a premature infant's due date, or the holidays. Some children's hospitals periodically hold memorial services for all children who have died during the previous month, quarter, or year. This is an important ritual not only for families but also for staff. Support should continue beyond discharge from the labor and delivery area or nursery. However, many institutions lack adequate resources for organized follow-up.

Many factors may influence how the family grieves the death of the child. In trying to effectively assist them, it is important to note such things as

- how the family has coped with prior losses;
- whether the family has experienced the death of another child;
- how effective the family's support system is; and
- whether the family has a spiritual grounding or religious faith.

One goal of many hospice and palliative care programs is to assist the family in preparing for the death. Many hospice and palliative care professionals speak about a "good" death. However, for family members facing the death of a child, no death is good, and no one in the family is ever truly ready or prepared. The best that health care professionals can do is to assist the family in finding a way for the death to occur in a manner that reflects their goals, values, cultural practices, and religious and spiritual beliefs.

Health care providers must also understand that they are not the experts in showing families how to grieve. Just as the goals of care for the living child are mutually derived by the patient, family, and health care providers, the bereavement plan of care is directed by the surviving family members. The hospice and palliative care team serves as guide and fellow traveler on this uncharted journey, providing support when the family feels they are losing their way.

SUDDEN DEATH OF A CHILD

Although most children cared for in palliative care programs will die of an illness diagnosed sometime in the past, palliative care programs must also address the grief and bereavement needs of families who lose a child suddenly. Consider the following:

- A 5-year-old is running across the street after his T-ball game. He is wearing his new baseball shoes with cleats, which cause him to slip in the street. An oncoming car does not see him in time.
- An 18-year-old boy was the valedictorian of his high school class. He is now a first-year student at a large state university. His first-quarter grades include one B. He is so distraught he jumps out his fifteenth-story dormitory window.
- A young couple wakes up one morning, well rested after their first complete night's sleep since the birth of their child, only to find their 4-month-old daughter lying lifeless on the Winnie-the-Pooh sheets in her crib.

Scores of children with equally gut-wrenching stories arrive at hospital emergency departments daily. Traumatic injury is the main cause of death in children ages 1 to 19; 88 percent of deaths in this age group result from trauma, including motor vehicle accident, homicide, suicide, and drowning. Among children who die before the age of 1 year, 11 percent die of sudden causes, including sudden infant death syndrome, homicide, and accidents (Guyer et al. 1999). Although these families interface with the health care system for only a brief time, palliative care principles can be applied in the care of these children to improve the long-term outcomes of the surviving family members.

Because there has been some time for preparation in an anticipated death, such deaths may present less of an assault on the grieving parents' adaptive capacities than a sudden death (Rando 1993). However, interventions based on these anticipatory grief techniques can prevent problems in mourning in situations involving sudden death, as well. The impact of the care rendered in the emergency room or intensive care unit can be of enduring value to the family.

In sudden death, parents, who normally function as their child's protector, have entered the emergency department with feelings of helplessness, loss, and perhaps guilt, depending upon the circumstances. If the child lives after the initial emergency department care, the stunned family is most likely confronted with the choice of either "doing everything" or "doing nothing." Surrounded by caregivers who are most likely strangers to the family, and armed with the common misperception of the successfulness of cardiopulmonary resuscitation, many parents choose full resuscitation. Because the likelihood of a positive resuscitative outcome is low, anticipatory grief techniques can be used even if only minutes are available.

The goals of emergency department caregivers in this situation should be

- to provide as much time as possible for the family to internalize the seriousness of their child's plight;
- to communicate in a logical and sequential manner; and
- to move the family toward acceptance of the situation and to help them cope with the irrevocability of the eventual outcome (Mancini 1986).

Maximizing the time that parents spend with the child and providing as full and complete an amount of information as is desired in a compassionate manner may also be helpful in this setting. Mancini (1986) recommends providing grave information in the emergency department in small incremental steps (two to three contacts) over fifteen minutes. The first contact would leave the family with the knowledge that "the doctors are doing everything they can." The second visit with the family would present the fact that things are looking worse and nothing appears to be working. By giving the information gradually, in "doses," the family becomes prepared for the third visit with the physician, who will inform them that the child has died.

This same approach can also apply to a family with a child who has a life-threatening condition and is expected to die but does not die according to an anticipated timetable or in the expected way. If the parents are given a particular illness trajectory, they may not be mentally prepared for a death that occurs earlier than predicted. The parents may respond in a similar manner to parents whose child dies of an accidental or intentional injury. If a child is expected to die as a result of a specific complication, such as aspiration pneumonia, but instead dies of a different complication, such as diarrhea and dehydration, the parents may react with shock and disbelief. Parents of a child with a known terminal condition may function with some degree of denial and react like parents of a child who dies suddenly. They may even react to their child's expected death with shock, disbelief, or hysteria. Some parents secretly harbor the belief, or fantasy, that their child's outcome will be different, that he or she will somehow "beat the odds," even if they know at an intellectual level that this cannot happen. The death of the child assaults parents in their role as protector, and this is one of the major stressors of a child's death. Regardless of the cause of death, parents lament, "How could I have not prevented this from happening?"

GUILT

Guilt plagues all bereaved parents. Doubts about having made the right treatment decisions for the child can be addressed by honoring parents' frequent request to review the medical events of their child's illness and death with different members of the health care team. Parents may question medical decisions they made, concerned they have hastened their child's death or altered the treatment outcome. These conversations are often part of the life review process. Harper and Wisian (1994) have conducted a study with thirty-seven bereaved parents. Overwhelmingly, these parents wanted doctors to be available for discussion for at least one month after the death and to provide medical information regarding the illness, the cause of death, and the autopsy report.

Guilt is a frequent feature of bereavement, and this is especially true for bereaved parents. Guilt may arise from questions of having made the right treatment decisions for the child, from the decision to pursue palliative rather than life-prolonging treatment, or even from having conceived or given birth to a child who developed a terminal illness or having "genetically infected" the child with the disease. Parents' guilt may also derive from the perceived failure to protect their child from harm or from the feeling that they have abandoned other children or family members, either behaviorally or emotionally, while caring for the deceased child.

Bereaved parents sometimes have the need to blame someone for the death of their child, especially if the child died in an accident, by suicide, or by homicide. But the same can hold true for parents whose child dies of natural causes. When this need to blame is targeted toward a marriage partner or other family member, stress on the whole family system is increased. It is also possible for a family member, such as another child, to be viewed as a scapegoat after a death. Caregivers need to be aware of these dynamics and help families find appropriate ways to deal with anger and blame.

PROLONGED GRIEF

Long after the acute pain of a child's death has subsided, graduations, marriages, and births, and even simple observed activities such as children playing in a park, remind the bereaved of what might have been if the child had survived. These events bring about renewed pain. One grieving mother said, "This will go on for a long time, but I look forward to the day when the pain will not be so intense. I know that life will never be the same as it would have been if my child had survived, but I hope to one day make some sense of all of this and perhaps even find some meaning for what we are going through." By addressing the pain, seeking to feel understood and not judged, negotiating painful events, and perhaps discovering some meaning in the loss, grieving parents may find that life can return to normal—not normal as it was or would have been, but a new "normal."

SUPPORTING BEREAVED SIBLINGS

Health care providers can coach the family in explaining the death to siblings in developmentally appropriate language. Siblings mourning a deceased brother or sister often feel separated from their grieving parents, suffering thereby an additional loss. Siblings may be the most isolated and forgotten mourners.

A surviving child may take on the role the deceased child had in the family, such as the "good" child, the athlete, or the "funny" child. It is important to assure bereaved siblings that they are loved for themselves (Davies 1999, 4). Assisting families in finding ways to memorialize the deceased child will increase family members' understanding that the dead child cannot be replaced.

Siblings frequently misunderstand the cause of death, often attributing partial responsibility to themselves (Davies 1999). Concrete and developmentally appropriate information can do much to allay the fears and concerns of most siblings. Parents will need help in gathering and sharing such information with their children. Expressive arts (music, painting) and play therapies are especially helpful in reaching siblings. Siblings may exhibit expressions of sadness or changes in behavior with parents and caregivers or at school. It is important to inform these potential sources of comfort and reassurance of the death so that they are not ill prepared to offer support.

MOURNING

Many family members struggle with the first task of mourning—accepting the reality of the child's death (Worden 2002). They may appear to understand and accept the death but emotionally are not quite ready to do so. It is common for family friends and health care professionals, out of their own discomfort with death, to encourage the bereaved family to reconnect socially with others, return to work, and clean out the child's room and belongings.

Parents need to be reassured that they will know when they are ready to deal with these tasks and resume regular activities.

Expression of feelings is the second task of mourning and is influenced by personality, ego strength, and cultural and religious values; expression of feelings is an important goal of bereavement counseling. Rituals and other nonverbal means, such as keeping a journal, art activities, a balloon release or tree planting to commemorate special dates, are useful ways to express feelings. Children are especially comforted by rituals.

HELPING GRIEVING PARENTS

What can help bereaved parents adjust effectively to the death of their child? Spinetta, Swarmer, and Sheposh (1981) followed bereaved parents for three years following their loss. Parents who were doing better at the end of that time exhibited some common characteristics:

- They had a consistent philosophy of life that helped them find some meaning in the loss.
- They had viable and ongoing support.
- They had been able to give their dying child information and emotional support consonant with the child's needs.

Parents whose children died after longer illnesses were not uniformly doing better after the death, though there was a trend in that direction.

Grieving is a social phenomenon. For grief to progress and the tasks of mourning to be accomplished, it is important that grieving persons have the opportunity to share their grief and experiences with others. Such sharing includes talking about the events leading up to the death, including the diagnosis, treatment, and interactions with others and with the deceased. Some people feel uncomfortable around bereaved parents and may cut off such conversations. Grief may, in fact, be "disenfranchised" (Doka 2002). Support groups can be a safe haven in which bereaved parents can share their thoughts and feelings with others who have also lost a child.

Segal, Fletcher, and Meekison (1986) asked a group of bereaved parents what they would have wanted after the death of their child. Many parents said that they would have found it helpful to have more information as to the cause of death, regarding risks to their other children, and on grief. In dealing with grieving parents, several important considerations should be noted. Table 8.1 gives a list of recommendations for caregivers.

Table 8.1. Dos and don'ts when caring for grieving families

Do
- allow your own human caring and concern to show through; take the initiative to contact the bereaved.
- recognize that families are systems, and that a child's death affects everyone in the family, not just the parents.
- acknowledge the depth of family members' loss.
- reassure the parents they did everything they could have.
- recognize the dead child as a person; refer to the child by name.
- encourage collection of memories, mementos, and keepsakes.
- educate parents and other family members about the range of grief responses over time; allow them to express their grief over time.
- pay attention to individual differences among family members, taking into account cultural, religious, personality, and other differences.
- give practical help.
- repeat information as needed, realizing the stress of the situation may preclude parents and others from grasping facts the first time.
- be available to listen and follow up.
- attend the funeral or memorial service or send sympathy cards.
- give attention to the surviving siblings.
- refer the parents to other bereavement resources.
- develop a plan to help the school and community cope with the child's death.
- pay attention to your own needs for emotional support.

Don't
- minimize their loss ("At least you have your other children [your big brother]" or "You can always have another child").
- judge parents' grief reactions or minimize their need to grieve.
- hurry their grieving process ("It has been months. Aren't you over it yet?").
- expect expression of grief to fit a protocol or to be uniform.
- interfere with the father's demonstrations of grief by reinforcing the male stereotype of strength.
- tell them what they "should" feel or do.
- offer platitudes or artificial consolation.
- avoid them because you feel helpless or uncomfortable.

Fathers' Grief

Although the death of a child greatly affects the entire family, the mother and child subsystem within the family commonly receives the most attention from society. This attention begins with concern for the mother's health during pregnancy and continues with a focus on the mother-child relationship. This emphasis is reflected both within clinical practice and in the literature, as studies of mothers and children are by far more common than studies of fathers. It is not surprising, then, that this emphasis can also be detected within the world of bereavement, in which studies of mothers' grief abound in comparison with studies of fathers' grief. When fathers are included in bereavement studies, they are commonly compared with mothers, whose perceptions are taken as the norm (Cook 1988).

Many fathers state that their perceptions and emotions during bereavement have been disregarded by health care professionals and by society in general. Instead of being asked about his reaction to the loss of his child, frequently the father is asked how his wife is doing and how she is dealing with her loss. Societal expectations thrust the father into the role of the family's protector; fathers are not encouraged to experience and express their own emotions, because they are expected to be "strong" for the sake of other family members. "When is it my turn to cry?" one father asked, and then he offered his own answer: "I'm not sure society or my upbringing will ever allow me a time to really cry, because of the reaction and repercussion that might follow. I must be strong for my wife because I am a man. I must be the cornerstone of our family because society says so, my family says so, and, until I can reverse my learned nature, I say so" (quoted in DeFrain et al. 1991, 112). This father's statement illustrates society's perspective on fathers' grief and raises the question of how the perception of fathers' experiences affects clinicians as they care for bereaved fathers.

There is some evidence to suggest that mothers and fathers grieve the loss of their child differently. Several studies have shown that bereaved mothers grieve more intensely and are more distressed than bereaved fathers (Lang and Gottlieb 1993; Moriarty, Carroll, and Cotroneo 1996; Murphy et al. 1998). However, other studies have found that the intensity of fathers' grief is equal to that of mothers but their ways of grieving can be incongruent; parents do not grieve in the same ways or over the same period of time (Hunfelt et al. 1996). These perceived gender differences depend on which measures are used as indicators of grief (Vance et al. 1995a). If only measures of anxiety and depression are used, the loss of a child appears to be more disturbing to women than to men. However, when measures of alcohol use are included as a reaction to stress, the difference in response becomes much smaller or disappears entirely.

Some explain the difference between mothers' and fathers' ways of grieving by looking at the nature of the relationship between each parent and the child (Lang and Gottlieb 1993; Gamino 1999). This is particularly relevant when newborns die. Gamino (1999), whose infant son died a few hours after birth, reports that his grief differed from his wife's grief because each was attached differently to the baby. For him, the relationship was more abstract, while for his wife, Marla, it was more physiological. Owing to the fetus's small size, Gamino felt his son move in utero only a couple of times. Marla, on the other hand, often felt the baby kick her internal organs and had a stronger sense of his aliveness; this lived experience of her child sometimes gave her comfort in her grief, while her husband was more often sad.

EMOTIONS IN FATHERS' GRIEF

Clinicians and researchers specializing in men's grief agree that men's emotional life exhibits a tension between the need to express unhappy feelings and fear of the consequences of doing so. Pollack (1998) claims that historical, cultural, and economic forces affect parenting styles in such a way that boys experience a premature psychic separation from both maternal and paternal caregivers. This may later become problematic for men as they unconsciously try to protect themselves from further loss by blocking expression of all strong emotions except anger. Consequently, their ability to grieve and mourn is impaired, as they are unable to tolerate feelings of vulnerability or to express and bear sadness. Moreover, men must confront the competing demands of the societal expectation that men should comfort their wives and the cultural notion that healthy grieving requires the sharing of feelings. A female bias in conceptualization and measurement of grief and in bereavement interventions makes fathers' grief invisible to both clinicians and researchers.

However, men seem to work hard at their "grief work." Their coping strategies commonly emphasize suppressing and blocking thoughts about the death, controlling upsetting emotions so as not to hurt others, and earnest attempts to deal with their wives' need for their husbands' expressiveness. Though they seem less affected by the loss, when assessed through various measures, bereaved fathers exert considerable effort in managing their emotions (Cook 1988). Rather than expressing their grief directly, men are more likely to be active and to keep themselves busy by working long hours or physically exhausting themselves through participation in sports (Worden 1996; Wood and Milo 2001). Nevertheless, there is room for individual differences in the response to the loss of a child. Some fathers are silent and stoic, avoiding open expression of their emotions; other need to talk about and express their emotional responses to facilitate their own healing. The two cases that follow illustrate the range of fathers' grief reactions (Davies and Gudmunds-dottir 2002).

Mike's 12-year-old son, Alex, died of brain cancer despite several treatments, including treatment in another state. Mike had a win-lose perspective of his family's battle with cancer. He became angry when the cancer relapsed, "chewing the cancer out" at his son's deathbed. In the three years since Alex's death, Mike has never cried; his strongest emotion is anger. He is less tolerant of other people's struggles and admits that a hard, protective shell has grown around him. The only people who can penetrate it are his wife and daughter. From the beginning, Mike felt the need to be strong for his family. Though he has wanted to cry, as soon as he feels tears approaching he unconsciously "shuts them off" by changing his thoughts, talking himself through the sorrow, or going somewhere else. When asked how and when he had learned to prevent himself from crying, he said, "I guess we were brought up that guys never cry," while at the same time admitting that his wife and daughter believe crying would help him in his grief. Mike even sought bereavement therapy for one and a half years but was still unable to cry. He is keenly aware of his restricted emotional repertoire. Though he believes that it would be better for him to express his hidden emotions, he is not ready for that yet.

Andrew lost his 15-year-old son, Daniel, to lymphocytic leukemia. Andrew initially believed that he needed to be strong, resourceful, and confident for his family. However, he also realized that this experience could destroy his family and discovered that he needed and wanted to talk about it. Moreover, his wife needed him to show his fears, worries, and sadness as they lived through this challenging time together, and, he says, "I learned to get over my sort of Rock of Gibraltar routine." Andrew's way of dealing with his newfound need to talk honestly about how he felt was to tell anyone who asked exactly what was troubling him, instead of saying that he was doing fine.

Andrew also finds comfort in his faith and spirituality. He describes himself as having an "ecumenical or postdenominational outlook on religion," but he says his life experience has brought him in touch with his own spirituality on a much deeper level than before his son's illness.

He learned to pray anew; and as he sat on his son's deathbed, holding his hand and reading aloud from the *Tibetan Book of the Dead,* he realized that his son was not just his child but was "a soul in his own destiny." Andrew's spirituality continues to nurture him two years after Daniel's death. His life without Daniel is bittersweet, but he says that he still has love to give and receive. He believes that celebration of life honors the memory of his son.

IMPLICATIONS FOR HEALTH CARE PROVIDERS

There is much to learn from these two fathers. Mike fits the stereotype of a man who has a difficult time expressing his emotions. Andrew learned that it helped him and his family to open up and to learn to express his emotions—a process characteristic of "women's ways" of coping with sorrow.

It is important to emphasize that no one way of grieving is better than another. However, clinicians need to be aware of and open to the many ways in which men express their grief. By accepting differences among men, clinicians will be better able to support bereaved fathers as they grieve for their children in their own unique ways.

Clinicians might help fathers by acknowledging the particular way a father is grieving. For example, fathers who are trying to be strong for the sake of their families need to be complimented for their endeavor. It may also be important for other family members, such as the wife, to understand that her husband's limited emotional expression may represent his inherent need to protect his family.

Mike saw his inability to cry as a deficit. For him, acknowledging that he may not be the kind of person who cries when faced with a tragedy and talking about the strong feelings he has—namely, his anger and frustration—and how his child's death impacts his own life may be more therapeutic. Andrew perceived the importance of his spirituality in his ability to cope. Helping fathers evaluate their strengths and using them to heal is an important way to help.

Attendance at support groups is often recommended to the newly bereaved, but many fathers do not find them helpful, and if they go, they frequently do so only to support their wives (Worden and Monahan 2001). This behavior may emanate from their gender socialization and their common need to be more private about their grief (Cook 1988; Murphy et al. 1998). As we learn more about the unique ways in which fathers live with the loss of a beloved child, we will be better able to offer care that is attuned to the special needs of fathers and thereby provide optimal care to all members of the family.

Perinatal Loss

Each year in the United States, nearly a million families are affected by birth tragedies. How does the loss of the fetus or newborn affect these families, and how can we as health care providers influence the experience of the families and support them through the difficult times ahead? Consider the following situation:

> Miranda is a 23-year-old woman who was weeping inconsolably at work. It was the one-year anniversary of the death of her baby, James, who had died at 5 days of age of prenatally diagnosed congenital heart disease. Although Miranda was given bereavement support group literature, she attended no meetings. She rarely speaks about James and had thought she was "over it." While she used to find solace in prayer, she finds that she can no longer pray. She is now twenty-two weeks pregnant and has sought no prenatal care. She is fearful that her current baby has heart disease and will also die.

Each year there are nearly nineteen thousand neonatal deaths; about one in two hundred of these deaths occurs before the child reaches twenty-eight days of age (Ventura et al. 2001). This underestimates the scope of perinatal loss, as there are close to a million fetal losses each year (16% of all pregnancies end in a miscarriage or stillbirth [Ventura et al. 2001]). Before the late 1960s, these losses were considered inconsequential in society's view (Hoeldtke and Calhoun 2001) and were rarely discussed. Even between mothers and fathers, reactions to perinatal losses were seldom shared. Since the 1970s, there has been increasing awareness of the grief associated with perinatal loss and the need for strategies to aid families to cope with or validate the loss.

Parental emotions after perinatal loss may encompass shock, denial, anger, depression, and acceptance, similar to other grief responses (Murray et al. 2000). Some families find ways to integrate the child's short life into the fabric of the family; others never speak of the baby again; still others mourn for a long time. Parental attachment clearly precedes the birth of an infant, making even an early miscarriage a significant loss for many parents (Weiss, Frischer, and Richman 1989). Recognition of the loss is reinforced by the burgeoning technology available to "connect with one's baby" with ultrasound, head phones to hear the heartbeat, and even three-dimensional imaging. The intensity of grief over a perinatal loss can be as great as that experienced at the loss of a spouse or close relative and may persist for years. In the early months after the death, grieving parents report frequent emotional and somatic signs of distress, including aching arms, feeling the presence of the baby, hearing baby sounds, and hallucinations of the dead baby. Parents may experience not only loss of the wished-for baby but also diminution of self-esteem, loss of confidence in their role as parent, and a feared inability to produce a healthy child (Weiss, Frischer, and Richman 1989). Guilt may arise owing to genetic issues or because of a maternal sense of responsibility for the death. Grieving mothers must also contend with engorged breasts, healing wounds, and physical exhaustion and then face a home, family, and community readied for a new baby.

Although early pregnancy losses may produce less intense grief than stillbirth or neonatal loss, grief intensity and complications are highly personal responses, unrelated to birth weight, gestational age, parental age, or participation in decisions to withdraw support. Depression and anxiety are more common in the first six to eight months (Vance et al. 1995b) but sometimes persist in a less intense form for twelve to sixteen months following the pregnancy loss. Although mood levels improve over time, there is significant interpersonal variability. Parents may benefit from understanding the range of anticipated emotional responses.

One-fifth to one-third of parents experience pathological grief one to two years following the loss (Rowe et al. 1978). Pathological grief is a continued inability to work through the sense of loss, with resultant continued feelings of self-hatred and deflation of self-esteem, extreme isolation, inability to return to work or previous activities of daily living, severe depression, and suicidal ideation. Diagnostic clues include the intensity, duration, or rigidity of the grief symptoms. Factors predisposing a parent to prolonged grief include an inability to hold the baby, the presence of a surviving twin, crises or ambivalence during pregnancy, lack of spousal, social, or family support, and a history of prior mental health problems (Rowe et al. 1978; Murray et al. 2000). Grief can be adversely affected by the behavior of family, friends, and health care providers. Referral to a mental health professional who has expertise with bereaved parents may be indicated in some cases.

Attitudes and actions of health care providers are powerful factors that may impede or facilitate future grief work (Weiss, Frischer, and Richman 1989). Support of the family is critical, regardless of the timing of the loss. When the fetus dies before it is born, parents may be left to grieve in an isolated, misunderstood way (Weiss, Frischer, and Richman 1989). Fetuses are not viewed as members of the family and community, and there are few rituals with which to recognize the loss. As technology and scientific advances create greater opportunities for information, testing, and screening during pregnancy, parents often learn of the potentially lethal condition long before delivery. In an instant, the parents begin saying good-bye even before they have had a chance to say hello. These parents not only experience the pain of loss but also may need to make difficult decisions (Weiss, Frischer, and Richman 1989). Two-thirds of the parents of a fetus with lethal conditions elect to terminate the pregnancy (Hassed et al. 1993). The grief response of parents electing termination is as intense as parents experiencing stillbirth or neonatal loss (Weiss, Frischer, and Richman 1989; Hoeldtke and Calhoun 2001), yet often this grief goes unacknowledged by the woman herself or by medical professionals. The need for support can be just as great, however. Parents may continue the pregnancy because of uncertainty about the probability of death, because of the desire to share what remains of the life of their child, or for personal or religious reasons.

For these parents, there is much that health care providers can do to help. Caregivers can provide emotional support, facilitate decision making and advance care planning, help the mourning process, and give parents permission to grieve (Weiss, Frischer, and Richman 1989). Perinatal hospice care is an emerging concept that can be offered as an adjunct or alternative to pregnancy termination (Hoeldtke and Calhoun 2001). It is a compassionate, structured program that provides a context in which parents can find meaning in the intimate experience of the life and death of their child. The concurrent themes of hope and sorrow, welcoming and mourning, require sensitivity and keen awareness in the health care professionals caring for the parents.

The hospice team generally consists of the obstetrician, pediatrician, social worker, nurse, chaplain, and others as indicated. The team reduces feelings of fear and loneliness during the pregnancy, delivery, and death of the baby and through bereavement. Anticipatory guidance and the development of an advance care plan or "birth plan" allows the family to have a sense of control over significant details, participate in decision making, and establish an understanding of what might happen in the event of a live birth. The advance care plan might include an obstetrical plan (mode of delivery, response to fetal distress or preterm labor), plan and preparation for the birth (site of care, delivery room management), and, potentially, the care of a surviving baby and the possible discharge to home or alternate setting. The hospice team collaborates with inpatient staff to help facilitate the wishes and goals of parents, preventing the initiation of undesired interventions. The focus of care turns to attention to the dignity of life regardless of duration. This may be the only opportunity for the mother and father to feel like parents to their fragile newborn.

Subsequent pregnancy poses unique challenges and concerns. A pregnancy initiated less than five or six months after the loss may cut short the mourning process, predisposing parents to mental disturbances (Rowe et al. 1978). While not all studies support adverse effects, most show that the next pregnancy can be fraught with mental, emotional, and physical challenges. Failure to mourn a dead child may have dire consequences for mothering a subsequent child. There may be overprotective and replacement feelings with the next child. With the birth of a new child, the family may feel disloyal toward the dead child. The new child may be perceived as having more health and behavior problems than actually exist. Problems are especially acute if the birthday is near the anniversary of the death of the earlier baby, if grief is not resolved, if the mother is more anxious than is normal, or if there is poor social support.

On the other hand, if the parents have been able to grieve in a healthy manner and are trying to work through the loss issues, the perceptions and rationale for another baby may be positive in the context of the individual family. Conceiving again and the subsequent birth may lessen grief, bring the couple closer, have positive effects on siblings, and integrate the memory of the dead child into the family experience. Interconceptual counseling might be indicated to answer remaining questions about the cause of death, rule out recurrent pregnancy risks, and allow informed decisions regarding future pregnancies. The health care provider can support the mother during pregnancy, relieve anxiety, validate the normal progression of pregnancy, and reinforce the health of the new baby (Weiss, Frischer, and Richman 1989).

Health care providers can play a role in the management of grief and loss. Silence is not always golden. Health care providers can compassionately affirm the death and ensure that individual family members' needs are expressed and met and that the family makes a seamless connection to bereavement follow-up care. Caregivers can be sympathetic listeners and sensitive informants. They can facilitate continued communication between the family and its the obstetrician and pediatrician. As nearly one-third of parents choose another physician after the death of a child, satisfaction with care is an important issue. Parents' satisfaction with health care positively correlates with the availability of providers, access to the appropriate medical information, being given help in addressing denial, and receiving grief counseling (Harper and Wisian 1994).

Support programs are effective in improving the understanding of autopsy findings and burial options, increasing confidence in a future pregnancy, and paternal involvement (Murray et al. 2000). Psychological and spiritual support, either professional or from a peer support group, can assuage anger and hostility, physical symptoms, depression, and intensity of grief, particularly in the first six months after the loss (Murray et al. 2000). This support is particularly important in the absence of family and social support. The higher the parents' risk, the greater is the benefit of the support and the satisfaction with the support program. As there are few societal rituals surrounding fetal loss, it may be particularly important to support parents experiencing miscarriage, stillbirth, or pregnancy termination.

There are many ways to be supportive in anticipation of a neonatal death or delivery of a stillborn infant (Weiss, Frischer, and Richman 1989). Providers can encourage the family to name the baby and hold, rock, or bathe the baby. Religious rituals such as baptism and pastoral counseling are frequently positive influences and should be prepared for in anticipation of the birth. Professionals should be open to unusual requests that might create meaning for the family. They can give concrete evidence of the baby's brief existence and foster memories by providing ultrasound pictures, photographs (especially of the infant in the parents' arms), handprints or footprints, bracelets, crib cards with measurements, birth or death certificates, and locks of hair. Baby clothes kept in a ziplock plastic bag may retain the baby's scent. If the family declines the offers of such mementos, the staff can save them in case they are desired in the future.

Doctors and nurses can facilitate decision making regarding who is present at the delivery, interventions desired or declined for the baby, autopsy, disposition of the body, and funeral arrangements. They can promote a sense of control in as many aspects of the process as possible (who cuts the umbilical cord, holds, rocks, or dresses the infant, and so forth). It is important to note that the actual death of the infant may not occur in the hospital but in some cases may be at home. The advance care plan or discharge plan may include home hospice or nursing care and should also address bereavement issues following the infant's death.

After discharge, there should be follow-up contact, referral to support groups, and continuity of care, if possible, with the next pregnancy. Parents often find it painful to reach out for help, so ongoing contact is important. As noted in chapter 10 of this volume, hospitals inexperienced in perinatal loss may need consultation and support from the tertiary care center if a baby with a condition incompatible with prolonged life is delivered in the community. Parent bereavement support groups are important resources for families experiencing perinatal loss, especially fetal loss.

BEREAVEMENT INTERVENTIONS

Bereavement intervention begins before the death of the child. Caregivers need to be aware of several goals for such intervention. Specific techniques of intervention can be tailored around these goals, depending upon the age of the child, the illness, the family, and the type of care setting and program. These goals include the following:

- *Help the family stay connected with their child until death.* While relatively easy for some, many families who see their child declining find it a most painful situation, and they may have trouble staying connected with the child until the end. One mother whose son was born with major congenital defects found living with him during his six years to be demanding and difficult to manage. During his final hospitalization, his mother was not there with him; afterward, she developed serious clinical depression related to guilt feelings because of having "abandoned" him. It took considerable therapy to help her work through her feelings.
- *Facilitate communication.* This involves communication not only between the family and the care giving staff but also among family members themselves. Being sensitive to what a parent, patient, or

sibling wants to know or does not want to know is an important part of good care. Helping parents say to their child what they need to say before the child dies may preclude regrets after the death.

- *Help the family develop memories that they can cherish long after the death.* Pictures and videotapes of the child with other family members are concrete memorials that the family will cherish and replay over the years.

- *Help parents negotiate the medical system.* Some parents are well skilled in this and do not need help. Others are more intimidated by the system and are hesitant to ask questions or to assert their preferences. Helping parents to develop these skills through role playing and providing them encouragement to do what they need to do can be an important part of prebereavement counseling.

- *Provide respite care.* The demands of caring for a sick child are many. They often fall on the mother's shoulders. Hospice volunteers are typically good resources for this type of respite care, allowing the parent to take a break from his or her caregiving responsibilities. However, the closer to death the child is, the more the family may want to be with the child.

- *Help parents with the concept of "appropriate death."* An appropriate death, according to Weisman, Worden, and Sobel (1997), is a death consonant with the goals, values, and lifestyle of the individual. Although the concept is more often used with adults, it can also be useful in dealing with children, particularly adolescents. One girl in late adolescence wanted to spend her final weeks of life out of the family home, in an apartment near the seashore. Although her parents would have preferred to have her at home, they helped her to find such living quarters, where she could experience a degree of autonomy, express the individuation appropriate to her age, and be with her friends—all values that were important to her.

- *Help parents talk about choices for the funeral or memorial service in advance, if they choose to do this.* Although such discussion is often difficult, it allows the parents and the child, if old enough, to plan a service that reflects the uniqueness of their child. Including family members such as siblings in this activity can be a worthwhile activity. For some parents, this activity may not be acceptable as, for them, it connotes a loss of hope and a too-early admission that their child will die. Parents whose children receive hospice care tend to be more open to funeral planning in advance of the death. (Worden and Monahan 2001)

An important distinction needs to be made between two types of bereavement support: the nonclinical support offered by trained bereavement volunteers and the clinical services provided by professional counselors. Some researchers believe that a normal life-cycle event, such as death, has been made pathologic to the point that bereaved individuals may be told they need a counselor to "get through it." Wolfelt (1997) describes "companioning" as an effective way to provide support to the bereaved that does not require clinical intervention. Wolfelt suggests that most bereaved individuals will successfully complete the bereavement tasks with or without the assistance of a counselor. They can benefit from a "friendly neighbor" or companion who will be their partner on this journey.

Bereavement

The Daniels family provides an example of a family who benefited from ongoing contact with a bereavement volunteer provided by their local hospice.

John and Sharon Daniels made the difficult decision to accept hospice services for their 3-year-old daughter, Jackie, who was born with a rare metabolic defect, nonketotic hyperglycinemia. During the two and a half years that Jackie was a hospice patient, John and Sharon received counseling services from a pediatric hospice counselor. They also intermittently participated in an ongoing parent support group. Jackie's older sibling, an 11-year-old brother, participated in a monthly sibling support group. As Jackie's physical status rapidly deteriorated, the family reconnected with their faith community and received the spiritual support they wanted.

During the first counseling appointment after Jackie's death, John and Sharon asked the counselor to maintain monthly phone calls with them. They attributed their feelings to normal grief and stated the anticipatory grief work the pediatric counselor did with them had been very helpful. John and Sharon articulated a desire to "just be able to talk about Jackie" without feeling that their emotions were pathological. Their counselor offered the services of a bereavement volunteer, and they agreed. Three months later, the Daniels reported satisfaction with the bereavement volunteer, noting that "she is like a friendly neighbor or family friend who listens to us without judging us or making us feel that we're going crazy." The counselor maintains weekly telephone contact with the volunteer, who alerts the counselor about any concerns she might have.

PROFESSIONAL BEREAVEMENT COUNSELORS

For other families, the loss of a child is so painful that they cannot complete the journey alone and may benefit from the assistance of a trained bereavement counselor who is knowledgeable about current bereavement theory, counseling goals, and interventions. Bereavement professionals must also have knowledge of family systems, with special awareness that families with young children may extend widely, including out-of-town grandparents and other family members. Understanding multigenerational needs is also important in providing proper support to grandparents. Grandparents grieve for at least two different reasons: they mourn the death of their grandchild, and they suffer emotional pain seeing their adult child in such distress.

COMMUNITY RESOURCES

Following a child's death, the child is gone but not forgotten. Keeping an updated list of supportive resources in the community available can be an important contribution to the long-term resolution of grief. The reference should include specific contact information. Not all families benefit from support groups; families should be encouraged to seek other forms of support, such as through Internet connections or church-related activities, as appropriate.

Bereavement support providers can offer one or two small booklets or printed handouts of relevant information and a list of appropriate books and booklets for the time when family members may feel ready to read them. The family can also be given the name of one person in the hospital (or a related agency) whom they can phone should they wish to ask a question or follow up on some advice that has been given. Many families feel a special bond with the professionals who cared for their child at the end of his or her life; this bond needs to be allowed to be released gently to avoid the family's feeling abandoned and isolated. In the words of a message from the support group Mothers in Sympathy and Support, "It is our hope that you discover the enormity and depth of the love you have for your child; a love that transcends time and distance, heaven and earth, life and death."

Conclusion

The death of a fetus, infant, or child has a profound and lifelong impact on parents, siblings, grandparents, and sometimes the larger community. Each person touched by the death has individual ways of expressing his or her grief. Adequate information, an effective prenatal program for an anticipated death, and prebereavement counseling are among the protective factors enabling successful bereavement. However, our society frequently ignores the grieving and bereavement needs of those who are most profoundly affected. Parents of unborn children who die, families of children who die of sudden causes, and fathers, siblings, and grandparents bereaved of infants and children need informed attention to their concerns. They require affirmation and support through direction to resources, continued contact with designated health professionals, peer group supports, professional counseling, or companioning. While it may be difficult to provide ideally for all of the needs of a family bereaved of a child, simple measures that depend only on one individual can make the experience significantly better for the majority of families. Health care professionals have the opportunity to heal through awareness of how to help.

References

Attig, T. W. 1996. *How we grieve: relearning the world.* New York: Oxford University Press.

Cook, J. A. 1988. Dad's double binds: rethinking fathers' bereavement from a men's studies perspective. *J Contemp Ethnogr* 17:285–308.

Davies, B. 1999. *Shadows in the sun.* Philadelphia: Brunner/Mazel.

Davies, E., and M. Gudmundsdottir. 2002. Fathers' experiences of pediatric palliative care. Unpublished manuscript. University of California, San Francisco.

DeFrain, J., L. Ernst, D. Jakub, and J. Taylor. 1991. *Sudden infant death: enduring the loss.* Lexington, Mass.: Lexington Books.

Doka, K. J. 2002. *Disenfranchised grief: new directions, challenges, and strategies for practice.* Champaign, Ill.: Research Press.

Gamino, L. A. 1999. A father's experience of neonatal loss. *Forum* 3:14–15.

Guyer, B., D. L. Hoyert, J. A. Martin, S. J. Ventura, M. F. MacDormanet, and D. M. Strobino. 1999. Annual summary of vital statistics: 1998. *Pediatrics* 104:1229–46.

Harper, M. H., and N. B. Wisian. 1994. Care of bereaved parents: a study of patient satisfaction. *J Reprod Med* 39:80–86.

Hassed, S. J., C. H. Miller, S. K. Pope, P. Murphy, J. F. Quirk, and C. Cunniff. 1993. Perinatal lethal conditions: the effect of diagnosis on decision making. *Obstet Gynecol* 82:37–42.

Hoeldtke, N., and B. Calhoun. 2001. Perinatal hospice. *Am J Obstet Gynecol* 185:525–29.

Hunfelt, J. A. M., M. M. Mourik, D. Tibboel, and J. Passchier. 1996. Parental grieving after infant death. Letter to the editor. *J Fam Pract* 42:622–23.

Lang, A., and L. Gottlieb. 1993. Parental grief reactions and marital intimacy following infant death. *Death Studies* 17:233–55.

Mancini, M. E. 1986. Creating and therapeutically utilizing anticipatory grief in survivors of sudden death. In *Loss and anticipatory grief,* ed. T. Rando. Lexington, Mass.: Lexington Books.

Moriarty, H. J., R. Carroll, and M. Cotroneo. 1996. Differences in bereavement reactions within couples following death of a child. *Res Nurs Health* 19:461–69.

Mothers in Sympathy and Support (The MISS Foundation). www.missfoundation.org (accessed March 31, 2004).

Murphy, S. A., C. Johnson, K. C. Cain, A. D. Gupta, M. Dimond, J. Lohan, and R. Baugher. 1998. Broad-spectrum group treatment for parents bereaved by the violent deaths of their 12- to 28-year-old children: a randomized controlled trial. *Death Studies* 22:209–35.

Murray, J. A., D. J. Terry, J. C. Vance, D. Battistutta, and Y. Connolly. 2000. Effects of a program of intervention on parental distress following infant death. *Death Studies* 24:275–305.

Pollack, W. S. 1998. Mourning, melancholia, and masculinity: recognizing and treating depression in men. In *New psychotherapy for men,* ed. W. S. Pollack, 147–66. New York: Wiley.

Rando, T. 1993. *Readings in pediatric psychology.* New York: Plenum.

Rowe, J., R. Clyman, C. Green, C. Mikkelsen, J. Haight, and L. Ataide. 1978. Follow-up of families who experience a perinatal death. *Pediatrics* 62:166–70.

Segal, S., M. Fletcher, and W. G. Meekison. 1986. A survey of bereaved parents. *Can Med Assoc J* 134:38–42.

Spinetta, J., J. Swarner, and J. Sheposh. 1981. Effective parental coping following the death of a child from cancer. *J Pediatr Psychol* 6:251–63.

Vance, J. C., F. M. Boyle, J. M. Najman, and M. J. Thearle. 1995a. Gender differences in parental psychological distress following perinatal death or sudden infant death syndrome. *Br J Psychiatry* 167:806–11.

Vance, J. C., J. M. Najman, M. J. Thearle, G. Embelton, W. J. Foster, and F. M. Boyle. 1995b. Psychological changes in parents eight months after the loss of an infant from stillbirth, neonatal death, or sudden infant death syndrome: a longitudinal study. *Pediatrics* 96:933–38.

Ventura, S. J., W. D. Mosher, S. C. Curtin, J. C. Abma, and S. Henshaw. 2001. *National Vital Statistics Reports* 49(4):1–10.

Weisman, A. D., J. W. Worden, and H. J. Sobel. 1997. Psychosocial screening and intervention with cancer patients. Final report of the Omega Project (CA19797). Bethesda, Md.: National Cancer Institute.

Weiss, L., D. Frischer, and J. Richman. 1989. Parental adjustment to intrapartum and delivery room loss: the role of a hospital-based support program. *Clin Perinatol* 16: 1009–19.

Wolfelt, A. 1997. *Healing the bereaved child: grief gardening, growth through grief and other touchstones for caregivers.* Champaign, Ill.: Companion.

Wood, J. D., and E. Milo. 2001. Fathers' grief when a disabled child dies. *Death Studies* 25:635–61.

Worden, J. W. 1996. *Children and grief: when a parent dies.* New York: Guilford.

———. 2002. *Grief counseling and grief therapy.* New York: Springer.

Worden, J. W., and J. Monahan. 2001. Caring for bereaved parents. In *Hospice care for children,* ed. A. Armstrong-Dailey and S. Zarbock, 122–39. 2d ed. New York: Oxford University Press.

The Other Side of Caring: Caregiver Suffering

Cynda H. Rushton, D.N.Sc., R.N., F.A.A.N.

Caring for children with life-threatening conditions and for their families can be a source of profound satisfaction, renewal, and affirmation. Sharing the journey with sick and dying children and their families is a privilege that only a few experience. For these caregivers, suffering for and with is an integral dimension of caring.

By definition, to care includes to suffer with, to share solidarity. Suffering for and with another person ignites our innate capacities for compassionate action. Caring for others signifies concern or interest in them as persons and in their well-being. It involves creating and sustaining relationships, emotional involvement, and a commitment to act on behalf of another; it connotes a strong sense of responsibility to attend to the holistic needs of another and, in the case of health care professionals, to provide needed services.

The act of caring for seriously ill and dying children demands compassion, sympathy, and empathy, three closely related responses. *Compassion* involves sharing and being touched by another's experience. *Sympathy* includes concern for the welfare of another, and *empathy* implies identification with the experience of another. For the caregiver, each response has the potential to create meaning, satisfaction, and renewal. But another side of care and caring must also be acknowledged: caring so much carries a cost.

Professionals who witness the pain and suffering of children and their families may also experience pain and suffering themselves. Health professionals may experience frustration and anguish as they observe the struggles of children against formidable odds and of parents grappling with some of the most difficult decisions a family can ever confront. Children bear the consequences of disease, injury, and medical technology in an often-hectic health care environment. Professionals face demands that are at times unrelenting, and they accomplish their tasks under high personal and professional tension. Ethical dilemmas grow as some children's lives end before their potential is reached and other children suffer too long before dying.

Caring for these children and their families requires specialized knowledge and skill, sustained relationships, and courageous advocacy. It draws on tremendous physical, emotional, and spiritual energies from health care professionals. When demands exceed their resources, their sense of integrity and self-worth is threatened. They begin to wonder what threshold of suffering they will be asked to endure. Clearly, when suffering becomes so great that it threatens the professional's sense of identity and integrity, it can no longer be justified (Rushton 1992). Health care professionals are not expected to be martyrs or to sacrifice their own well-being to carry out their caregiving roles. Nor can they be expected to deliver high-quality care when their integrity has been shattered.

A high school junior, 16-year-old Mark has a four-year history of osteogenic sarcoma of the leg subsequently recurring in several other locations. Mark is an attractive, gregarious adolescent who excels in everything he attempts. Each recurrence of his cancer has been treated with extensive surgical resection and multiple chemotherapeutic regimens. Most recently the tumor recurred in the spine. It was surgically debulked; stabilization rods and radiation implants were inserted. After the initial treatment, he was referred for an autologous bone marrow transplant as the best option for possible cure. During the preparation phase, the tumor continued to enlarge, causing spinal cord compression that required aggressive surgical intervention. After several weeks, the bone marrow transplant was performed. Recurrent infections, medically managed renal failure, and wound dehiscence have complicated the posttransplant period. Mark became bedridden because of the neurologic impairment of his spine, the large back wound that required frequent cleaning, debridement, packing, and constant diarrhea. He is often in pain that is treated with patient-controlled analgesia.

Mark has always been an independent youngster; always meticulous about his appearance, he prided himself on his self-sufficiency. Mark's dependence on the nurses and his family for care of his basic human needs is devastating for him. He often apologizes for needing to be cleaned up, one more time. The nurses caring for him empathize with his suffering and respond with compassion to the indignity of the disease and the assault of treatment on his self-image. They treat him with the utmost respect, physically and emotionally. They take aggressive measures to restore his dignity by whatever means possible—by maintaining his privacy, allowing him choices, and honoring the coping mechanisms he uses to deal with his treatment and disease. They aggressively advocate for management of his pain and spend time with him, listening to his concerns while keeping silent in order to honor him.

Anna, an 8-month-old infant with perinatally acquired HIV, has been hospitalized repeatedly with a variety of HIV-related health problems, including opportunistic infections, recurrent fever and sepsis, thrombocytopenia, impaired myocardial function, chronic diarrhea, encephalopathy, failure to thrive, and developmental delay. Six weeks ago, she was admitted to the hospital with respiratory distress, poor oxygenation, and failure to thrive. Her respiratory compromise worsened, and she was electively intubated and placed on mechanical ventilation. Her liver and spleen were greatly enlarged; myocardial function diminished secondary to cardiomyopathy. Over the next week, she required maximal ventilatory support and oxygen supplementation and was unable to wean from the ventilator. She also experienced pain from muscle aches, mouth sores, candidiasis, hepatosplenomegaly, and frequent painful procedures.

When Anna was 5 months old, her 19-year-old mother died of AIDS-related complications. Anna had been placed in foster care as a newborn because of her mother's age and history of drug abuse and Anna's positive toxicology screen at birth. Anna's grandmother was unable to care for her because of her own history of schizophrenia and because she was the focus of an active protective service case for child neglect. Because no other relatives were available to assume her care, Anna became a ward of the state. She was initially cared for by her specially trained foster mother, but as Anna's condition worsened, it became necessary to admit her to a chronic care facility for children.

As Anna's condition continues to deteriorate, controversy regarding the goals of her treatment is emerging among the health care team. On admission to the intensive care unit, she is treated aggressively for respiratory failure and multisystem organ failure. Multiple therapies have been instituted, some unsubstantiated in the treatment of AIDS-related syndromes in children. Some members of the health care team believe that, since their understanding of the trajectory in children with AIDS is evolving, it is imperative that she be treated aggressively. The nurses caring for Anna are increasingly concerned about the level of her pain and the extent of painful interventions to maintain her life. After numerous attempts to provide adequate analgesic relief, they believe that Anna is still undermedicated for her pain. The nurses believe that Anna is dying and that the interventions they are providing are merely prolonging her suffering.

The situation is further complicated because the state is Anna's legal guardian and must therefore be involved in any decisions to initiate or forgo treatment. Decision making thus is compromised by the bureaucratic process and by the fact that her primary nurse, primary health provider, and social worker have all assumed major roles in acting as advocate for Anna in the absence of an individual who has an ongoing relationship with her and can advocate for her interests. As long as there is controversy among the members of her care team, the state is unlikely to decide to withhold or withdraw treatment. (Adapted from Rushton et al. 1993)

Shared human encounters give rise to an empathetic identification by the health care professional with the patient's suffering. In Mark's case, these encounters are perceived as compassionate responses to his condition. His caregivers are able to honor him as a person and to believe that their actions are congruent with their professional values and ideals. In contrast, moral tension and distress among the care team, whose members disagree on what will best serve the patient, mark Anna's case. Some of Anna's caregivers feel that they are being asked to act against their moral beliefs, thereby diminishing their integrity. In the absence of a single advocate for Anna's interests, moral tension is heightened by conflicts among those acting as surrogates. Certainly, each clinical situation would ideally have outcomes similar to Mark's case, yet the ideal is often difficult to achieve.

Several factors seem to influence clinical experiences, particularly those involving children with life-threatening conditions. First, the context for providing palliative and end-of-life care is fraught with the ambiguities that accompany such conditions. Decisions regarding treatment for these children inevitably must be made under conditions of uncertainty. Determining the child's best interests can be particularly difficult when the diagnosis, prognosis, or disease trajectory is unclear. In such cases, assessing the benefits or burdens that will result from treatment or nontreatment admits of no easy solution.

The unpredictability of a child's response to treatment may motivate caregivers or parents to try to reduce the uncertainty by pursuing additional diagnostic studies and innovative therapies. This creates ambiguity and controversy about whether the child's condition is reversible or represents the terminal phase of the disease. Depending on how the uncertainty is viewed, either as threat or opportunity, caregivers or parents may be willing in some instances to accept a greater degree of burden to give the child an opportunity for a longer life and the possibility of future beneficial treatments (Mischel, Shoda, and Peake, 1988). At times, however, the quest for absolute certainty may result in disproportionate burden on the patient. In cases like Anna's, nurses or other health care professionals may experience frustration and ridicule if they question the plan or suggest that the burden of treatment has exceeded the benefit of sustaining life or that the desire to innovate or scientific curiosity has supplanted patient goals.

Second, technological achievements in neonatal and pediatric care have created unanticipated dilemmas as powerful diagnostic techniques, sophisticated surgical procedures, effective drugs, and expedient therapeutic interventions have interrupted the usual course of illness and disability. Problems are magnified because life can be sustained for a significant period if the patient accepts dependence on a specific procedure or machine. The uncertainties and ambiguities that result from disease, injury, and the use of technology often force health care professionals to demand cure in the absence of otherwise compelling evidence to choose a different course.

Even in providing routine care, health care professionals must balance competing obligations to their institutions, their co-workers, and themselves as individuals. Situations can and do arise in which the safety and quality of care are jeopardized as a result of institutional policies, lack of administrative support, interprofessional and intraprofessional conflicts, or legal constraints. Cases like Mark's and Anna's, in which patient acuity and the intensity of interventions are high, carry increased risk of provider errors (Institute of Medicine 2000). Institutional decisions to admit every critically ill patient despite limited resources exacerbate such risks and create intense moral distress among health care professionals. The end result—despite efforts of caregivers to put on a professional face and appear "strong"—is all too often a downward spiral of mistakes, guilt, diminished self-esteem, and suboptimal patient care. The provision of care that is incongruent with the core values of health care professionals threatens their self-image and integrity.

In addition to the conflicts within health care itself, Anna's case illustrates the convergence of societal ills in one troubled inner-city family beset by poverty, drug and alcohol abuse, illness, violence, and grief. In the face of these overpowering misfortunes, Anna's caregivers struggle to make a difference in her life and to protect her interests. No small task, this requires that they balance their values as professionals with the realities of Anna's care, while only the state is allowed to speak on her behalf. They must also acknowledge that the medical model is inadequate to address social problems such as those facing Anna, and they struggle to find some way to accommodate the tensions that result from this fact.

Suffering

DEFINITION

The experiences of suffering and loss are intrinsic and inevitable dimensions of caring for children with life-threatening conditions. According to Reich (1989), suffering is "an anguish experienced as a threat to our composure, our integrity, the fulfillment of our intentions, and more deeply as a frustration to the concrete meaning that we have found in our personal experience. It is the anguish over the injury or threat of injury to the self and thus the meaning of the self that is at the core of suffering." This construct clarifies why professionals caring for critically ill children feel threatened if they get too close to the child and allow themselves to experience grief. At the most profound level, they fear that this level of intimacy will threaten their ability to continue to function in their professional roles (Barnard 1995).

In such instances, caregivers struggle to find the place of integrity in their relationships so that they do not suffer for and with others to the point of their own demise. As they fulfill their obligations and expectations as professionals, they may encounter threats to their ideal of their profession and professional goals, their self-image, moral character, and personal identity. They may judge themselves harshly if the hoped-for outcomes do not occur, if they are treated with disrespect or punished by other health care professionals or the institution in which they practice, or if they fail to act because they lack skills or courage. The assault on their basic values—their understanding of life, death, disability, and relationships—may compromise how they perceive the meaning of their work. Disruptions may emerge as changes in the health professional's autonomy, moral well-being, character, or self-esteem and can manifest themselves in many ways in the care the professional provides.

Whether real or imagined, caregivers' powerlessness—the inability to cause or prevent change—contributes to their suffering and undermines moral agency. A health care professional's perceived inability to minimize or eliminate tragic outcomes brings on feelings of powerlessness and help-lessness. These feeling are magnified when professionals feel that they have no control over their practice, no input into the treatment plan, or no recourse in carrying out a plan they find morally objectionable, such as providing painful treatments to dying patients. In short, if they believe that they receive little, if any, legitimization by other members of the health care team or the institution in which they practice, their moral agency is threatened. Enforc-ing rules or imposing policies that limit or discount the legitimate role of nurses or other health care professionals in the decision-making process ren-ders them powerless, suppresses their values, and ultimately undermines their capacity for compassion (Rushton 1995).

Understanding these threats is the key to understanding caregivers' suf-fering. Underlying them all is a threat to the individual's integrity, that inter-nal state of wholeness in all dimensions of a person's being—physical, emo-tional, and spiritual. Integrity relies on the balance and harmony of the various dimensions of human existence. Because we are whole beings, suf-fering occurs at the level of the whole being (Singh 1998). Threats to bodily integrity, for instance, can manifest as disease, injury, or illness. For caregivers, the occurrence of physical symptoms may reflect their own suffering within their professional roles. In like manner, psychological integrity may be under-mined by a disintegration of the self by psychopathology or threats to person-hood. The self-image of health professionals can be undermined by various threats, from unrealistic expectations, suppressed feelings that mute the authentic self, and maladaptive coping to dysfunctional relationships and communication. Because spiritual integrity involves an integration of moral character, adherence to moral norms, and coherent and consistent behavior within a set of principles or commitments, it too is vulnerable to disruptions. For caregivers, treatment decisions may threaten their understanding of jus-tified and unjustified burdens, obscure or extinguish the meaning of their work, or even lead to a crisis of faith. Consider the two cases described earlier in this chapter: in Mark's case, caregivers' integrity was promoted; in Anna's case, it was fractured.

Among the threats to the integrity of health care professionals are arbitrary or capricious decisions that are made and acted on. Such actions may alienate them from their convictions and cause them to neglect what matters most—in many cases, their sense of being a "good" physician, nurse, social worker, or other professional. When caregivers act in a way they believe to be wrong, their loss of integrity results in suffering. Physicians, nurses, child-life specialists, social workers, chaplains, and others may struggle to determine whether they did all they could to help a child or whether they missed any signs or symptoms that could have altered the outcome, were inaccurate in diagnosis, or did not fulfill their professional obligations or the dictates of their moral code. Their expectations and desire to alleviate or improve the patient's condition often frame their sense of what is required in their role. They may believe that if they "try hard enough" or are "smart enough," they can accomplish the outcomes they desire. When death is the outcome, their self-image may be altered, their integrity compromised because the outcome is incongruent with the ideals of their profession (Rushton 1995).

The health care professional's sense of doing the right thing may also be challenged, particularly in the face of significant ambiguity and uncertainty. The questions that may arise include the following:

- Am I helping or harming this child by the treatments I am providing?
- Can I live with the image of myself as a doctor, nurse, and so on if I carry out a particular action?
- Can I live with the choices that I have made on behalf of this patient?
- Can I live with my participation in implementing the choices made by others (health care professional, parents, and administrators)?

Each of these questions reflects a concern about acting in a way that undermines the health care professional's sense of integrity.

Suffering can arise intermittently or be sustained over long periods. The intensity of Mark's suffering increased when procedures were performed that caused the loss of his bodily, psychological, and spiritual integrity. Through their responses, Mark's nurses transformed his suffering into compassionate action and healed their own threatened integrity. By contrast, Anna's caregivers were unable to transform their suffering into compassionate action.

The repeated threats to their integrity resulted in a sense of alienation from their self-identity, the goals of treatment, and the integrity of their work.

Tattlebaum (1989) differentiates suffering from painful feelings; suffering is the "persistence of painful feelings long after they were provoked." In other words, suffering results when pain leaves an indelible imprint on the psyche of the person experiencing it. We are hardwired, it seems, to remember our pain; integrating its details into both conscious and unconscious parts of our psyche. Caregivers often can recount the events surrounding a situation that caused them suffering many years later, with more vivid detail than they can give for an event occurring only a few days previously. When a suffering experience is unprocessed or unresolved and remains in the unconscious, the response to it will most likely reappear whenever similar experiences of pain or grief occur or may appear as inappropriate or disproportionate responses to other situations.

The experience of suffering often leaves the person feeling exposed and vulnerable. At its root is the sense of having no control over one's destiny, of submitting to or being forced to endure some particular set of circumstances (Hauerwas 1986). This view of suffering as a passive process tends to leave the person feeling victimized and powerless; it is often reinforced by a view of suffering as an inevitable part of certain experiences, diseases, or roles. Some believe that suffering has redemptive value and "builds character"; others hold that it reveals, rather than builds, character. Regardless of the meaning assigned to the experience of suffering, both positive and negative consequences are possible.

RELATED CONCEPTS

Several concepts—burnout, compassion fatigue syndrome, and moral distress—are related to the concept of caregiver suffering. The terms *burnout* and *compassion fatigue syndrome* describe the sense of being disconnected from oneself that characterizes caregiver suffering. Burnout is "a state of physical, emotional, and mental exhaustion caused by long-term involvement in emotionally demanding situations" (Pines and Aronson 1988, 9). It emerges gradually and is a result of emotional exhaustion and job stress. In contrast, compassion fatigue is characterized by a sense of helplessness, confusion, and isolation from supporters and can have a more rapid onset and resolution than burnout (Figley 1995).

Moral distress occurs when an individual is unable to translate his or her moral choices into action (Jameton 1993). Acting in a manner contrary to

Table 9.1. Factors that may threaten caregiver integrity

Internal	External
• Powerlessness	• Institutional policies, priorities, or values
• Competing obligations	• Lack of administrative support
• Value conflicts	• Interprofessional and intraprofessional conflicts
• Inability to articulate the ethical problem or source of suffering	• Interpersonal disrespect
• Conscience violations	• Disintegrated models of care delivery
• Lack of knowledge or skill	• Legal, regulatory, or financial constraints
• Lack of confidence	• Politics of "being in the middle"
• Lack of awareness	• Responsibility without authority
• Misplaced guilt, blame, or shame	

personal or professional values undermines the individual's sense of integrity. When health care professionals cannot live up to their personal values by acting in an ethical manner, their suffering is compounded by moral distress.

Initially, persons in moral distress may experience feelings of frustration, anger, and anxiety in response to the obstacles and conflicts with others about important values. Once the need for action is recognized, they then respond to their real or perceived inability to act on their initial moral distress. This process involves an appraisal of how the situation and the actions taken or not taken promote or undermine integrity or result in participation in actions that they view as wrong (Jameton 1993).

At the core of each concept is the sense of loss—loss of integrity, self-image, relationships, and hopes for the future—and of grief in the face of loss. For health care professionals, this includes threats to their integrity when they cannot resolve core issues. They may feel unable to honor their core commitments to their patients, for example, or incapable of seeing dignified death as a healing act.

Many interrelated factors may undermine the integrity of health care professionals, cause moral distress, and ultimately result in caregiver suffering. Many of the factors listed in table 9.1 have also been associated with burnout and compassion fatigue syndrome. For instance, institutional policies and politics may lead to a sense of powerlessness; in like manner, other external causes of moral distress work their way through to internal manifestations.

This dynamic may exist between and among internal and external factors threatening integrity; for example, a lack of confidence might result in interprofessional and intraprofessional conflicts.

THE EXPERIENCE

By nature subjective and unique to the person experiencing it, suffering is intensely personal and private. With its potential to transform or destroy, suffering can be the catalyst for self-understanding and growth or it can erode a person's sense of integrity and undermine physical, emotional, and spiritual health. Suffering can signify a sense of endurance, perseverance, and courage rather than disintegration and degradation. The cause of suffering, according to Tattlebaum (1989), is not the situation or its consequences but rather the way the individual views and responds to the situation.

A compassionate response to suffering fosters empathy and connection rather than alienation or isolation. Health care professionals witness the suffering that accompanies illness or injury—the indignities and the damage to the patient's self-image, the depletion of financial and human resources, the stress of parents who desperately hope for their child's recovery, and the anxiety born of the sense of powerlessness in a situation beyond their control. Health care professionals suffer because they understand and identify with the sufferings of the patient and family.

Nurses experience this suffering in a particularly intimate way. Their roles place them in the most sustained proximity to the patient, and they directly carry out the treatment plan. They witness the impact of their ministrations on the child and family and sometimes struggle to make sense of interventions they may view as harmful or senseless. This intimate connection gives nurses the opportunity to confront their own mortality and losses. Nurses and other health care professionals who are parents confront the fragility of their own children's lives and their inability to protect them from disease or injury. Caring deeply and genuinely for patients as individuals involves identifying with their experiences while acknowledging their independent existence and experience. Nurses demonstrate compassion by their presence, their attunement to the patient, and the actions they take to relieve the patient's physical, emotional, or spiritual distress.

Parents and health care professionals experience an unspeakable sense of grief and failure when a child is dying. This often leads them to try to eliminate any uncertainty surrounding treatment. When interventions do not yield the desired outcome, health care professionals question whether they have done everything within their power to help the child. They may compartmentalize the child's care into organ systems and examine the evidence for any suggestion of progress; they may consider interventions and approaches that have not been proved useful in a particular population. If health care professionals view death as a failure, then doing everything becomes the modus operandi to forestall the inevitable threat to their integrity. In such instances, efforts to avoid "failure" may contribute to clinical practices that result in premature declarations of futility or, alternately, overtreatment that is burdensome to the patient.

Feelings of guilt have many dimensions. For parents, such feelings may manifest themselves as the guilt of helplessness, survivorship, and ambivalence, perceived misdeeds, shame, or codependence (Miller and Ober 1999). While some of these are particular to parental grief, Miller and Ober's (1999) data suggest that health care professionals may manifest similar forms of grief, although clearly of a lesser magnitude. For example, professionals may experience feelings of guilt at their inability to prevent the child's death. This guilt often results in blaming self or others for the failure of medical interventions or in expressions of regret and remorse. Health care professionals may also feel the guilt of ambivalence about their responses to the child and his or her family, their advocacy efforts, or their attentiveness to the child or family. In some cases, this ambivalence leads to shameful feelings and loss of self-esteem. For professionals, as for parents, the most profound form is causal guilt, guilt that accompanies an unspoken suspicion that in some way they caused the child's death—either by contributing to, failing to prevent, or figuratively causing the death through acts of omission or commission. At its core, this is the guilt of perceived responsibility for the child's death.

RESPONSES

Caregiver suffering may present itself through a wide array of symptoms, as shown in table 9.2. These symptoms, or responses, cluster in four main categories: physical, emotional, behavioral, and spiritual. Individual caregivers display varying patterns of responses to suffering. Distinctions among the categories are not always clear; for example, fatigue and depression may be closely linked. Distinctions between emotional and behavioral responses are even more difficult to draw. Sarcasm may be considered a distancing behavior, and resentment an avoidance response. It may be helpful to identify emotional responses as feelings, internal in nature, and behavioral responses as actions, or external.

Table 9.2. Common symptoms of caregiver suffering

Physical	Emotional	Behavioral	Spiritual
• Fatigue	• Fear	• Addictive behavior	• Crisis of faith
• Exhaustion	• Guilt	• Controlling behavior	• Loss of control
• Lethargy	• Resentment	• Shaming others	• Hopelessness
• Hyperactivity	• Sorrow	• Offended behavior	• Loss of self-worth
• Weight gain	• Depression	• Victim behavior	• Disrupted religious practices
• Weight loss	• Grief	• Depersonalization	• Disconnection with people,
• Persistent physical ailments	• Anxiety	• Apathy	work, community
(headaches, gastrointestinal	• Confusion	• Indifference	
disturbances)	• Sarcasm	• Avoidance	
• Impaired sleep	• Emotional outbursts	• Boundary violations	
• Impaired mental processes	• Emotional shutdown	• Erosion of relationships	
• Susceptibility to illness	• Feeling overwhelmed		
	• Cynicism		

Some individuals may find themselves seeking a physician's help with persistent gastrointestinal problems, for example, while ignoring their underlying suffering. Others may find anger "easier" than emotionality or the admission of suspect behaviors. Professionals who feel they were constrained from taking the moral actions they believed to be right may respond with resentment. Others may experience guilt because they believe they lacked the courage to do what they knew was right. In cases like Anna's, caregivers experience guilt when they believe they have inflicted pain and suffering on their patient. In some instances, health care professionals experience emotional shutdown and become so disconnected from their own emotions that they no longer feel capable of compassion or engagement with others.

Like physical and emotional symptoms, behavioral responses take many different forms. Avoidance behaviors are common among professionals who feel victimized and powerless. These include avoiding contact with the patient or family, developing a pattern of absenteeism, and making frequent job changes. Addictive behaviors range from self-medication with drugs or alcohol to gambling or other less overtly destructive activities, such as compulsive shopping and workaholism.

Another category of behavioral response involves shaming or victimizing others. For example, some individuals adopt attitudes of arrogance or superiority based on their credentials, expertise, or role and use their status to disrespect, discount, or minimize the expertise or contributions of others. Some adopt "offended" behaviors to protect themselves at the expense of others, making themselves essentially impenetrable to human dimensions and situations. Some professionals resort to focusing on the behaviors of others rather than taking responsibility for their own behavior or participation; this may contribute to a failure to engage in moral discourse with others, undermining community integrity. Beyond these, there may be a pervasive expression of indifference and cynicism.

Boundary violations, either constricted or diffuse, can be another issue for caregivers. Health care professionals may employ constrictive controlling behaviors to create a sense of safety from the uncertain and unpredictable events inherent in caring for children with life-threatening conditions. Their rigidity may manifest itself in lack of flexibility in their own actions and thought or as criticism of others who do not practice in the same way or share the same beliefs and values.

This rigidity often presents with distancing behaviors, such as emotional withdrawal, physical isolation, and superficial or cool interactions with patients,

patients' families, and colleagues. Other distancing behaviors include rage, hostility, or distraction in a flurry of activity (keeping busy to avoid experiencing the feelings). For health care professionals who believe death represents failure, distancing behaviors may be an attempt to avoid situations that arouse feelings of guilt, sorrow, or grief.

Diffuse boundary violations are also indicative of caregiver suffering. They include patterns of overinvolvement with patients and their families to meet personal needs and behaviors that have been labeled as codependent. Inappropriate disclosures and interactions, including breeches of confidentiality, are also symptoms of diffuse boundary violations. Whether diffuse or constricted, boundary violations can undermine relationships is every sphere—personal, professional, and community.

Threats to one's spiritual integrity may manifest as feelings of loss of meaning in one's role or work, relationships, or life in general. Health care professionals who experience cumulative suffering may search for meaning in their work in the face of pain and suffering. Some individuals may experience a crisis of their faith in God or a higher being. Questions about how and why the suffering of children is permitted may arise. Loss of spiritual integrity can also result in a disruption in religious practices and disconnection with relationships, work, or community. Feelings of hopelessness, loss of control, and diminished self-worth pervade threats to spiritual integrity.

When suffering becomes severe and unacknowledged, the result can be described as soul pain, "the experience of an individual who has become disconnected and alienated from the deepest and most fundamental aspects of himself or herself" (Kearney 1996, 63). The intense distress inherent in soul pain creates an overwhelming need to do something to alleviate painful feelings. This need may manifest itself in the symptoms and behaviors discussed earlier. When soul pain and its manifestations lead to the loss of confidence, erosion of self-esteem, and loss of integrity, individuals may compensate by constantly seeking the approval of others or compartmentalizing themselves.

The physical symptoms arising from underlying suffering may intensify and fail to respond to usual treatments. Behavioral responses, at least initially, tend to be characterized by denial. Because it is too threatening to accept that some children will not benefit from their efforts, health care professionals deny that the treatment they are providing may be overly burdensome or may compromise important values. Instead, they narrowly focus on the functioning of individual body systems of the patient rather than integrate efforts to address the holistic needs of the patient and family. The temporary reassurance this gives ultimately results in alienation and disconnection as the evidence of impending death escalates. Denial of the possibility of death and the impact of the death on the caregiver can give way to feelings of emptiness, hopelessness, numbness, and meaninglessness. Unable to experience feelings, they no longer respond to the suffering of others and of themselves. In essence, they deny—or, more precisely, try to deny—the existence of suffering.

Strategies to Address Caregiver Suffering

The suffering of health care professionals in their caregiving roles is real. The framework of integrity provides a roadmap for preserving and reclaiming the integrity of the persons providing care to children with life-threatening conditions. If integrity is the goal, health care professionals and the institutions in which they practice must share a vision of the behaviors and character traits they value. In such an environment, persons of integrity consistently exhibit the virtue of integrity, honoring the integrity of self and others. They understand that integrity encompasses autonomy but is not synonymous with self-determining actions or the exertion of their will on others. As persons of integrity, they are willing to subject their views to scrutiny and criticism. They engage in a process of assessing good and bad reasons for making concessions in situations in which values conflict. They are committed to revising or reassessing principles based on an open process of analysis that leads to justifiable moral modifications. Persons of integrity cultivate trust through their trustworthy behaviors, relationships, and commitments; they honor the boundaries and limits of relationships (Pellegrino 1990).

Creating an environment that allows caregivers to practice with integrity is no simple task. Strategies to promote the integrity of the person being cared for, that person's family, the health care professional, the institution, and the community require multipronged efforts. Only through a commitment to a shared vision can health care professionals and institutions successfully affect the experience of suffering and its effect on the quality of patient care.

The process of addressing this important issue involves much more than individual interventions. Initially, single-discipline sessions may help create trust and illuminate the issues. For interdisciplinary sharing and problem solving to occur, the entire care team needs to participate in interdisciplinary forums in which they can discuss suffering and define coping strategies.

To accept and understand the suffering of others, health care professionals must first acknowledge the existence of it and relate to their own suffering and emotions with compassion, tenderness, and forgiveness. The ability to identify the sources of and responses to suffering can ease the process of transforming suffering into meaning. Although sharing suffering makes it bearable, it involves participation in the entire process not only in an isolated moment of pain. This entails recognizing the suffering of others and being willing to enter into a dynamic process with them to help give meaning to the experience. For health care professionals, making sense of situations that undermine their integrity requires an environment of trust: they must feel free to honestly express what they think and feel, without censoring their comments and obscuring who they really are.

The Latin root of the word *suffering* means "to allow" or "to experience," yet our natural inclination is to try to relieve ourselves of feelings of sadness, anguish, and despair. The most healing approach may be to simply reside with and experience the full pain of our loss and suffering. Although professionals are often unable to extinguish their own suffering or the suffering of others, bearing witness allows them to lend their nonjudgmental presence to others and to acknowledge their own suffering, which they might otherwise ignore. This can help them acknowledge suffering as an integral dimension of their practice—a reality that many may wish to deny.

DEVELOPING FORUMS FOR DISCUSSION, REFLECTION, AND SHARED UNDERSTANDING

Forums can help give voice to suffering. Small interdisciplinary and unidisciplinary groups can be an important strategy for building community and openness. Facilitated discussions in these forums can provide the freedom and the safety health care professionals need to discuss moral issues and the intense feelings associated with the experience of suffering. Creating a safe place in which to share the disappointments, fears, and concerns about patient situations can help caregivers as they struggle to identify the sources of suffering, responses, and ways of creating meaning. Telling their own stories and listening to their co-workers' stories can help them negotiate meaning and make sense of incomprehensible and confusing situations.

Stories help because the meaning an individual assigns to a particular situation is unique, derived from a unique set of influences that include social, cultural, familial, religious, and political values. Understanding this context gives insight into how meaning is derived, and the search for meaning can lead to understanding. This understanding does not simply mean "knowing" certain facts or concepts; rather, it requires integrating information into one's values, beliefs, and commitments. Finding meaning is a way for us to make sense of the experience of patients, their families, and ourselves, all of whom are served by our interdisciplinary teams.

Reich (1989) suggests four questions to guide professionals as they struggle to make sense of their own suffering and the suffering they witness and inflict on patients under their care:

- How can I see myself as a healer in the face of death and profound suffering?
- What gives meaning to me personally?
- What gives meaning to my work?
- How have I grown personally or professionally as a result of this experience?

Facilitators of groups aimed at addressing caregiver suffering must be respectful, skillful, and trustworthy with respect to the emotions and responses elicited by the suffering and grief of others. For this reason, it is desirable to have a person with specialized expertise in group facilitation who is not a direct member of the health care team but whom the team trusts to facilitate these discussions.

CREATING AN ENVIRONMENT OF RESPECT
FOR PATIENTS, FAMILIES, AND CAREGIVERS

Although health care professionals and organizations hold respect to be a core value, disrespect is often pervasive in the health care environment and can contribute to erosion of integrity and consequent caregiver suffering. Disrespect can arise within interactions with patients and families, with other health care professionals, and with administrators. When people are not treated with respect, it is less likely that they will treat others or themselves with respect.

Creating an environment of respect requires a robust understanding of the needs of individuals and the institutions in which they practice. Respect is an intentional act of acknowledging the integrity of another person. It involves valuing the knowledge, skill, and diversity of each person, whether patient, family member, health care professional, or other. Respect invites us to see beyond the characteristics, personality, role, title, or discipline of others to appreciate the essence of who they are. An environment of respect creates norms of behavior that breed trust and integrity.

Respect does not imply agreement on every decision, value, or behavior. Rather, it is demonstrated in how one deals with conflict and diversity. Respect cannot be demanded; it must be earned through trustworthy actions. Respect requires that members of an organization respect themselves, since without self-respect externally imposed norms or structures are unlikely to create respect for others.

FOSTERING RESPECTFUL COMMUNICATION, DECISION MAKING, AND CONFLICT RESOLUTION

Creating norms of communication and decision making based on respect and integrity provides the foundation for addressing suffering. Caregivers are more likely to experience the negative dimensions of suffering when they perceive that they are marginalized from the process of decision making. The same is true when the goals of care are communicated unclearly or left unsaid and when there is no mechanism for resolving conflicting goals and values within the team in a respectful manner.

One "safe" way to foster dialogue about palliative and end-of-life care and caregiver suffering is to establish regular interdisciplinary care rounds. Medical and nursing leadership can play an important role in establishing, and making routine, ongoing discussions of this type. Palliative care and ethics rounds, or educational events using a case-based format, can focus on the source of suffering, the varied responses, and ways of creating meaning. They can also provide forums in which health care professionals can discuss challenging patient care situations and engage in problem solving and care planning to address potential threats to integrity in a proactive manner. In addition, integrating indicators of the quality of palliative care into morbidity and mortality conferences can help diminish the intensity and frequency of situations that threaten the integrity of health care professionals. When particular cases are creating caregiver suffering, patient care conferences and institutional mechanisms for examining and resolving conflict, such as ethics consultations, can provide supportive structures and processes for caregivers.

CREATING MECHANISMS FOR ACKNOWLEDGING AND PROCESSING GRIEF AND LOSS

Responses to patients' deaths affect health care professionals both personally and professionally in caregiver suffering and responses to grief. Papadatou identifies special considerations for health care professionals facing the death of pediatric patients. These include the level of investment in the relationship with the patient and family, expectations of the health care professional's identity and roles, and personal or social constructs. Each death can affect one or more levels of loss:

- loss of the relationship with the patient
- loss owing to identification with the pain of the patient's family
- loss of unmet goals and expectations of the professional self-image
- loss of beliefs and assumptions about self, life, and death
- past unresolved or future anticipated losses
- the death of one's own self (Papadatou 2000)

Interventions to address health care professionals' needs to acknowledge and process their own grief and loss will be necessary to promote healthy grieving and restore integrity. Such interventions would be aimed at several tasks:

- managing their emotional responses to the death in ways that work for them
- restoring or maintaining their professional integrity
- finding meaning in the death
- transcending the present suffering so that they might reinvest in life (Sanders and Valente 1994; Papadatou 2000)

Approaches that are aimed at providing information, clinical reviews, and emotional support facilitate meaning making. Activities such as debriefing sessions after a child dies can help create a space for grief and provide caregivers with opportunities to reflect on the events leading to a child's death, the meaning of the child's life and death to the health care professionals, personal responses, and self-care strategies. Debriefing sessions also provide health care professionals an opportunity to identify things that went well and opportunities for future changes in practices and structures.

TRANSFORMING SUFFERING BY CREATING MEANING

In the search for meaning, the critical task is to transform suffering into an act of healing. This transformation requires nurturing compassion rather than yielding to the negative and destructive dimensions of suffering. Accomplishing this depends in large part on the recognition that compassion can affect the experience of suffering. The search for meaning requires that physical, emotional, psychosocial, and spiritual needs be addressed. Individuals will often need additional support and encouragement to move beyond their denial of these manifestations of their suffering and to begin to engage in activities that will assist them in their own process. Resources such as employee assistance programs and referrals to personal coaches and mental health professionals should be made available. Beyond this lies an opportunity for "depth" work to achieve an experience of soul. Meditation, bodywork, working with imagery and dreams, and participation in creative arts or music can help the soul reconnect with significant and meaningful aspects of living. Mindfulness meditation programs for health care professionals or programs that focus on restoring meaning to professional work can be particularly helpful.

Meaning making can also be supported through memorial rituals, be they formal services or creation of a living memorial, such as a butterfly garden. Many institutions have annual tribute services to honor and remember the children who have died in their care. Similarly, some institutions are developing regular memorial services and rituals, enabling the staff to acknowledge the children they care for and to create opportunities for closure, especially when it is not possible for them to attend the funeral or family memorial service.

DEVELOPING SELF-CARE PRACTICES

Health care professionals need to develop self-care practices for themselves and their colleagues. Practices as simple as regular exercise, leisure activities with friends and family, solitary time for reflection and renewal, or reaching out to other professionals with a kind word and compassionate query have great value. All too often, professionals look to their own needs last. They must remember that they have certain duties to themselves, duties that must be given moral weight within the boundaries of professional responsibility. A newly added plank in the American Nurses Association's (2001) Code of Ethics for Nurses includes such recommendations and should help nurses as they work to lessen caregiver suffering within their profession.

Institutions must begin to invest in the health and well-being of their employees. This includes deliberate attention to aspects of the work environment that may exacerbate the suffering of health care professionals. Attention to work load, reward systems, decision-making authority, and organizational ethics are essential to an environment that promotes integrity. So too are measures that contribute to the development of personal self-care practices, including allowing employees time for self-care in the workplace. One critical care unit engages a massage therapist to give weekly seated chair massages to the staff.

CULTIVATING HEALTHY BOUNDARIES

Health care professionals caring for children with life-threatening conditions are particularly vulnerable to boundary violations. Developing processes to monitor personal and team involvement and responses to patient care situations can help them protect their integrity while allowing them to connect with others and to say no when appropriate. These efforts require the development and use of support systems to assess involvement and responses. Although it is possible to exercise advocacy without compassion, the act of caring necessitates a measure of sacrifice and suffering within appropriate boundaries. For health care professionals, this means setting proper limits for compassion and self-sacrifice for their patients and their families—and for themselves.

ADDRESSING VIOLATIONS OF INTEGRITY

Health care professionals cannot ignore violations of their integrity. Although they must make compromises, they must be able to make them conscientiously, assessing which are moral and which are not. Acting in opposition to moral principle involves self-betrayal. Integrity demands that professionals, on occasion, raise a conscientious voice and make a conscientious refusal. In some instances, this may entail responsible whistle-blowing or a conscientious exit.

Fortunately, such circumstances are relatively rare. Jameton (1993) suggests that caregivers, when confronted with an issue that threatens their integrity, ask themselves the following key questions:

- What is possible for me to do?
- What is the extent of my responsibility?
- When others are not meeting their responsibilities, what is the extent of my responsibility to compensate for their omissions?
- What personal risks are health care professionals obligated to take for patients? for their profession? for themselves?
- When I assist others who are making decisions, and the decisions prove harmful to patients, to what extent do I share the blame?

Asking these questions can clarify issues and roles in situations that threaten professional integrity. Answering them can guide caregivers in their choice of actions and support them in knowing their consciences as professionals and their own hearts as individuals.

Conclusion

Caring for sick and dying children and their families is a privilege that carries profound responsibilities and offers great rewards. By understanding and accepting suffering, caregivers are better able to deal with painful cases. The ability to recognize their own suffering empowers them to adopt strategies that protect their patients and preserve their own professional integrity.

Our capacity to feel grief and to identify with the misfortune of others is the basis of our humanity. Without the recognition of suffering, there can be no compassion, for children with life-threatening conditions and their families or for their caregivers.

References

American Nurses Association. 2001. *Code of ethics for nurses with interpretive statements.* Washington, D.C.: American Nurses Association.

Barnard, D. 1995. The promise of intimacy and the fear of our own undoing. *J Palliat Care* 11:22–26.

Figley, C. R., ed. 1995. *Compassion fatigue: coping with secondary traumatic stress disorder in those who treat the traumatized.* New York: Brunner/Mazel.

Hauerwas, S. 1986. *Suffering presence: theological reflections on medicine, the mentally handicapped and the Church.* Notre Dame, Ind.: University of Notre Dame Press.

Institute of Medicine. 2000. *To err is human.* Washington, D.C.: National Academy Press.

Jameton, A. 1993. Dilemmas of moral distress: moral responsibility and nursing practice. *AWHONN'S Clin Iss Perinatal Women's Health Nurs* 4:542–51.

Kearney, M. 1996. *Mortally wounded.* New York: Scribner.

Miller, S., and D. Ober. 1999. *Finding hope when a child dies: what other cultures can teach us.* New York: Simon and Schuster.

Mischel, W., Y. Shoda, and P. K. Peake. 1988. The nature of adolescent competencies predicted by preschool delay of gratification. *J Pers Soc Psychol* 54:687–96.

Papadatou, D. 2000. Caring for dying children: a comparative study of nurses' experiences in Greece and Hong Kong. *Cancer Nurs* 24:402–12.

Pellegrino, E. 1990. The relationship of autonomy and integrity in medical ethics. *Bull PAHO* 24:361–71.

Pines, A. M., and E. Aronson. 1988. *Career burnout: causes and cures.* New York: Free Press.

Reich, W. T. 1989. Speaking of suffering: a moral account of compassion. *Soundings* 72:83–108.

Rushton, C. H. 1992. Caregiver suffering in critical care nursing. *Heart Lung* 21:303–6.

———. 1995. The Baby K case: the ethics of preserving professional integrity. *Pediatr Nurs* 21:367–72.

Rushton, C. H., E. E. Hogue, C. A. Billet, K. Chapman, D. Greenberg-Friedman, M. Joyner, and C. D. Parks. 1993. End-of-life care for infants with AIDS: ethical and legal issues. *Pediatr Nurs* 19:79–83; 94.

Sanders, J., and S. Valente. 1994. Nurse's grief. *Cancer Nurs* 174:318–25.

Singh, K. 1998. *The grace in dying.* San Francisco: HarperCollins.

Tattlebaum, J. 1989. *You don't have to suffer: a handbook for moving beyond life's crises.* New York: Harper and Row.

PART III

SPECIAL CARE ENVIRONMENTS
AND PATIENT POPULATIONS

10

The High-Risk Newborn

Suzanne Toce, M.D., Steven R. Leuthner, M.D., M.A., Deborah Dokken, M.P.A., Brian S. Carter, M.D., F.A.A.P., and Anita Catlin, D.N.Sc., F.N.P.

Even in the highly technical environment of the neonatal intensive care unit (NICU), where intensive, invasive, and at times aggressive life-saving or life-prolonging interventions are the norm, palliative care has a role. Integrating principles of palliative care into the care of newborns and their families is not only possible but necessary. Newborns and their families, as well as the NICU staff, benefit from palliative care addressing pain and symptom management, family support, and optimization of quality of life for critically ill newborns and their families during their hospitalization, regardless of the outcome of care.

Any parent whose newborn requires resuscitation or admission to the NICU experiences numerous losses and grieves over the wished-for healthy, full-term baby (Sydnor-Greenberg and Dokken 2000), premature loss of the pregnancy, and the loss of self-esteem. Past losses may resurface, and the family may anticipate the possible death of their ill newborn. These families all need emotional, psychosocial, and spiritual support. For the nearly nineteen thousand families in the United States who experience the death of their newborn each year (Hoyert et al. 2001), these needs are intensified.

> Baby Amy was born precipitously at home before the midwife could arrive and was profoundly depressed. At the community hospital, the parents were grief stricken when the neurology consultant suggested that Amy had suffered severe brain damage, resulting in the inability to suck and swallow. After careful consideration, they requested cessation of mechanical ventilation. When Amy continued to breathe on her

own, the parents requested that artificial nutrition and hydration also be withdrawn. After the hospital's legal counsel recommended against their proposal, arrangements were made to transfer Amy to the tertiary care center. The care plan included intensive comfort care but no artificial hydration or nutrition. Amy's parents spent nearly every minute at the hospital, holding their daughter until she died a few days later. They expressed their gratitude for the support that the NICU staff had provided for them and for Amy. Several months after Amy's death, her parents and three siblings attended the annual memorial service at the tertiary care center. At the end of the event, along with other families, they released a balloon in Amy's memory.

Perinatal hospice is an emerging concept, first described in 1982 (Whitfield et al. 1982). Clinicians practicing neonatal intensive care can and should create an environment in which high tech and high touch coexist and complement one another. While most neonatal units consider themselves family centered and competent to care for infants whose death is imminent, there are numerous opportunities to improve the provision of palliative care for dying newborns. This will require that health care professionals attend to the following questions:

- For which infants should we consider palliative care?
- What barriers exist that limit the provision of palliative care in the NICU?
- What constitutes optimal care for the neonatal patient and his or her family?
- What is a reasonable approach to decision making and advanced care planning that incorporates the family's goals, values, and preferences and ensures that we always act in the newborn's best interest and minimize suffering?
- How can we optimize pain and symptom management in the NICU?
- What is the optimal site of care, and how can we modify the environment to make it more family and infant friendly?
- How do we support the needs of families?
- How do we support the needs of the health care providers?
- What are the needs in the community, and how do we develop community resources so that family-centered care and excellent palliative care are ensured, regardless of the site of care?

The Selection of Newborns for Palliative Care

Despite remarkable strides in neonatal survival, some newborns still die. In 1999 there were 18,728 neonatal deaths (4.73 per 1,000 live births) (Hoyert et al. 2001). The fetal mortality rate in 1998 was 6.7 per 1,000. The infant mortality rate in the United States has remained unchanged since the mid-1980s, at approximately 7.1 deaths per 1,000 live births; many of these deaths are the result of perinatal illnesses (Hoyert et al. 2001). Hence it is rare for any health care provider associated with all but the smallest labor and delivery service or nursery to have escaped the experience of dealing with perinatal death and bereavement.

> Baby Elizabeth was a full-term infant diagnosed prenatally with anencephaly. The obstetrician proposed termination of the pregnancy, but the mother's religious values prohibited this practice. The mother was introduced to a neonatal and palliative care consultation service. She continued her prenatal care there with an accepted plan of comfort care for Elizabeth after birth. Elizabeth was born alive and remained with her mother in the delivery room. She was provided warmth, comfort, and sublingual morphine as needed for distress. She never cried and was only fed small amounts of oral feedings. She went home with her family on her second day of life, and the palliative care team provided follow-up services. Elizabeth died after three days at home. The family reported that they highly valued these three days with their child and that the care the palliative team offered had made the experience as comfortable as possible for all concerned.

> Angela was a 520-gram, twenty-three-week female delivered to a 25-year-old multigravid woman. The parents did not want their baby to suffer and had previously declined resuscitation in the event of delivery before twenty-four weeks' gestation. As labor progressed, the nursery team, including the chaplain, provided "comfort care" for the premature newborn and also psychosocial and spiritual support for the family. The baby was baptized in the delivery room and spent the next hour in the family's arms until she died. The family received information about bereavement support services in their community as well as regular phone calls from the care team.

As illustrated by these cases, there are three general categories of indications for hospice or palliative care to be considered and discussed with families: newborns born at the limit of viability, newborns with congenital anomalies that are incompatible with prolonged life, and newborns with overwhelming illness who are not responding to aggressive life-sustaining medical treatment or for whom continued treatment may prolong suffering (Catlin and Carter 2002). There is debate in the neonatal literature about what constitutes viability (American Academy of Pediatrics 1995b), but most would argue that infants born at less than twenty-three weeks are considered nonviable and that, given low survivability and high morbidity, a prevailing approach of palliative care should be offered as an alternative or in addition to life-prolonging interventions for those born before twenty-three or twenty-four weeks. Many anomalies associated with potential mortality can be diagnosed before birth. When the fetus has a condition incompatible with prolonged extra-uterine survival, postpartum palliative care can be offered as an alternative to pregnancy termination. If resuscitation is undertaken in the delivery room while the child's prognosis is uncertain, palliative care should be provided concomitantly.

Death or severe neurological impairment is difficult to predict for an individual newborn. Provision of palliative care concurrent with life-prolonging care is appropriate for many newborns with severe but potentially treatable conditions (for example, infants with extremely low birth weight, congenital diaphragmatic hernia, or hypoplastic left heart syndrome). Although survival in such cases is possible or probable, morbidity is high, and attention to the physical comfort of the baby and the emotional and spiritual needs of the family should be the standard. Parents should understand that some of these newborns will fail to benefit from attempts to prolong life and that transition to exclusively palliative care goals may be appropriate.

Joshua was a full-term infant born with Goldenhar syndrome, presenting with esophageal atresia–tracheoesophageal fistula, severe tracheobronchomalacia, aqueductal stenosis, and hydrocephalus. A complicated repair of the esophageal atresia was attempted to meet the initial goal of supporting growth. However, because of severe airway problems, the plan was modified to include gastrostomy tube, tracheostomy, and mechanical ventilation. A ventriculoperitoneal shunt also became necessary, the presence of which would complicate the other procedures. Although the family hoped for survival, they realized that death and morbidity were likely and Joshua faced significant burden from the multiple surgical procedures. They agreed to a palliative care consultation for comfort measures concurrent with life-prolonging treatment, if the baby improved, and agreed to a transition to palliative care as the main treatment goal if Joshua's condition deteriorated.

The timely initiation of a discussion about palliative care as the primary goal may be prudent in a number of circumstances. Neonatal conditions in which a newborn is likely to die despite available treatment include complex and multiple birth defects, severe neurodevelopmental sequelae and very poor quality of life (for example, severe hypoxic-ischemic encephalopathy), inability to survive free of parenteral nutrition (for example, severe short-gut syndrome), or inability to wean off extracorporeal membrane oxygenation (ECMO). In these cases, the burdens of continued life-prolonging treatment might outweigh the benefits. Palliative care and attempts to cure or prolong life are not mutually exclusive. In cases in which death is likely or becomes inevitable, "treatment" may only prolong suffering, and transition can be made to palliative care as the main goal of treatment.

Barriers to the Provision of Palliative Care in the Neonatal Intensive Care Unit

THE ENVIRONMENT OF CARE

The environment of the NICU itself is a challenge to the provision of excellent palliative care (Catlin and Carter 2002). Quiet, dim lighting, and privacy are scarce. This high-tech, busy, noisy, crowded environment may contribute to the family's stress and uncertainty concerning their ability to parent their ill newborn. Considering the NICU as the only site of care for critically ill newborns becomes a barrier to family-centered palliative care (Catlin and Carter 2002).

TECHNOLOGY

The personnel attracted to working in this stressful environment apply their considerable energy to fighting for survival on behalf of their tiny patients. Death may be viewed as a failure. The ready availability of technologically sophisticated machines may contribute to the perceived technologic imperative: If it is there you must use it. The real issue is not the value of the technology but whether the newborn can benefit from the technology. Is the health care team doing something *for* the baby or *to* the baby? The question ought to be not "Can we use it?" but "Should we use it?" (Hoeldtke and Calhoun 2001). Unfortunately, by publicizing the stories of "miracle" babies the media has contributed to denial of infant death and the public's expectation that all babies will be cured and survive (Carter and Stahlman 2001).

OBSTACLES TO FAMILY PARTICIPATION

The high-tech environment and culture of the NICU can present many barriers to family-centered care (Harrison 1993). Families may feel that the child's treatment and care are out of their hands, that they have no role in parenting their child, or that their presence is not welcome (Peabody and Martin 1996). While giving parents choices and support is important, parents may feel burdened if they are solely responsible for difficult decisions about discontinuing medical treatment. If life prolongation is not possible or is deemed too burdensome to the child, the health care team should recommend the option of adjusting the goals of care to an exclusive approach of palliative care.

ETHICAL AND LEGAL ISSUES

In conjunction with amendments to the Federal Child Abuse Statutes known as the Baby Doe regulations, concerns about malpractice liability have influenced physicians' attitudes toward withholding or withdrawing life-prolonging interventions, even when they feel such actions are appropriate (Goldsmith, Ginsberg, and McGettigan 1996; Peabody and Martin 1996; Sexson and Overall 1996; Boyle and Kattwinkel 1999). The Baby Doe regulations (U.S. Child Abuse Protection and Treatment Amendments of 1984, Public Law 98-457) permit limiting or withdrawing life-sustaining measures in cases of

- chronic and irreversible coma;
- treatment that merely prolongs dying, is not effective, or is otherwise futile in terms of survival; and
- treatment that would be inhumane.

While all three of these considerations speak indirectly to quality-of-life judgments, infant suffering and outcome are not specifically addressed. Some physicians mistakenly feel that the regulations mandate treatment until death is certain and that, as clinicians, they are placed at increased liability when life-sustaining treatment is withdrawn. Case law, however, has generally supported the right of parents to withhold or withdraw life-sustaining treatment (Goldsmith, Ginsberg, and McGettigan 1996). It must be understood that the Baby Doe regulations are intended not to guide physicians and parents but to guide state social services receiving funding for child protective services. (The regulations do not allow for medical professional or health care institution liability.) There has never been a legal case against a physician or hospital based on the Baby Doe regulations, and no state has lost federal funding based on a lack of their enforcement. Efforts to overcome the misconceptions regarding Baby Doe must be pursued to prevent the loss of opportunities to provide appropriate excellent palliative care to newborns.

Decision Making in Neonatal Medicine

The primary ethical principle guiding treatment decisions in neonatal intensive care is to act in the newborn's best interest (American Academy of Pediatrics 1995b). Admittedly, newborns do not have the cognitive capacity to retain any interests themselves. Thus others must make decisions for an infant who has not had an opportunity to live within any value system or to develop or express its own interests. Decision making that is dynamically shared with parents ensures that decisions incorporate parental values in determining their infant's best interests. The requirement that someone other than the patient make decisions combined with the lack of certainty of prognosis in neonatal care make it a challenge (Peabody and Martin 1996) to minimize inappropriate treatment of the newborn (American Academy of Pediatrics 1995a).

In general, health care professionals in the United States try to base best-interest decisions on an individualized prognostic approach (American Academy of Pediatrics 1995a). Care is provided at the appropriate level based on expected outcome at the time care is initiated. Prognosis should be reassessed frequently, based on the best available information in conjunction with the changing condition of the individual infant, the physician's judgment, and parental values. This requires not only a review of the medical literature with consultation of any experts, as needed, but also an assessment of family values that determine the *meaning* of the child's outcome within the family. It must be recognized that parents and health care providers may have different values systems and may view benefits and burdens of treatment quite differently (Saigal 2000; Sydnor-Greenberg and Dokken 2000). Difficulties arise when prognosis is uncertain and treatment may be burdensome, painful, expensive, or cause prolongation of suffering (Goldsmith, Ginsberg, and McGettigan

1996; Niermeyer et al. 2000). In the presence of uncertainty, decisions become value laden. Families should have the primary role in determining the values guiding care, unless they appear to be going against some important societal norm or standard of care. Inherent in this approach is the willingness of the medical staff to admit to uncertainty and to explore not only the values of the parents but their own values as well (Sydnor-Greenberg and Dokken 2000; Leuthner 2001).

The following guidelines help frame decision making in the care of high-risk newborns:

- The role of the parents as proxy decision makers for their child is clear but not absolute.
- The concept of parental permission is pertinent.
- This does not mean that parents' interests outweigh those of the newborn.
- It is rarely appropriate to override a parent's decision, and, in almost all cases, it is inappropriate to exclude a parent from the discussion.
- In cases of disagreement, the physician has the duty to prove that parents are not acting in the best interests of the child. (Goldsmith, Ginsberg, and McGettigan 1996; Peabody and Martin 1996; Boyle and Kattwinkel 1999)

Physicians are not obligated to provide care that they consider to be futile in terms of survival (for example, resuscitation of a twenty-two-week fetus or an infant with anencephaly).

Physicians are not obligated to withhold care that they feel is medically indicated (for example, resuscitation of an otherwise healthy twenty-eight-week fetus).

Generally, overriding parental autonomy is warranted only in cases of medical certainty or deviation from some standard of beneficial care. Attempting to define medical certainty or a particular standard of care is often challenging. Cases that proceed to the courts for deliberation have resulted in decisions that are inconsistent, at best. In all such cases, the weight of parental, health care professional, or legal professional values have done more to determine decisions than any real degree of medical certainty or standard of care. A general preference has evolved to avoid turning to the courts for conflict resolution unless all other avenues have been exhausted (Boyle and

Kattwinkel 1999; Leuthner 2001). Clear documentation of family involvement in decision making and the informed consent process, as well as documentation of the resulting plan of care, is important. Discussions concerning palliative care as the main treatment goal occur at four points in time: during a perinatal visit, at delivery, during ongoing NICU care, or at home (Goldsmith, Ginsberg, and McGettigan 1996; Hoeldtke and Calhoun 2001).

PRENATAL DECISIONS

A decision made in advance to forgo resuscitation is generally reserved for children whose conditions can be reliably diagnosed in the prenatal period and are inevitably incompatible with life beyond infancy (Hoeldtke and Calhoun 2001). These conditions include anencephaly, hydranencephaly, holoprosencephaly, trisomies 13 and 18, triploidy, renal agenesis–pulmonary hypoplasia, sirenomyelia, lethal short-limbed dwarfisms, and some other syndromes (Goldsmith, Ginsberg, and McGettigan 1996). Decisions made prenatally regarding resuscitation of a preterm infant at the limits of viability are difficult because of the limited accuracy of gestational age determination and the variability of birth weight at each gestational age (American Academy of Pediatrics 1995b; Boyle and Kattwinkel 1999). Accurate early obstetrical dating (through first-trimester ultrasound or knowledge of the exact date of conception) is more accurate than late-second- or third-trimester ultrasound dating measures or a neonatologist's exam and could contribute to a decision before birth to provide only palliative care. Additional considerations for the preliminary plan of care might include the site of delivery, the level of obstetrical care, and the level of care available in the delivery room (Finer and Barrington 1998; Hoeldtke and Calhoun 2001; Catlin and Carter 2002).

DELIVERY ROOM DECISIONS

Finer and Barrington (1998, 645) have referred to delivery room resuscitation as "an unusual team sport in which the only player who never swings the bat is also the only one who can strike out. Decisions regarding appropriate resuscitation and treatment of the extremely low-birth-weight infants should neither be the triumph of hope over reason nor the victory of ego over uncertainty." The delivery room may not be the best place to make a decision about withholding resuscitation (Stevenson and Goldworth 1998). Whether because of a precipitous delivery or lack of prenatal care, at times there are inadequate data at the time of delivery to determine the prognosis or future potential of the expected newborn. While it would be ideal to have prenatal discussions between the family, obstetrician, and the pediatrician, it is not always possible.

In cases of prenatal uncertainty, the family must be aware that the treatment plan depends on verification in the delivery room of the infant's condition. Because withholding resuscitation may not result in death, and delay will most certainly result in increased disability, resuscitation will generally proceed if there is a reasonable chance of survival without severe disability (Goldsmith, Ginsberg, and McGettigan 1996; Boyle and Kattwinkel 1999; Niermeyer et al. 2000). If, on the other hand, after stabilization the newborn assessment indicates with certainty a lethal anomaly or a nonviable preterm infant, the information is reviewed with the family, a consensus is formed, and the goals may be shifted to exclusively palliative care. The Neonatal Resuscitation Program guidelines acknowledge that resuscitation is not always appropriate: "noninitiation of resuscitation in the delivery room is appropriate for infants with confirmed gestation of less than twenty-three weeks or birth weight of less than four hundred grams, anencephaly, or confirmed trisomy 13 or 18" (American Academy of Pediatrics and American Heart Association 2000, 7-19). The guidelines also note that discontinuation of resuscitation may be appropriate if spontaneous circulation does not return within fifteen minutes. A poor response to resuscitation (for example, an Apgar score of less than 3 at fifteen minutes) from an infant in whom mortality or severe disability is expected is also a reason to consider the discontinuation of support.

NEONATAL INTENSIVE CARE UNIT DECISIONS

Most applications of palliative care in neonatology will probably be within the NICU after a trial of life-sustaining treatment for the borderline viable preterm infant or the severely depressed or asphyxiated newborn (Goldsmith, Ginsberg, and McGettigan 1996; Sexson and Overall 1996; Stevenson and Goldworth 1998; Boyle and Kattwinkel 1999). However, given the possibility of nonresponsiveness to resuscitation, palliative or comfort measures for both the mother and her nonviable newborn may be initiated in the delivery room or postpartum area. Palliative care may also be provided after the limits of life-extending or cure-oriented care have been met and a neonatal patient who is days to weeks old is declining in health and suffering more burden than benefit from interventions that are being applied. The role that neonatal caregivers play in these settings may vary across institutions. Some are adept at handling all such considerations and decisions to change the goals of care from cure to comfort. Others may enlist the help of an ethics consultant or a palliative care consultant or team.

Components of Palliative Care for the Newborn

The goals of care in neonatology must be expanded (Pierucci, Kirby, and Leuthner 2001). Rather than seeking merely survival, the concept of success must also include supporting the family to find meaning in their baby's life, however long or short that life might be. Death of the infant is not failure; rather, failure should be seen as unnecessary suffering for infants and their families. Prevention of suffering includes attention to the physical environment and to the needs of the newborn, including during procedures, and provision of a family-centered approach that both facilitates and supports decision making and advanced care planning. Social and spiritual support is also integral to the palliative care approach.

THE ENVIRONMENT OR SITE OF CARE

Bright lights, loud noises, and sleep interruptions are all sources of discomfort for neonates. Scheduling that maintains low levels of noise and light at night can be introduced. Staff can teach parents how to touch their infant and participate in care. Positioning is important. Encouraging parents to provide toys and family pictures to place at the bedside and tapes of their voices can make even the NICU a family-centered environment, benefiting both the baby and his or her family (Harrison 1993; Sydnor-Greenberg and Dokken 2000). Visiting restrictions should be minimized or eliminated so that siblings and other family members, as well as family-chosen support persons, feel welcome and included in the care.

If the newborn is likely to die in the NICU, care may be relocated to a family or parent care room where the baby can remain on life support for a time, surrounded by parents and extended family. In some hospitals, the baby is moved to a quiet room outside of the NICU. Whatever the setting, family access to their newborn, privacy, quiet, and support by the current team of health care providers is optimal (Sydnor-Greenberg and Dokken 2000).

In cases in which the decision not to resuscitate is made in advance, the family may prefer delivery in their local community hospital instead of in a distant tertiary specialty center, to be within familiar surroundings with easy access to support from family, friends, or religious community. In cases of uncertain diagnosis or prognosis, options might include on-site consultation by neonatologists, geneticists, or other subspecialists, telemedicine linkages, or transfer to the tertiary care center. If the newborn has been transferred to the tertiary care center, transfer back to the community hospital may be possible following confirmation of a condition incompatible with prolonged survival. Maternal transport before delivery may be preferred if the diagnosis is uncertain or the likelihood of survival is long or if the community hospital personnel are uncomfortable with the care plan. In some cases, the infant may be moved to the home with provision of hospice and palliative care support. The parents should be fully informed and supported in deciding their preferred site of care. Whatever choice is made, comprehensive palliative care should be provided to the newborn and family by competent caregivers sensitive to the needs of the newborn patient and the unique aspects of perinatal loss for the family.

THE NEWBORN

Pain Management. It is clear that newborns experience pain. Pain results in physiologic, metabolic, and behavioral changes. It has been said that newborn infants never cry without legitimate cause. But a lack of behavioral response does not mean the newborn is not in pain (Scanlon 1991; Lynn, Ulma, and Spieker 1999; American Academy of Pediatrics 2000). Untreated, severe, or prolonged pain increases mortality and morbidity.

Several acute pain scales have proved useful in assessing pain in the full-term and preterm neonate (Lawrence et al. 1993; Krechel and Bildner 1995; Stevens et al. 1996; Buchholz et al. 1998); one such is Buchholz and colleagues' (1998) modified infant pain scale presented in table 10.1. Use of one of these pain scales should be incorporated into routine assessment. Procedural pain, including that associated with surgery, and discomforts associated with ventilation are frequent in infants. Regular use of appropriate pain and other symptom assessment tools will help caregivers gauge and manage pain in neonates (American Academy of Pediatrics 2000). In general, efforts should be made to prevent, limit, or avoid painful stimuli. Table 10.2 presents a list of appropriate pharmacologic and nonpharmacologic analgesic interventions. Nonpharmacologic interventions such as swaddling, positioning, nonnutritive sucking, holding with skin-to-skin contact, and oral milk or sucrose may modify mild pain (Lynn, Ulma, and Spieker 1999; Anand 2001). When avoidance is not possible, appropriate analgesia must be provided. It is critical that

Table 10.1. Modified infant pain score

Behavior	Behavior score[a]		
	0	1	2
Sleep during last hour	None	Five- to ten-minute naps	Less-than-ten-minute naps
Facial expression: brow bulge, open mouth, chin quiver, stretch mouth vertically, stretch mouth horizontally, nasolabial furrow, eye squeeze	Marked	Less marked	Calm
Quality of cry	Screaming, high pitched	Modulated; infant can be distracted	No cry
Spontaneous motor activity	Incessant agitation, thrashing	Moderate	Normal
Excitability and responsiveness to stimulation	Tremulous, clonic movement, spontaneous Moro reflex	Excessive reaction to any stimulus	Quiet
Flexion of toes and fingers	Pronounced and constant	Less marked, intermittent	Absent
Sucking	Absent or disorganized	Three to four sucks, stops with crying	Strong, rhythmic; pacifies
Overall tone	Strong, hypertonic	Moderately hypertonic	Normal tone
Consolability	None after two minutes of comforting	Quiet after one minute of effort	Quiet within one minute
Sociability (eye contact) in response to face or smile	Absent	Difficult to obtain	Easy and prolonged

Source: Adapted from Buchholz et al. (1998).
[a]Total score 0 (severe pain) to 20 (complete comfort).

Table 10.2. Suggested approaches to analgesic

Procedure	Prevent, limit, or use alternative	Swaddling, tucking	Nonnutritive, milk, or sucrose sucking	Anesthetic				Other
				Topical	Injection	NSAID	Opioid	
Heel stick	Consider	Consider	Consider	NA	NA	NA	NA	Use automated lancet
Venipuncture, IV insertion	NA	Consider	Consider	NA	NA	NA	NA	NA
PICC insertion	NA	Consider	Consider	Consider	Consider	NA	NA	NA
Peripheral cutdown	NA	Consider	Consider	Consider	Consider	NA	Consider	NA
Umbilical catheter placement	NA	Consider	Consider	NA	NA	NA	NA	NA
Lumbar puncture	NA	NA	Consider	Consider	Consider	NA	Consider	NA
SQ or IM injection	IV if possible	Consider	Consider	Consider	NA	Consider if multiple	NA	NA
Non-life-threatening intubation	NA	Consider	NA	NA	Consider	NA	Consider	Atropine, sedative, or analgesic, paralytic
Endotracheal tube suctioning	NA	Consider	NA	NA	Consider	NA	Consider	NA

260

NG-OG suctioning	NA	NA	NA	NA	NA	NA	NA	NA
Circumcision	NA	Consider	Consider	Consider	Dorsal penile nerve or ring block	Consider before and after	NA	Mogen less painful than Gomco; nerve blocks more effective than topicals
Ongoing analgesia for routine care and procedures	NA	Consider	Consider	NA	NA	Consider	Consider, especially for ventilated baby	Reduce environmental stress
Postoperative	NA	NA	NA	NA	NA	NA	Consider continuous	Monitor ventilation vitals and pain scales rigorously

Source: Adapted from Anand (2001).

the health care provider be able to understand the unique dosing and safety issues of the analgesic drugs (Lynn, Ulma, and Spieker 1999; Young and Mangum 2001). Cardiorespiratory monitoring of the newborn and availability of trained staff may be needed.

Procedural pain for bedside procedures such as insertion of a chest tube can usually be managed by infiltration with local anesthetics such as lidocaine with or without analgesics (Scanlon 1991; Lynn, Ulma, and Spieker 1999; American Academy of Pediatrics 2000; Anand 2001). Lidocaine-prilocaine 5 percent (EMLA) can be safely applied topically one hour in advance of procedures such as lumbar puncture, venipuncture, and peripheral intravascular catheter placement. Unfortunately, EMLA does not always eliminate pain associated with heel-lance procedures (Lynn, Ulma, and Spieker 1999; Anand 2001). As use of an indwelling catheter or venipuncture is less painful than heel lance, these alternatives should be considered where appropriate.

The limited data available suggest that nonsteroidal anti-inflammatory drugs (NSAID) and acetaminophen may be helpful for mild to moderate pain and as an adjunct to opioid medications (table 10.3). Data on ibuprofen in the neonate are limited (Lynn, Ulma, and Spieker 1999).

Opioids are effective for moderate to severe pain for procedures, during surgery, for postprocedural pain, and for medical conditions that are painful, such as necrotizing enterocolitis (Anand 2001). The dose may need to be adjusted as the pharmacokinetics in the newborn, and especially the premature newborn, are different from those of older infants. Opioids are generally given orally and by intermittent or continuous intravenous (IV) infusion. Although infants and children can be given opioids intramuscularly (IM), subcutaneously (SC), sublingually, and rectally, there are few data concerning safety in neonates. In general, intramuscular injections should not be used, as they are unnecessarily painful and provide no advantages. Continuous infusions result in fewer variations in drug levels and may be preferred if long-term use is necessary. Inappropriate health care provider fears of addiction, tolerance, dependence, and adverse effects such as respiratory depression (incidence probably less than 1%) may contribute to inadequate dosing (American Academy of Pediatrics 2000). These issues are indications for vigilance and availability of skilled personnel, not the withholding of appropriate medication.

Noxious environmental stimuli result in behaviors indistinguishable from pain responses and may result in similar morbidity; thus minimization of noise, light, and other negative stimuli should be a goal in the NICU. When stress is unavoidable and nonpharmacologic measures are insufficient, sedatives and anxiolytics may be required (American Academy of Pediatrics 2000). Muscle relaxants have no analgesic or anxiolytic properties and should not be used alone (American Academy of Pediatrics 2000; Anand 2001). As with opioids, tolerance and dependence result from long-term use of muscle relaxants. Thus if use is no longer required, the medications should be tapered. Of the benzodiazepines, midazolam is approved for use in neonates and is preferred over long-acting benzodiazepines such as diazepam. Potential adverse effects such as cardiorespiratory depression and possible neurologic complications warrant close monitoring and may be exacerbated by combination with opioids. Because of a paucity of data in premature infants and concern about neurologic sequelae, midazolam cannot be recommended as a routine sedative in the NICU (Anand 2001). Chloral hydrate may be used in the short term; it has been well studied and appears to be safe. In summary, assessment and treatment of pain, stress, and anxiety in the neonate should be routine in the NICU.

Symptom Management and Care. Most terminally ill newborns die in the NICU soon after cessation of mechanical ventilation. A few newborns survive despite withdrawal or withholding of medical treatment and can be cared for at home with the support of hospice or palliative care services. It is optimal for care to be provided by professionals skilled in neonatal care as well as palliative care. This care may include elements of normal newborn care, such as cord care, bottle-feeding, and diaper changes, but is often more skilled. Symptoms such as dyspnea, nausea, and seizures should receive prompt attention. Poor skin integrity can be treated with lotions. Dry mouth can be improved with glycerin swabs. Petroleum jelly may help dry lips. These symptoms may be particularly challenging as the baby is dying.

Artificial means of feeding, while not necessarily required or recommended, may be preferred by parents, and therefore appropriate services should be available. However, while the medical goal for nutrition and hydration is typically growth and maturation, under palliative care the goal is comfort for the child and his or her nurturing parents (Carter and Leuthner 2003).

THE FAMILY

Family-Centered Care. Care is optimally tailored to the individual needs of each family (Harrison 1993). While confidence in the care of their infant is important for the family, palliative care also entails supporting the family's

Table 10.3. Medications for neonatal palliative care

Drug	Category	Starting dose (per kg body weight)	Route and interval	Comments
Acetaminophen	Analgesic, antipyretic	24 mg load 10–15 mg 45–50 mg load 20–30 mg	PO once PO every 4–8 hrs PR once PR every 6 hrs	Inhibits prostaglandin synthesis. Reversible liver dysfunction at high doses.
Chloral hydrate	Sedative, hypnotic	10–25 mg 25–75 mg	PO, PR every 6–8 hrs PO, PR single dose	Conjugated hyperbilirubinemia, gastric irritation, CNS depression. Renal failure with prolonged use.
EMLA (lidocaine-prilocaine 5%)	Topical anesthetic	A thin layer of cream	Topical, 1 hour before procedure; cover with occlusive dressing	Methemoglobinemia with prolonged use (preemies at higher risk). Not effective for heel lance procedures. Skin must be intact.
Fentanyl	Opioid analgesic	0.5–4.0 mcg 0.5–5.0 mcg/kg/hr	IV (or IM) every 2–4 hrs Continuous IV	Respiratory depression, hypotension reversed by naloxone. Stiff chest more likely with bolus; reversed by paralytics. Fewer gastrointestinal effects than morphine.
Furosemide	Diuretic	1–2 mg	IV, PO, IM every 12 hrs	Hypokalemia, hypochloremia
Glycopyrrolate	Anticholinergic drying agent	0.01 mg	IV, PO, IM every 4–8 hrs	Thickened airway secretions
Lorezepam	Benzodiazepine sedative, anxiolytic, anticonvulsant	0.05–0.1 mg	IV every 4–8 hrs	Respiratory depression, hypotension reversed by flumezanil. Limited data in neonates.
Methadone	Opioid analgesic	0.05–0.2 mg	IV, PO every 12–24 hrs	Long duration of action, ileus, delayed gastric emptying

Metoclopromide	Antiemetic, promotility	0.03–0.1 mg	IV, PO, IM every 8 hrs	May improve feeding tolerance. Dystonic reactions at high doses.
Midazolam	Benzodiazepine sedative, anxiolytic	0.05–0.15 mg 0.01–0.06 mg/kg/hr 0.3–0.5 mg	IV, IM every 2–4 hrs Continuous IV PO	Respiratory depression, myoclonus, hypotension reversed by flumezanil. Decrease dose if concurrent opioids. Use with caution, particularly in the premature infant.
Morphine	Opioid analgesic, decreases dyspnea	0.05–0.2 mg 0.2–0.5 mg 0.1–0.2 mg/kg/hr	IV, IM, every 2–4 hrs PO every 4–6 hrs IV continuous infusion	Respiratory depression, hypotension reversed by naloxone. Decreases gastrointestinal motility. May also be given rectally or sublingually.
Naloxone	Opioid antagonist	0.1 mg 0.001 mg/kg/hr	IV, IM, SC, per ET IV infusion	May precipitate withdrawal if prolonged opioid use
Sucrose 12–25%	Analgesic	1–2 ml	PO	Stimulates endorphins. Safety not demonstrated in premies.

Source: Adapted from Lynn, Ulma, and Spieker (1999); Young and Mangum (2001).

spiritual and psychosocial needs. An interdisciplinary team, including at a minimum physicians, nurses, social workers, and a chaplain, is critical to meet all these needs. Parents particularly value recognition of their role as parents. Orientation to the NICU, discussions in quiet rooms, and information about the roles of the various health care providers and how to obtain information will be helpful. More important, staff should explore with parents their expectations of health care providers, how they want to be involved in the care of their ill newborn, their goals for their baby, their support systems, and their values concerning death and disability (Sydnor-Greenberg and Dokken 2000; Catlin and Carter 2002). Staff should be sensitive to unique personal, cultural, ethnic, and religious differences that affect each family's way of coping. The team may help parents deal with natural feelings of guilt and self-blame while supporting feelings of control, competence, and self-esteem. Child-life specialists can help parents explore how siblings are dealing with death and how the parents can best assist those siblings.

Members of the care team can do many things to be supportive in anticipation of a neonatal death. Baptism, other religious rituals or traditions, and pastoral counseling are helpful to many families. The comfort of memories and mementos such as the armbands and crib card is also important (American Academy of Pediatrics 1995b; Catlin and Carter 2002). Even if the baby dies in the delivery room, the parents can name, hold, and photograph their baby, take hand and foot impressions and locks of hair, if desired. This has recently been emphasized in the event of multiple gestation in which loss may occur to one or more of the newborns (Pector 2004). Even in the presence of severe anomalies, parents should have the opportunity to view and hold their newborn. Sensitively pointing out the beauty of the child's normal features may be appreciated.

Many questions (often unspoken) will need to be addressed by caregivers providing palliative care, including the following:

- What did I do to make this happen?
- Why did this happen to my baby?
- What did the health care professionals do to make this happen?
- Why did this happen to me?

Because guilt, particularly on the part of the mother, is common, it is frequently helpful to review the prenatal history and specifically address whether the condition was preventable or might recur in future pregnancies (Catlin and Carter 2002). Referral to a genetic counselor may be helpful.

Grief Support. Some centers provide a bereavement packet including a disposable camera, baby clothes and a blanket, a baby book to record memories, and information about bereavement, including contact information for community-based support groups. After the baby's death, walking the family to their car with a bereavement packet or stuffed animal to fill their empty arms aids the transition out of the NICU for the last time (Catlin and Carter 2002). In some locations, laws allow parents to transport their infant's body themselves. Staff should support the parents in choosing those activities that are consistent with their values, religion, and culture.

Advance Care Planning. Once a decision has been made to allow a natural death, the team must begin advance care planning. This includes anticipatory guidance, including an explanation of what the death may look like, the possibility of survival after discontinuation of life support, and the need for contingency planning. The advance care plan might address such issues as withholding or withdrawing life-sustaining support, resuscitation, site of care, transition to home, availability of support persons, continuing treatments, pain and symptom relief, use of community resources such as a hospice or palliative care center, and whether to call emergency medical services in the event of an emergency. A letter explaining the diagnosis, prognosis, and mutually derived goals of care for the infant should be provided for families who go home with their young infant receiving palliative care. This may assist them, and others, should an emergency arise.

THE STAFF

The fact that U.S. society is largely a death-denying culture is nowhere more evident than in the neonatal intensive care unit. Family members are not alone in suffering a loss. Many NICU staff members who have cared for an infant feel great loss, too (Catlin and Carter 2002). Health care providers may feel a profound sense of failure, frustration, and sadness when a newborn dies. Physicians, who bear much of the responsibility for directing care and treatment decisions, can find the death of a newborn patient particularly stressful (American Academy of Pediatrics 1995a; Catlin and Carter 2002). Nurses bear much of the responsibility for bedside care and interaction with the family but, in some centers, may have limited involvement in the decision-making process. Feelings of helplessness, moral distress, and spiritual suffering may be seen in health care providers in these difficult situations (Catlin et al. 2001). Involvement of all key staff in interdisciplinary decision making can diffuse the feelings of powerlessness. Spiritual support may be appreciated by some NICU personnel (Catlin et al. 2001). Staff education and training in neonatal hospice principles may reduce stress, but other support is necessary as well (Catlin and Carter 2002). Some centers have formal neonatal hospice courses, interdisciplinary mortality review, small group discussion, or formal debriefing (Whitfield et al. 1982; Reddick, Catlin, and Jellinek 2001; Catlin and Carter 2002) during which reactions to the death, and good and problematic aspects of the care, can be discussed. When palliative care results in a peaceful death for the newborn, the staff can feel a great sense of professional and personal fulfillment.

COMMUNITY RESOURCES

When a dying newborn remains in the local community hospital, is transferred from a tertiary care center, or is cared for at home, collaborative consultation from the tertiary specialty center may be needed to render the seamless, family-centered care appropriate to a dying newborn. Neonatal palliative care protocols, policies, and consultation and ongoing communication are effective tools for facilitating such transitions of care (Carter and Bhatia 2001; Pierucci, Kirby, and Leuthner 2001; Catlin and Carter 2002).

One model for community-based palliative care for children with life-limiting conditions is the Footprints program (www.footprintsatglennon.org) at Cardinal Glennon Hospital in St. Louis, Missouri. Advance care planning and documentation, care coordination, and a continuity physician from the tertiary care center ensure seamless community-based continuous care after discharge. Nearly all community caregivers in the St. Louis area, including physicians, nurses, and the emergency medical services, agree to abide by the advance care plan. Program staff provide education about pediatric palliative care to the community health care providers at the time of the baby's transition from hospital to home. Despite the large numbers of newborns who die following discontinuation of life support in the NICU, one-quarter of the children in the Footprints program were referred when they were less than six months old.

Care When Prolongation of Life Is No Longer the Goal

The expected length of survival is immaterial to the grief of the family. If hospice or palliative care principles are initiated at the time of admission, the infrastructure will be in place at the time of dying (Whitfield et al. 1982).

In many intensive care nurseries, more than 70 percent of deaths occur following the withdrawal or withholding of life-sustaining treatment (Wall and Partridge 1997). Several recent reviews describe the use of palliative care consultation and protocols in the NICU (Carter and Bhatia 2001; Pierucci, Kirby, and Leuthner 2001; Catlin and Carter 2002), assisting staff to focus not on what cannot be done ("cure" the baby, prevent death, spare the family anguish) but on what can be done (provide compassion, comfort, warmth, humane care, provide for a "good death") (Pierucci, Kirby, and Leuthner 2001). The health care team provides continual assessment and management of pain and other physical symptoms as well as coordination of the plan of care. Intensive comfort or supportive care is continued, frequently in a different, more private and quiet, setting (Whitfield et al. 1982). Emotional and spiritual support for the family is intensified. Treatments not consistent with the primary goals of palliative care, such as vital signs monitoring, lab tests, mechanical ventilation, transfusions, and artificial nutrition and hydration, may be discontinued. Secure, reliable intravenous access or a nasogastric tube should remain in place for analgesic, anticonvulsant, and sedative medications, if needed.

The time before discontinuation of life-sustaining treatment is frequently the first opportunity the parents have had to hold their fragile newborn and provide normal parenting functions, such as bathing and dressing their infant. Family involvement and rituals should be individualized, and staff should be open to unusual requests, especially those based in cultural and religious traditions that may be different from the mainstream. When the family is ready for the child to be extubated, the infant should be suctioned, and intensive management of symptoms ensured. Analgesics and sedatives should be titrated to relief, and it is common for doses to be doubled to effectively treat pain, agitation, and dyspnea (Burns et al. 2000). The definition of a "good death" is child and parent specific, and strategies that help the family prepare and define for themselves the circumstances of their child's death should be implemented (Pearson 1997).

The Role of the Health Care Provider

After discontinuation of life support, the baby will generally die peacefully within minutes to hours. Many parents hold the child at this time; some want to be surrounded by loved ones, others prefer solitude. Clinicians can facilitate decision making and planning for autopsy, organ donation, disposition of the body, and funeral arrangements and can thus promote the family's sense of control. Sensitivity to cultural and religious perspectives is again critical here. Autopsy is forbidden in some traditions, as is organ donation. The newborn is rarely a suitable donor for tissues other than the cornea or heart valves; the regional transplant organization can be a resource concerning what tissues are appropriate for donation or other questions. Nonetheless, dialogue with parents about these issues is important and may even be required in some jurisdictions. Autopsy continues to provide valuable insights into the cause of the newborn's death as well as possible genetic factors that may be of importance in future family planning. Finally, in addition to filling out the death certificate and any other required paperwork, the physician should contact the referring obstetric and pediatric physicians concerning the death of the baby.

Conclusion

Applying palliative care principles to the care of the high-risk newborn is not only possible, it is necessary if health care professionals are to provide optimal family-centered care for newborns and their families. Clinicians and staff across all pertinent disciplines can cooperate to provide an environment in the delivery room and the neonatal intensive care unit in which palliative care principles are integrated into care regardless of whether the treatment goal is cure, prolongation of life, or exclusively palliation until expected death. Whatever the site of care, treatment must be in the best interest of the newborn, consistent with the goals and preferences of the family, compassionate, and humane. Care should focus not only on the physical comfort of the baby but also on the emotional, psychosocial, and spiritual needs of the entire family, including siblings and grandparents.

The process can begin prenatally with identification of fetal conditions that may potentially limit the life of the newborn or contribute to a family's sense of loss. There exists a need to expand available data so that evidence-based, ethically sound, multidisciplinary, family-centered decision making before and after birth will become the standard. Following death, bereavement support should be provided to enable the family to integrate the loss into their lives and to return to a functional existence (see chapter 8 in this volume). Finally, health care professionals should not forget to care for themselves and their colleagues in the NICU and in the community so that they may continue to provide compassionate care for all high-risk newborns and their families.

References

American Academy of Pediatrics and American Heart Association. 2000. *Textbook of neonatal resuscitation,* ed. J. Kattwinkel. 4th ed. Elk Grove Village, Ill.: American Academy of Pediatrics.

American Academy of Pediatrics, Committee on Fetus and Newborn. 1995a. The initiation or withdrawal of treatment for high-risk newborns. *Pediatrics* 96:362–63.

———. 1995b. Perinatal care at the threshold of viability. *Pediatrics* 96:974–76.

———. 2000. Prevention and management of pain and stress in the neonate. *Pediatrics* 105:454–61.

Anand, K. J. 2001. Consensus statement for the prevention and management of pain in the newborn. *Arch Pediatr Adolesc Med* 155:173–80.

Boyle, R. J., and J. Kattwinkel. 1999. Ethical issues surrounding resuscitation. *Clin Perinatol* 26:779–92.

Buchholz, M., H. W. Karl, M. Pomietto, and A. Lynn. 1998. Pain scores in infants: a modified infant pain scale vs. visual analogue. *J Pain Symptom Manage* 15:117.

Burns, J. P., C. Mitchell, K. M. Outwater, M. Geller, J. L. Griffith, I. D. Todres, and R. D. Truog. 2000. End-of-life care in the pediatric intensive care unit after the forgoing of life-sustaining treatment. *Crit Care Med* 28:3060–66.

Carter, B. S., and J. Bhatia. 2001. Comfort/palliative care guidelines for neonatal practice: development and implementation in an academic medical center. *J Perinatol* 21:279–83.

Carter, B. S., and S. R. Leuthner. 2003. The ethics of withholding/withdrawing nutrition in the newborn. *Sem Perinatol* 27:480–87.

Carter, B. S., and M. T. Stahlman. 2001. Reflections on neonatal intensive care in the U.S.: limited success or success with limits? *J Clin Ethics* 12:215–22.

Catlin, A., and B. Carter. 2002. Creation of a neonatal end-of-life palliative care protocol. *J Perinatol* 22:184–95.

Catlin, E. A., J. H. Guillemin, M. M. Thiel, S. Hammond, M. L. Wang, and J. O'Donnell. 2001. Spiritual and religious components of patient care in the neonatal intensive care unit: sacred themes in a secular setting. *J Perinatol* 21:426–30.

Finer, N. N., and K. J. Barrington. 1998. Decision-making in delivery room resuscitation: a team sport. *Pediatrics* 102:644–45.

Goldsmith, J. P., H. G. Ginsberg, and M. C. McGettigan. 1996. Ethical decisions in the delivery room. *Clin Perinatol* 23:529–50.

Harrison, H. 1993. The principles for family-centered neonatal care. *Pediatrics* 92: 643–50.

Hoeldtke, N., and B. Calhoun. 2001. Perinatal hospice. *Am J Obstet Gynecol* 185:525–59.

Hoyert, D. L., E. Arias, B. L. Smith, S. L. Murphy, and K. D. Kochanek. 2001. Deaths: final data for 1999. *National Vital Statistics Reports* 49(8):1–114.

Krechel, S., and J. Bildner. 1995. CRIES: a new neonatal pain measurement score: initial testing of validity and reliability. *Pediatr Anesth* 5:53–61.

Lawrence, J., D. Alcock, P. McGrath, J. Kay, S. B. MacMurray, and C. Dulberg. 1993. The development of a tool to assess neonatal pain. *Neonatal Netw* 12:59–66.

Leuthner, S. R. 2001. Decisions regarding resuscitation of the extremely premature infant and models of best interest. *J Perinatol* 21:1–6.

Lynn, A. M., G. A. Ulma, and M. Spieker. 1999. Pain control for very young infants. *Contemp Pediatr* 16:39–66.

Niermeyer, S., J. Kattwinkel, P. Van Reempts, V. Nadkarni, B. Phillips, D. Zideman, et al. 2000. International guidelines for neonatal resuscitation: an excerpt from the guidelines 2000 for cardiopulmonary resuscitation and emergency cardiovascular care. *Pediatrics* 106:e29.

Peabody, J. L., and G. I. Martin. 1996. From how small is too small to how much is too much. *Clin Perinatol* 23:473–89.

Pearson, L. 1997. Family-centered care and the anticipated death of a newborn. *Pediatr Nurs* 23:178–82.

Pector, E. A. 2004. Views of bereaved multiple-birth parents on life support decisions, the dying process, and discussions surrounding death. *J Perinatol* 24:4–10.

Pierucci, R. L., R. S. Kirby, and S. R. Leuthner. 2001. End-of-life care for neonates and infants: the experience and effects of a palliative care consultation service. *Pediatrics* 108:653–660.

Reddick, B. H., E. Catlin, and M. Jellinek. 2001. Crisis within crisis: recommendations for defining, preventing, and coping with stressors in the NICU. *J Clin Ethics* 12:254–65.

Saigal, S. 2000. Perception of health status and quality of life of extremely low-birth-weight survivors: the consumer, the provider, and the child. *Clin Perinatol* 27:403–19.

Scanlon, J. W. 1991. Appreciating neonatal pain. *Adv Pediatr* 38:317–33.

Sexson, W. R., and S. W. Overall. 1996. Ethical decision making in perinatal asphyxia. *Clin Perinatol* 23:509–18.

Stevens, B., C. Johnston, P. Petryshen, and A. Taddio. 1996. Premature infant pain profile: development and initial validation. *Clin J Pain* 12:13–22.

Stevenson, D. K., and A. Goldworth. 1998. Ethical dilemmas in the delivery room. *Semin Perinatol* 22:198–206.

Sydnor-Greenberg, N., and D. Dokken. 2000. Coping and caring in different ways: understanding and meaningful involvement. *Pediatr Nurs* 26:185–90.

Wall, S. N., and J. C. Partridge. 1997. Death in the intensive care nursery: physician practice of withdrawing and withholding life support. *Pediatrics* 99:64–70.

Whitfield, J. M., R. E. Siegel, A. D. Glicken, R. J. Harmon, L. K. Powers, and E. J. Goldson. 1982. The application of hospice concepts to neonatal care. *Am J Dis Child* 136:421–24.

Young, T. E., and B. Mangum. 2001. *Neofax: a manual of drugs used in neonatal care.* 14th ed. Raleigh, N.C.: Acorn.

11

Palliative Care in the Pediatric Intensive Care Unit

Marcia Levetown, M.D., Stephen Liben, M.D., F.R.C.P., and Marylene Audet

As sickness progresses toward death, measures to minimize suffering should be intensified. Dying patients may require palliative care of an intensity that rivals that of curative efforts. Even though aggressive curative techniques are no longer indicated, professionals and families are still called on to use intensive measures—extreme responsibility, extraordinary sensitivity, and heroic compassion.

Wanzer et al. (1989, 847)

Pediatric palliative care is care of the mind, body, and spirit of children with life-limiting conditions and their families. Intensive care units are designed to bring to bear the full force of science and technology with the aim of extending life and curing disease as much as possible. The intensive care unit (ICU) usually conjures images of a high-tech, sterile, hectic environment in which teams of specialized professionals are engaged in a pitched battle against life-threatening illness. In contrast, conceptions of palliative care evoke images of a quiet, peaceful, homelike environment in which people minister to the body and spirit of a loved one in preparation for the voyage toward death. Given that both of these images are exaggerations of the varied realities of intensive care and palliative care, the question remains: How can a bridge be built between the seemingly disparate goals of intensive care (to fight death, strive for cure, and prolong life at all costs) and palliative care (to promote comfort and acceptance of death as an outcome)?

Before exploring how to bridge intensive care and palliative care, it will serve to first explore why both types of care need to be integrated in the care of children with life-threatening conditions. Intensive care can have the objective of the greatest comfort possible, including physical, psychological, and spiritual realms, for both the patient and his or her family. These goals can exist in the ICU either exclusively or in conjunction with efforts to prolong life.

In North America, the majority of children who die do so in hospitals, most often in neonatal and pediatric intensive care units (McCallum, Byrne, and Bruera 2000). This should not be surprising, given the epidemiology of childhood death (see chapter 1 of this volume) and the strong drive of parents and professional caregivers to "save" or extend the life of the child, coupled with medicine's increasing ability to do so, whether or not the child is benefiting from such interventions. In both neonatal and pediatric intensive care units, the full complement of medicine's technical advances is concentrated, usually with the sole purpose of sustaining life at all costs (financial, physical, emotional, and psychological). In many cases, this goal is appropriate; for instance, extremely premature children, many of whom may have a good quality of life, cannot initially survive outside of the neonatal ICU setting (see chapter 10 of this volume).

Among children who die between the ages of 1 and 18 years, the cause of death is most often trauma. In this situation, previously healthy children are suddenly injured; thus the initial use of all resuscitative measures is generally entirely appropriate, and care occurs in the pediatric intensive care unit (PICU). In other cases, previously healthy children become suddenly ill from an overwhelming illness that may threaten their very survival, such as a viral cardiomyopathy; these patients, too, will be cared for in the PICU.

Many of these patients derive the full benefit of ICU care and have the hoped-for outcome. While they are receiving this care, exquisite attention must be paid to the physical, social, emotional, and spiritual needs of the patient and his or her family. Similarly, attention must be paid to signs that the outcome will not be good, and an openness to changing the goals of care must be maintained. Fewer than half of the children over the age of 1 year who die do so of chronic illnesses; of these, many die of rare disorders with trajectories that are difficult to predict. Like Enrique in the case below, they have made numerous visits to the PICU, and the timing of the final visit, the one that will end in death, cannot always be discerned in advance. Pediatric intensive care units will therefore inevitably be the location of death for the majority of children who die of sudden injury, acute overwhelming illness, or chronic conditions. In fact, 4.6 percent of PICU admissions end in death (Levetown et al. 1994). Despite the initial apparent incongruence between the principles of palliative care and intensive care medicine, it is precisely because of the frequency of death in this setting that PICU staff must be prepared to provide palliative care, including effective and compassionate communication, symptom prevention and control, and ethical decision making. Care must include the entire family from the time of admission, when the grief associated with the realization of the seriousness of the life-threatening injury or illness first strikes, through and including bereavement following the child's death.

Enrique was born at term after an uncomplicated pregnancy. His parents noted weak cries at 1 week of age. By the age of 1 month Enrique was intubated for respiratory distress. He suffered a cardiac arrest from a drug reaction, was resuscitated, and admitted to the PICU. After many tests, including a nerve biopsy and an electromyogram, he was diagnosed alternately with congenital multiple axonal neuropathy, a diagnosis with a very poor prognosis and an average life expectancy of less than one year, and then Guillain-Barré syndrome, a frequently curable disease. Following therapies directed at treating Guillain-Barré syndrome, he was weaned off the ventilator and sent home.

At the age of 3 months, Enrique was again intubated and ventilated, but this time he remained hospitalized for weeks owing to labored respiration and associated failure to thrive. His parents tried to normalize his childhood by bringing him home on a weekend pass, but he required ventilation within two days and was never again able to breathe on his own.

At 6 months of age, Enrique was finally diagnosed with spinal muscular atrophy, type 1, a degenerative genetic disease characterized by progressive muscle weakness with an average life expectancy of two years. Even on mechanical ventilation, Enrique was a smiling, babbling, happy baby. After many discussions with the PICU health care team, Enrique's parents decided to continue treatment, on the condition that should Enrique's quality of life deteriorate past the point of benefit of life-extending care, from their perspective, they would have the right to change goals. In addition, his parents requested that no attempts to resuscitate him should be made in the unlikely event of cardiac arrest.

Enrique underwent surgery for the placement of tracheostomy and gastrostomy tubes for transfer to an intermediate care unit for ventilator-dependent children. His parents received care training and support from both hospital and community health agencies, enabling Enrique to spend weekends at home. During the weekdays in the intermediate care unit, he was cared for by a team that acknowledged the family as the unit of care. Enrique's 4-year-old brother had play therapy sessions with child-life therapists. His mother was taught basic massage therapy skills. Enrique benefited from music therapy, hydrotherapy, and daily physiotherapy. Volunteers were recruited to ensure that Enrique would not be alone when his parents were not present. A speech therapist taught Enrique the basics of sign language; an occupational therapist facilitated the purchase of a specially adapted wheelchair that allowed him to travel out of the hospital with his respirator secured. At the age of 19 months, Enrique was introduced to a local day care center to interact with other children.

By the age of 23 months, Enrique's condition had deteriorated significantly. He had lost the ability to smile and was losing the ability to make sounds. He began to withdraw, deriving little enjoyment from anything other than being rocked or watching television; he cried or appeared distressed most of the time. His family felt that his quality of life had become unacceptable and that the burden of life-extending technologies had become greater than their benefits. His distress and anxiety were treated with oral and rectal medication, and all efforts were made to optimize his daily quality of life.

On his second birthday, Enrique had a massive pulmonary hemorrhage, requiring deep sedation to control the dyspnea. After one week, his parents felt that, given the toll on their son's body and soul, it was time to let him go. At the family's request, Enrique was liberated from the ventilator, at a time when their primary care physician could be present. Medications were titrated to keep him comfortable, and he died a few hours after extubation, surrounded by family and staff of the PICU. One of the PICU nurses who had known Enrique well agreed to provide bereavement follow-up to the family.

Enrique's life story raises several issues that must be addressed in the care of children living with a life-threatening condition, before or during a stay in the PICU:

- the timing and appropriateness of discussions of limitations of medical interventions, including cardiopulmonary resuscitation
- the need for recurrent review and revision of joint decisions regarding the relative value and burden of life-prolonging treatments
- the use of invasive and high-technology procedures to improve quality of life even in the face of a shortened life span (including the

availability of trained pediatric home care personnel and continuity of care)

- the need for flexible admission and discharge policies to maximize desired time at home
- the need for a functioning interdisciplinary team
- the provision of effective symptom control at the end of life
- the appropriate elective removal of life support when the associated burdens outweigh the benefits
- the means to systematize such a mutually respectful, comprehensive, patient- and family-centered course of care
- the availability of mechanisms to ensure the needs of parents and siblings are addressed during the life of the child and through bereavement

Background

Most children who die in a pediatric intensive care unit do so after a decision has been made either to withhold or to withdraw life-extending therapies, including ventilators, antibiotics, intravenous fluids, and other potentially life-prolonging technologies (Vernon et al. 1993; Levetown et al. 1994). Faced with decisions that challenge the very essence of the parenting role, parents of children in the PICU for whom withdrawal of life support has been recommended need to hear assurances that the health care team has not made this recommendation lightly. Certainly, there also needs to be acknowledgment of the value of the individual child and the sorrow and lifelong pain that such decisions evoke for parents (Greig-Midlane 2001). Parents also need to be assured that their child will not suffer and that all efforts will be made to control symptoms and allow the family to be with the child as much as desired and feasible.

Parents know little of the outcomes of life-support technologies. Numerous studies document the desire of most parents to be given more and clearer information (Garwick et al. 1995; Levinson 1997; Levi et al. 2000). There is also evidence that, among adult patients, factual information alters the decisions made about cardiopulmonary resuscitation (O'Donnell et al. 2003). The outcome of cardiopulmonary resuscitation in children already receiving life support, or those who require resuscitation after prolonged respiratory compromise, is particularly poor (Schindler et al. 1996; Torres et al. 1997; Slonim 2000).

Awareness of these facts can lessen the guilt and grief associated with the decision-making process in pediatric cases. Providing this information well before the time of cardiac arrest, allowing for calm and reasoned decision making, is an essential duty of the health care team. Unlike physicians, whose greatest priority is prolongation of life at all costs, most parents see as their goal the prevention of a prolonged death and unnecessary suffering (American Academy of Pediatrics 1995).

Enrique's parents made these things abundantly clear in their decision-making process, and in this respect they are representative, not unusual. What was unusual, perhaps, was the continuity of care provided to Enrique, the clear information they were given, and the health care team's respect for the decisions they made. This partnership is also important for the survival of the family (Contro et al. 2002).

Patients' Needs

Children cared for in ICU settings have a variety of diagnoses, giving them and their families greater or lesser ability to participate in the care they receive. The spectrum within a given ICU can range from a previously healthy toddler, now unconscious from a hypoxic insult (for example, drowning) to a teen with multiply relapsed cancer who is fully aware of his prognosis and course. In between these patients are those who are chronically ill, with profound developmental delay and recurrent pneumonia, young infants and children with congenital heart defects or the sequelae of extreme prematurity, and children, like Enrique, with normal intelligence and a profound physical disability leading to technology dependence throughout their short lives, much of it in a PICU setting. Most children cared for in an ICU setting receive sedation, which also compromises their ability to participate actively in their own care and care decision making.

Each child, regardless of age or circumstance, needs to be cared for first and foremost as a child, next as a member of a family, and third as a patient, even in a PICU environment. Children need respect as demonstrated by compassionate, child-centered, individualized care and the presentation of choices, where practical and desired by the patient and his or her family. Much of the decision making for chronically ill pediatric patients should take place in advance of an ICU admission. This requires anticipation of future deterioration, potential care goal options, and the burdens associated with achieving the hoped-for benefits as well as clear explanations of the likelihood of recovery and further compromise. These options should be presented to parents and children, when the child is able and desires to participate (American Academy of Pediatrics 1995). The idea that the child is protected by being kept unaware of his or her future, including death and deterioration of health status, has been refuted (Bluebond-Langner 1978). Outcomes for the child and the family are optimized when the child's perspectives and preferences are included as an essential part of the decision-making process (Mastroyannopoulou et al. 1997). Guidance from the health care team about situations that lie ahead and gentle reminders to consider preferred outcomes will enhance the process.

Children want to know that they will not be forgotten. Reassurance of their importance, their legacy, and continued love are important aspects of parenting dying children. For a child whose potential death can be anticipated, such as a cancer patient, taking steps to create memories during times of relative health, continued affirmations that they are loved and will not be forgotten, are important. For a child who dies suddenly, such as a trauma victim, innovative approaches may include creating a mold of the child's hand (thereby always having the child's hand to hold), saving a lock of hair, or taking photos and videos at the time of family visitation with the child. Those entrusted with the care of a dying child should try to provide opportunities to create legacies.

However, as stated earlier, this luxury is not available to most of the children who die in the PICU and their families. Generally, care must focus on the essential needs of the child. All children will benefit from effective prevention of pain and distress, batching of procedures, and minimization of sleep disruption. Alert children may wish to listen to music or have a favorite movie played. More important, critically ill infants and children need access to their supporters, including parents, siblings, and friends. At times this may take the form of creative options to go home for care, whether for short periods of time, as Enrique did, for longer periods of time, or for the final chapter of the child's life. Owing to practical and financial circumstances, however, most PICU patients who die will not be able to leave the ICU environment. Accommodation must be made, through liberalized visitation policies or other creative options, such as a "home away from home" setting within the hospital (Levetown 1998).

All ill children require meticulous attention to their physical concerns, with their needs anticipated and addressed proactively. Examples of symptoms commonly encountered by children in the PICU include pain associated with procedures and with injury or illness, including dyspnea, cough, seizures, constipation, pruritis, and skin irritation. Nonphysical symptoms often seen include depression, insomnia, and the syndrome of ICU psychosis. Only relatively recently has the frequency of these symptoms and the importance of assessing and treating them received attention (Wolfe et al. 2000). Awareness of the potential for symptom distress is essential to diagnosis and successful intervention. This is best accomplished by routine assessment by nursing and other interdisciplinary personnel and by making the resolution of such symptoms a priority. Yet even today, few if any pediatric critical care fellowship programs address symptom assessment and interventions. The concept of continued intervention until the resolution of the symptom, or titration to effect, is also widely absent from practice and training.

Much work remains to be done in validating assessment tools and treatment protocols for symptoms other than pain. As with many elements of pediatric medicine, the stopgap measure is to follow and modify adult measures for children. Research tailored to children's disease processes and physiology is needed but may never be complete, owing to the financial implications of research on children. In the meantime, fears of creating harm by treating symptoms are frequently misguided; in fact, one study has demonstrated statistically significant improvement in life expectancy with opioid treatment for dyspnea management in premature infants who were removed from mechanical ventilation (Partridge and Wall 1997). Interdisciplinary care, including the input of physician, nurse, social worker, mental health professional, and child-life, respiratory, and physical therapists, as well as protocols for symptom assessment, intervention, and reassessment, will enable more routine and effective relief of these concerns for the PICU patient.

Research on child-specific tools for the diagnosis and treatment of symptoms is desperately needed.

Evidence suggests that the presence of family during the numerous medical, diagnostic, and therapeutic procedures faced by PICU patients is beneficial both for the child and the family (Leith and Weisman 1997). To be effective, parents need training regarding their role—not to monitor the procedure but to assist the child with distraction or other psychological therapies, providing support and reassurance as well as affection. An increasing body of evidence demonstrates the benefits of preventing pain during procedures (Porter, Grunau, and Anand 1999). Patients recover more readily and avoid such devastating consequences as disseminated intravascular coagulopathy (DIC), intraventricular hemorrhage (IVH), possibly permanent intellectual and mental health impairments, and even death (Anand and Hickey 1987) when local anesthetics, pain relievers, psychological techniques such as distraction or guided imagery, and sedatives (as needed) are used appropriately.

Children and parents often benefit from parental presence during invasive procedures.

The child is the one most affected by his or her illness or condition and its treatment. The child alone knows the physical pain, the pain of falling behind peers, and the pain of isolation, as well as individualized perceptions of quality of life and desire to press on with life-extending, if not curative, interventions. The knowing child's preferences and perceptions must be solicited and incorporated into the creation of the goals of care and the resulting plan of care (American Academy of Pediatrics 1995). Unfortunately, it is not uncommon that the child's perspective is either ignored or overruled, particularly if the child prefers not to continue to prolong life. Children can have a variety of reasons for refusing therapy, and these reasons must be explored and respected rather than rejected outright. In many instances, the child's assessment of risk and benefit may be wiser than that of the caregiving adults.

Incorporate the child's perspectives into the plan of care.

Most of the deaths of children in the ICU occur following withdrawal or forgoing of medical interventions (Levetown et al. 1994). This often entails discontinuation of mechanical ventilation. Obviously, there is a high risk of respiratory distress and dyspnea associated with this situation. Measures to prevent this distress include stopping intravenous fluid administration, suctioning the endotracheal tube (ETT) immediately before extubation, an immediate response with parenteral opioids if dyspnea is detected, and benzodiazepines for anxiety. These medications should be titrated to relief of distress, which may include inducing or maintaining unconsciousness, as was the case with Enrique. Some practitioners provide a large bolus of opioids or sedating medications before extubation, to preempt distress (Truog et al.

2001). However, others prefer to monitor the child closely and be ready to treat distress immediately, as some children do not experience distress following extubation, presumably related in part to the decreased discomfort associated with the removal of the endotracheal tube from the pharynx.

When the child is not heavily sedated, parents may have the opportunity to see their child smile and have open eyes before death, an experience that is sometimes greatly valued. Certainly, inducing paralysis at the time of extubation is unacceptable (Truog et al. 2000), as paralysis merely hides the distress from observers but exacerbates the distressing sensations for the patient. Some practitioners also wean the child from the ventilator but retain the endotracheal tube to prevent the noises associated with a lax airway. On the other hand, the presence of an endotracheal tube may be distressing to both the patient (heart rate and sedation needs change dramatically on removal of the tube) and the family. Intensive monitoring and aggressive treatment of symptoms can minimize distress for both the child and the family.

The environment and circumstances of a child who dies as a PICU patient may not be conducive to plying the child with kisses in the final moments of life. Privacy and family presence, if desired by the child and family, is another important aspect of providing comfort to both parties. The Butterfly Program, a joint program of a university hospital and a local hospice in Galveston, Texas, offers a range of services to children with life-threatening conditions, including those in ICU settings. Toward the expected end of a child's life, the program gives parents the opportunity to move the child to the Butterfly Room, a private room large enough to hold fifty family members or other supporters (fig. 11.1). After disconnecting monitors and discontinuing tests, vital sign measurements, fluids, and medications that do not promote the child's comfort, while maintaining vasopressors and the ventilator, parents and anyone of their choice are given the opportunity to support one another and celebrate the child's life as they choose, to hold the child during and following extubation, and to provide the child the comfort of a familiar touch, smell, and affection in perhaps their final moments.

Difficult as it may be to confront death in the ICU, children's needs *can* be met, even in this highly technical environment and even in the face of tragic, sudden loss. Interdisciplinary cooperation and respect, attention to the presence and relief of pain and other symptoms, and most important, responding in a manner that clearly acknowledges that each patient is still a child and a member of a grieving family constitute the pillars of the provision of palliative care in the ICU.

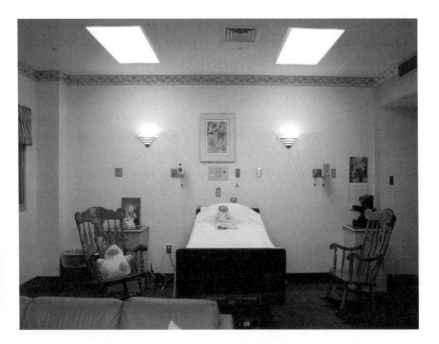

Figure 11.1. A spacious and comfortable place, the Butterfly Room in Galveston, Texas, allows for patient and family choice in setting the environment for end-of-life care.
Source: Provided by Dr. Marcia Levetown.

Family Needs

Parents of children who died suddenly of accidental or intentional trauma or of sudden infant death syndrome have testified at the Institute of Medicine about their wishes to be informed about their child's critical condition. Most parents state that they wanted to receive full information in person. Many expressed a desire to first receive a "warning shot" ("your child has been injured, please come to the hospital—yes, it is serious"). But some wanted to have full information as soon as possible. Parents' repeated insistence on being informed should certainly be honored. Parents need and want jargon-free information. Most of all, they need to be treated as an important part of the care team and respected as persons who have a life outside of the hospital.

Families of children who become suddenly ill, such as trauma patients, are plunged without warning into a frightening new setting. They are in a state of shock and disarray. Providing information about the ICU layout and policies and clarifying the roles of each practitioner is helpful. The parents of an ICU patient need to feel acknowledged as experts on their own child. This message is most clearly sent by soliciting their opinion and experience with medications and comfort preferences. It is also expressed when they are asked about ideas that constitute meaning and value, both from the child's and the family's viewpoint, provided clear information with which to make decisions, and encouraged and enabled to participate in the direct care of the child. Patiently, and often repeatedly, answering questions, acknowledging the personal distress and family disruption that this severity of illness creates, and finding ways to include siblings and, to a lesser extent, extended family is valued tremendously, according to bereaved families. Enrique's family benefited from the inclusion of his older brother in the hospital setting and in therapy directed at helping him cope with his brother's illness and eventual death.

Provide concrete information to orient parents to the ICU.

Solicit values to guide care.

Acknowledge parental expertise regarding their child.

Enable a parenting role by providing clear, empathetic answers to questions.

Acknowledge family distress and disruption.

Parents also state that addressing the practical needs incurred in such settings decreases the stress they experience. As an example, parents need to eat, but do not want to abandon their child. Solutions include enabling them to eat near the ICU or providing a pager to allow them to be immediately notified of any change or the arrival of the physician while they are out of the ICU, such as in the hospital cafeteria. Parents need to sleep, and the provision of comfortable bedding arrangements in or near their child's room helps in this regard. When the ill child has siblings, child care difficulties arise; supervised play areas for the other children, as well as therapeutic interventions for them, will also be appreciated. Unnecessary expenses, such as parking costs at the hospital and having to buy hospital food because there is no access to a refrigerator, combined with missed work and mounting financial pressures, can add to the pressure of having an ill child.

Minimize practical burdens on families.

The decisions parents make on behalf of their dying children are among the most difficult any person can face. Understanding that these decisions are the result of a process that takes time and consultation helps parents endure the situation. Parents need affirmation from health care providers and trusted advisers from other areas of their lives, including religious leaders, extended family members, close friends, and the child's home pediatrician, that they have made the right decisions. Access to a telephone for long-distance calls and to secure e-mail communication can help parents garner such support. Social workers and case managers often are well versed in finding ways to accommodate such needs. Parents also desire consultation with other parents who are in the same situation or who have previously faced such situations. Some hospitals have accommodated these needs by providing parent ambassadors. Concerns about legal liability and privacy issues have to be considered, but they must not be given undue weight in reaching reasonable solutions to such needs.

Ensure parental ability to communicate with trusted advisers.

Siblings' understanding of the ill child's situation may be inaccurate. Being invited into the ICU, after an orientation, ideally by a child-life therapist, about what the ICU and the sibling will look like, and knowing that they can leave if the visit becomes uncomfortable can lessen the amount of misinformation and the severity of distress. The visiting child can be offered opportunities to provide care as well. Suggestions about making a picture for the ill child, singing to or praying with him, watching a movie with him, or assisting in bathing or other physical care needs may be welcome. Parents can be of great help in knowing what would appeal to the healthy sibling.

Siblings need assistance to understand what is happening. Child-life specialists, social workers, and pediatric psychologists may enable a positive experience.

In addition, parents, siblings, other family members, and friends may need to spend the final moments with the dying child. Restrictive PICU visitation policies need thoughtful discussion and revision. Moreover, even if the parents are never able to accept the opportunity to withdraw life-sustaining medical interventions, evidence suggests that some families not only want but also benefit from the opportunity to be present during resuscitative efforts

(Robinson et al. 1998). Bereavement is less complicated for families who have witnessed their child's resuscitation attempt than for those who wanted to be present but were barred from the room.

> *Consider the impact of visitation restrictions and attempt to revise them as needed.*

According to parents, bereavement needs are best met by having continued contact with persons who knew their child, including hospital caregivers. Condolence cards, occasional phone calls and visits, or attendance at the funeral are healing to them (and often to caregivers as well). Simple measures of bereavement by others who cared for their child mean a lot to families.

Despite general expectations to the contrary, many parents appreciate the offer of an autopsy to ensure that the child was indeed irreversibly ill, that they did not give up too soon, and to clarify any risk for recurrence in their family. When autopsies are performed, parents want the results to be presented to them in a manner they can understand. Failure to provide results implies to the parents that the autopsy was performed not for their benefit but perhaps for another purpose. They feel at loose ends as they wait. The physician who cared for the child is in the best position to explain the results and how they affirm or add to what was known before the child's death. This conversation may be enriched by the presence of the pathologist, a social worker or chaplain, and a nurse with strong ties to the family. Face-to-face meetings provide opportunities to answer questions, respond to unspoken concerns expressed in the parents' body language, and determine how the family is coping with their loss and whether additional referrals and assistance are needed.

> *Consider offering autopsies. Be ready to explain the results of the autopsy in understandable language.*

Caregivers' Needs

Since most children who die in developed countries die in neonatal or pediatric intensive care settings, each of which functions with large numbers of multidisciplinary caregivers, a large number of professional personnel will recurrently be exposed to the deaths of children. All these deaths are felt to be tragedies. Some of the hardest to confront are those that result from abuse, murder, and suicide; staff will have conflicts regarding the need to comfort the bereaved family and the discomfort of suspicion and blame that the family was responsible in some way. Accidental death is problematic owing to exposure to the intensity of the families' grief and guilt related to the sudden death of a previously healthy child.

Probably the most disturbing cases for staff are the many patients who are well known to them from recurrent or prolonged ICU stays for life-threatening complications of diseases and congenital anomalies. Two scenarios commonly play out: in the first, the child seemed to be responding to therapy, then "suddenly" dies; in the second, the disorder never responded in the hoped-for manner, and the child endures progressively more invasive and less likely successful ("innovative") attempts to prolong life. In the former situation, the staff are surprised by the death; they had felt they were doing a good job, and when the death unexpectedly happens, they question their techniques, their skill, and their colleagues, looking for answers as to why the child died and what the perceived "avoidable cause" might have been. In the second case, when the therapies never seem to be effective, a tension can arise between those practitioners who feel that continued attempts to prolong life are harmful to the child and family and those who feel it is reasonable to keep trying. These differences of opinion result from differences in experience, personal philosophy and values, religious beliefs and their interpretation, poor communication, and, sometimes, misinformation.

Lack of respect between physicians of differing backgrounds, poor interdisciplinary communication, hierarchical lines of authority, and feelings of helplessness in morally troubling situations contribute to practitioner stress and burnout, perhaps more than the deaths of the children per se (Fields et al. 1995; Heffernan and Heilig 1999). These issues must be recognized and addressed proactively to prevent the loss of highly skilled practitioners. Examples of ways to improve the quality of work environment for practitioners in ICU settings include clear orders documented in the chart, as well as the following:

- scheduling routine interdisciplinary rounds
- creating and actively maintaining an atmosphere of open and respectful communication
- conducting ethics discussions on a routine basis
- assigning clinical mentors with whom it is safe to discuss concerns and emotional responses regarding the patient or the plan of care

- having care team debriefings after difficult deaths, providing access to crisis intervention teams, chaplains, or psychologists as desired
- conducting memorials after the deaths of some patients
- encouraging follow-up with bereaved families
- acknowledging grief associated with professional and personal losses
- acknowledging the value of excellence in the provision of palliative care

The pain of the death of a child is unavoidable in the ICU setting. However, acknowledgment and respectful, open discussion of the controversies, coupled with mutual support of one another and of the children and families served, will do much to lessen the stresses and increase the rewards associated with caring for children who die in the ICU.

Community Resources

Community resources for children like Enrique are hard to come by. Personnel trained specifically to care for children are difficult to find outside of a tertiary care center. For a technology-dependent child such as Enrique wanting to be discharged from an ICU setting and go home, the options are few. Such children are generally cared for by a pediatric home care service that provides nursing care alone, supplemented by government-provided benefits (such as provision of tube feedings and respiratory therapy). A comprehensive family-centered approach is lacking in this option. In the absence of hospice care, parents are often relegated to the role of case manager, dealing with vendors for durable medical equipment and with pharmacies, nursing agencies, and insurers or Medicaid offices. Parents of technology-dependent children often say they spend more time talking on the phone than parenting their child for the brief time he or she is alive.

The hospice alternative in the United States offers a comprehensive, family-centered approach, including case management and total assistance with managing medications, durable medical equipment, and bereavement care, but generally has no pediatric expertise and is very "low tech," owing to the structure of the Medicare-Medicaid benefit, which, in 2004, provides $120 a day to pay for all care given to the patient and his or her family. Moreover, hospices caring for patients receiving "life-sustaining measures" are deemed to be operating outside their license and are at risk of being fined for providing "fraudulent care."

There is generally low availability of respite care. In some areas, depending on the child's condition, transportation, and the availability of appropriate personnel, a child's school can serve as a respite for parents. However, schools and other care providers may be unwilling to honor parent-requested limitations of medical intervention, and parents may need to choose between school and the possibility of a death associated with unwanted invasive, nonbeneficial interventions. Support groups and other community resources that require the child to leave the home are rarely available to parents of technology-dependent children, nor can such children be left with a neighborhood babysitter. Sometimes nurses will volunteer to sit with the child for a few hours.

Families with access to the Internet can find chat lines and on-line support groups to assist them in learning more about their child's condition and to provide practical solutions as well as solace. With so few children with such needs, most of them spread far apart, there are no systematic answers for families whose child is afflicted with a life-threatening, technology-dependent condition. Creative families find solutions with their extended families and members of religious and philanthropic organizations, and once their savings are lost, some families may qualify for governmental assistance.

Primary care pediatricians in the community, as well as PICU physicians, often become local experts in the care of such children. They are valuable resources in providing continuity of care and in making decisions about medical care, which will shift with time as the child's condition deteriorates. Knowing the child well, understanding the parents' perspectives, and adding professional experience and judgment to the mix, the child's pediatrician can help ensure that the best decisions are made for the individual patient and family. Thus ICU physicians guiding end-of-life care should inquire about the resources in the family's community, draw on their experience, and acknowledge their roles in the care of this child and family, as well as the loss they will inevitably feel as the child's life draws to a close. As with Enrique's family, it may be important for community caregivers to be included in the withdrawal of interventions, to provide affirmation and support for one another.

Conclusion

Palliative care is not only consistent with critical care settings; it is essential to them. Routinely acknowledging the importance of the individual child, the context of the family, the impact of illness on physical, psychosocial, and spiritual realms, the need for clear information, respect, and the observation of meaningful rituals should be honored for all patients, particularly those in ICU settings, regardless of their outcome. Increased research on instruments to reliably assess symptoms in critically ill pediatric populations and research to ensure effective and safe treatment of these symptoms is urgently needed. In the meantime, simple, no-cost measures can markedly enhance the experience of children and their families receiving care in pediatric or neonatal intensive care units.

References

American Academy of Pediatrics, Committee on Bioethics. 1995. Informed consent, parental permission and assent in pediatric practice. *Pediatrics* 95:314–17.

Anand, K. J. S., and P. R. Hickey. 1987. Pain and its effects on the human neonate and fetus. *N Engl J Med* 317:1321–29.

Bluebond-Langner, M. 1978. *The private worlds of dying children.* Princeton: Princeton University Press.

Contro, N., J. Larson, S. Scofield, B. Sourkes, and H. Cohen. 2002. Family perspectives on the quality of pediatric palliative care. *Arch Pediatr Adolesc Med* 156:14–19.

Fields, A. I., T. T. Cuerdon, C. O. Brasseux, P. R. Getson, A. E. Thompson, J. P. Orlowski, and S. J. Youngner. 1995. Physician burnout in pediatric critical care medicine. *Crit Care Med* 23:1425–29.

Garwick, A. W., J. Patterson, F. C. Bennett, and R. W. Blum. 1995. Breaking the news: how families first learn about their child's chronic condition. *Arch Pediatr Adolesc Med* 149:991–97.

Greig-Midlane, H. 2001. The parents' perspective on withdrawing treatment. *BMJ* 323:390.

Heffernan, P., and S. Heilig. 1999. Giving "moral distress" a voice: ethical concerns among neonatal intensive care personnel. *Camb Q Healthcare Ethics* 8:173–78.

Leith, P. J., and S. J. Weisman. 1997. The management of painful procedures in children. *Pediatr Clin North Am* 6:829–42.

Levetown, M. 1998. Palliative care in the intensive care unit. *New Horizons* 6(4):383–97.

Levetown, M., M. M. Pollack, T. T. Cuerdon, U. E. Ruttiman, and J. J. Glover. 1994. Limitations and withdrawals of medical intervention in pediatric critical care. *JAMA* 272:1271–75.

Levi, R. B., R. Marsick, D. Drotar, and E. D. Kodish. 2000. Diagnosis, disclosure, and informed consent: learning from parents of children with cancer. *Int J Pediatr Hematol Oncol* 22(1):3–12.

Levinson, W. 1997. Doctor-patient communication and medical malpractice: implications for pediatricians. *Pediatr Ann* 26:186–93.

Mastroyannopoulou, K., P. Stallard, M. Lewis, and S. Lenton. 1997. The impact of childhood non-malignant life-threatening illness on parents: gender differences and predictors of parental adjustment. *J Child Psychol Psychiatry* 38:823–29.

McCallum, D. E., P. Byrne, and E. Bruera. 2000. How children die in hospital. *J Pain Symptom Manage* 20:417–23.

O'Donnell, H., R. S. Phillips, N. Wenger, J. Teno, R. B. Davis, and M. B. Hamel. 2003. Preferences for cardiopulmonary resuscitation among patients 80 years or older: the views of patients and their physicians. *J Am Med Dir Assoc* 4:139–44.

Partridge, J. C., and S. N. Wall. 1997. Analgesia for dying infants whose life support is withdrawn or withheld. *Pediatrics* 99:76–79.

Porter, F. L., R. E. Grunau, and K. J. S. Anand. 1999. Long-term effects of pain in infants. *J Dev Behav Pediatr* 20:253–61.

Robinson, S. M., S. Mackenzie-Ross, G. L. Campbell-Hewson, C. V. Egleston, and A. T. Prevost. 1998. Psychological effect of witnessed resuscitation on bereaved relatives. *Lancet* 352:614–17.

Schindler, M. B., D. Bohn, P. N. Cox, B. W. McCrindle, A. Jarvis, J. Edmonds, and G. Barker. 1996. Outcome of out-of-hospital cardiac or respiratory arrest in children. *N Engl J Med* 335:1473–79.

Slonim, A. D. 2000. Cardiopulmonary resuscitation outcomes in children. *Crit Care Med* 28:3364–66.

Torres, A., C. B. Pickert, J. Firestone, W. M. Walker, and D. H. Fiser. 1997. Long-term functional outcome of inpatient pediatric cardiopulmonary resuscitation. *Pediatr Emerg Care* 13:369–73.

Truog, R. D., J. P. Burns, C. Mitchell, J. Johnson, and W. Robinson. 2000. Pharmacologic paralysis and withdrawal of mechanical ventilation at the end of life. *N Engl J Med* 342:508–11.

Truog, R. D., A. F. M. Cist, S. E. Brackett, J. P. Burns, M. A. Curley, M. Danis, M. A. DeVita, S. H. Rosenbaum, D. M. Rothenberg, C. L. Sprung, S. A. Webb, G. S. Woody, and W. E. Hurford. 2001. Recommendations for end-of-life care in the intensive care unit: the Ethics Committee of the Society of Critical Care Medicine. *Crit Care Med* 29:2332–48.

Vernon, D. D., J. M. Dean, O. D. Timmons, W. Banner Jr., and E. M. Allen-Webb. 1993. Modes of death in the pediatric intensive care unit: withdrawal and limitation of supportive care. *Crit Care Med* 21:1798–1802.

Wanzer, S. H., D. D. Federman, S. J. Adelstein, C. K. Cassel, E. H. Cassem, R. E. Cranford, E. W. Hook, B. Lo, C. G. Moertel, P. Safar, A. Stone, and J. van Eys. 1989. The physician's responsibility toward hopelessly ill patients: a second look. *N Engl J Med* 320:844–49.

Wolfe, J., H. E. Grier, N. Klar, S. B. Levin, J. M. Ellenbogen, S. Salem-Schatz, E. J. Emanuel, and J. C. Weeks. 2000. Symptoms and suffering at the end of life in children with cancer. *N Engl J Med* 342:326–33.

12

Palliative Care in the Home, School, and Community

Bruce P. Himelstein, M.D., F.A.A.P., Stacy F. Orloff, Ed.D., L.C.S.W.,
Dale Evans, R.N., Ph.D., and Janice Wheeler, M.Ed.

"It's so nice to be at home with my family. Friends can come over, and it's just best to be home with your own things," said Terry, a 16-year-old girl who was dying from a rare form of leukemia. She had been undergoing treatment, including a bone marrow transplant, for twenty-two months. Even though she was in the last stage of her life, on parenteral nutrition and multiple medications for pain and symptom control, Terry was able to stay at home surrounded by family, pets, school friends, and members of a well-qualified interdisciplinary palliative care team.

A few months before her death, Terry agreed to appear in an educational film about palliative home care to "help others understand how important it is for kids." Shortly after that, she presided from her wheelchair as prom queen with a high school class that demonstrated a degree of compassion often seen when the school and community become involved with supporting children facing a life-threatening illness and their families. Terry's visible presence at homecoming reminded everyone that she was indeed living, even in the face of her impending death. Terry's school friends, teachers, neighbors, and the community as a whole had a strong desire to be helpful and often sought ways to be supportive of her and her family.

As Terry lived her final days, her friends sent special communications in the form of e-mails, personal letters, handmade cards, and "singing" telegrams. Her closest friends continued to spend time on the telephone with her and to make personal visits.

Terry kept a large jigsaw puzzle in her bedroom. "If you're going to come over to see me, you have to be willing to put a piece in the puzzle," she laughingly insisted. Terry's friends enjoyed the challenge, and this simple task helped the teenagers feel more at ease while visiting. Her friend, Brooke, remarked, "Sometimes I don't know what to do or say. But I can always find a piece in the puzzle."

Church members often delivered meals and ran errands for the family. Close family friends frequently included Terry's younger sister, Rachel, in their own family activities and outings. Rachel enjoyed these opportunities to go to the movies, visit the zoo, or take a walk in the park—simple pleasures that her parents could not often provide while caring for Terry at home.

As the holiday season drew near, the youth group from Terry's church gathered on her front lawn. Although too weak to come to the door, Terry could easily hear the caroling voices filling the evening air with a joyful song; and she welcomed Santa's bedside delivery of special gifts from the church.

Each special encounter with Terry was an active and effective way for members of the school and community to respond to, and later remember, their young friend. In early January, a large number of students and teachers attended Terry's memorial service. The following day, teachers allowed time for students to talk and share memories of Terry, recognizing that it could not be just another day at school. Students decided to dedicate the school yearbook to Terry, and graduation was held that spring in her memory.

Terry's case raises many questions about caring for children living with life-threatening conditions in an out-of-hospital setting, including the following:

- What are the principles of palliative care for children in the home, school, and community, and are they different from what might be required in an acute care setting?
- What are the elements of a successful model of care for children?
- What are the challenges to providing care in the community?
- What are some of the innovative approaches possible for out-of-hospital care for the child with a life-threatening condition?

There are many other important yet unanswerable questions to consider when reviewing palliative care plans for children at home, at school, and in the community. Finding answers to these questions requires an evidence base that does not yet exist. The questions are presented here as challenges to the pediatric palliative care community, to generate interest in the research required to answer them:

- What is the effect of home care on the frequency of hospital stay, intensive care admissions, and emergency room visits?
- Could more children die in the place of their choice if psychosocial support were offered earlier in the disease process?
- Does having control of day-to-day care and decisions improve the experiences and quality of life of ill children and their families?
- How are parents affected by being transformed into medical care providers?
- What outcome measures are available to help teams determine the most effective care modalities and the results of their interventions?

Principles of Palliative Care for Children in the Home, School, and Community

Hospice or palliative care programs for children living with life-threatening conditions should have an integrated model of care that includes service to all affected by the illness of the child (Levetown 2000). Services must be available in the home, in the acute care hospital, and in any other setting in which the family and child feel comfortable. Palliative care should begin with the child's involvement in the diagnostic process and should continue through bereavement. Responsible pediatric programs will address the needs made evident within the child's home, school, religious or faith communities, and service clubs as the child continues to live with his or her condition and ultimately dies from it. A comprehensive psychosocial assessment at the time of admission to the hospice or palliative care program will identify the important spheres of influence for the ill child and his or her siblings. The principles of practice of pediatric palliative care do not vary according to the setting.

Children and their families are part of an integrated system made up of many different parts. Together, these parts function like a finely tuned machine. If one part is not working well, the entire machine will be affected. Medical treatment of the ill child without consideration of the context of care is not effective. A child is part of a family, including extended family members, as well as a larger supportive community. Interventions must be practically available to all parts of the larger family system.

The home is generally considered the preferred site of living until death. In a study of parents who lost a child to a life-threatening illness, insurance coverage and home health care were ranked as the two most important services. Of all the services used by families during the course of their child's illness, families indicated the greatest satisfaction with home health or hospice care. Families viewed this service as the most critical in helping them to cope with their child's illness (Utah Department of Health 2001). Benefits to parents of home care also include greater freedom, more privacy, and less disruption to the family. Many families reported caring for their dying children as a positive experience (Collins, Stevens, and Cousens 1998).

Home-based palliative care for children facing life-threatening illness must be an option. Families should have unlimited access to their children, and no setting assures that as well as home care. In the home, parents are in control of their child's care plan. With sufficient support, most families can carry out even the most complex medical tasks. It is not uncommon for staff working with parents who have been caring for the child for a long period of time to realize that the parents know more than they do about the disease and the best treatments, medications, and equipment for that individual child.

Palliative care is best provided by an interdisciplinary team, whether the patient is in the home, at school, or in the community. Palliative care is philosophically, personally, and emotionally challenging. The skill sets and support of members of different disciplines and volunteers are critical to the care of the child and family as well as the effective functioning of the team. Depending on the child's medical and psychospiritual condition, essential members of the interdisciplinary team may include the following:

- the child's primary physician or specialist
- nurses and nursing assistants
- social workers
- pharmacists
- volunteers and respite workers
- pastoral care providers
- child-life and expressive therapists
- dieticians
- bereavement counselors
- teachers
- psychologists
- physical, occupational, and speech therapists

Care is directed by the needs of the child and family, as they define those needs, with the guidance of the palliative care team. A nurse must be available to the family twenty-four hours a day, seven days a week, with backup on-call physicians and pharmacists who know the child and his or her condition. Homemakers and respite caregivers supplement volunteers in providing needed support to parents and siblings as well as the ill child. When possible, home teachers or a school schedule should be maintained. Celebration of holidays, birthdays, and treatment milestones as well as the creation of memories through pictures, stories, hand molds, and memory books assist the child and family to maintain a degree of normality. Often, community groups can be of great assistance in providing resources for celebrations of the child's life. Anticipatory grief programs and bereavement care are essential components of any service model. Home care results in enhanced bereavement outcomes for family members who otherwise may have had limited access to the child.

Patients' Needs

The need for effective control of pain and symptoms is as important in the home as in any other setting. Many troubling symptoms may afflict chronically ill children, including psychological symptoms and disorders such as anxiety and depression. Symptoms are commonly underreported because children wish to protect their parents from the emotional pain of their illness and impending death and because of methodologic problems in pediatric palliative care delivery and research (Carr-Gregg et al. 1997; Collins et al. 2000, 2001; Wolfe, Klar, et al. 2000). These issues are addressed in greater detail in chapter 7 of this volume.

Medication doses and even routes of delivery for children differ from those for adults. In the absence of needed pediatric data, adult dose regimens are commonly extrapolated for children. Dignity issues, especially with adolescents, may require alternatives to rectal administration of medication. Many medications are not available in dose strengths small enough for the younger child unless a compounding pharmacy is available.

Frequently, pain and other symptoms are more effectively managed when the parents and child are in control of medications and treatment. Unlike the acute care setting, however, the local pharmacy is not necessarily available twenty-four hours a day; it may not necessarily stock needed medications; and getting prescriptions filled can be an onerous task for families dealing with a very sick child. Although many infusion companies support families with twenty-four-hour pharmacies, time must be allowed for the pharmacist to mix the medications and to have them delivered to the house. The best approach is to work with the pediatrician and available experts in palliative care to plan ahead; in many situations, symptoms are predictable. A child with a brain tumor, for example, may have seizures or pain from increased intracranial pressure. Having rectal diazepam or a similar anticonvulsant, as well as sublingual morphine drops, in the home in advance is a prudent preparation. In the worst-case scenario, the drugs will remain in the medicine cabinet, unused, until their disposal at the time of death.

Alternative treatment modalities such as massage therapy, play and expressive therapies, and guided imagery are an accepted and natural part of the home setting. The child's need to have as normal a life as possible and to accomplish developmental tasks occurs more easily when in familiar surroundings, among parents, siblings, friends, and pets. Open and clear communication with the child is critical and must be based on the child's ability to understand. With younger children, much of the communication is nonverbal, expressed in drawings and play. The child's wishes regarding continued treatment and rehospitalization must be considered; the door of return to an acute care setting must never be closed. Both parents and children should receive sensitive support to reach decisions that are in the best interest of the child's quality of life, free from pressure or guilt. In the home setting, the spiritual needs of the child can be addressed with pastoral care home visits or by providing information and support to the family's own spiritual or religious adviser.

Families' Needs

Children requiring palliative care in the home, at school, and in community settings have many conditions, often rare. Caring for such children requires a well-planned, well-coordinated, and well-communicated plan of care. Everyone involved in the child's care must have access to the same assessment information; medications prescribed by different specialists should be coordinated to avoid competing efficacies, dangerous interactions, or unnecessary side effects. A clear path to assessment and management must be available at all times. Families need a reliable, designated "quarterback" to help them navigate the health care delivery system to get what is required for the child's medical and psychospiritual care.

A care plan developed to meet the child's needs is an essential tool to help parents survive the demands of around-the-clock caregiving. The plan must be developed with the parents to best meet their unique needs. Although home care gives parents unlimited access to their child, the stress of performing care, coordinating and often transporting the child for treatments, interacting with insurance carriers, and meeting their responsibilities at work and with their other children can be overwhelming. Palliative care team members and volunteers can provide needed assistance with medical treatments, pain and symptom control, financial concerns, emotional support, counseling, and respite. Parents frequently are challenged by complex medical tasks that are constant and from which they have little relief. This is particularly true of parents with technology-dependent children.

The family's emotional life becomes centered around the ill child, with little energy left for maintenance of the marital relationship and for the child's siblings. Team members can be of assistance in providing supportive services to siblings, counseling to parents, and respite time for the family to engage in activities away from the home. Some families who have cared for the child at home prefer not to have the child die at home. For others, home care is not an option. Hospice options need to be explored for these families. Grief and bereavement services are critical to families and may often be unavailable because of financial reasons (no reimbursement of expenses) or lack of trained staff. Local hospices may provide these services to families—even to families that may not have used the hospice before the child's death. Grief and bereavement services may also be provided by community groups such as Candlelighters and Compassionate Friends.

Parents caring for a child with a terminal illness at home need to know what to expect. In a study of families who cared for a child with cancer who died at home, for example, several parents discussed the need for better preparation for the child's death and for better understanding of what to do after the death occurs (Sirkia et al. 1997).

Health Care Providers' Needs

"The medical professionals who enter the home of a terminally ill child must be exceptional individuals. These are people who are pivotal during the most painful experience of a lifetime, and who can have an influence so profound that the outcome of the whole experience can actually be positive and seem as a blessing" (Utah Department of Health 2001). The need for training in pediatric palliative care for home care and hospice workers and volunteers is clear. The training needs to include effective communication skills, pain and symptom management, and how to celebrate relationships. Pediatric care and hospice principles must be clearly understood. Institutional support must be available for the home care team to help them cope with the challenges of working with families and children facing life-threatening illness, long treatment protocols, remissions and relapses, and death. Research is needed to develop outcome measures appropriate to pediatric palliative care to help teams determine the most effective care modalities and interventions.

Educational opportunities do exist, but there is no mandate for education in home care practice for those caring for children in the home. For example, Neale, Hodgkins, and Demers (1992) established a three-month home health rotation for second- and third-year family medicine residents, combining experiential and didactic learning. Changes in resident attitudes, knowledge, supervisory assessment, and patient reactions to home visits were documented. Seligman and colleagues (1999) demonstrate that exposure to a clinical hospice experience during medical school training can have positive effects on physician self-assessments of knowledge, skills, and attitudes in their future practice. The use of standardized-patient protocols in the home setting has been studied to test the pain assessment skills of hospice nurses (Owens et al. 2000). All such programs, however, are both time and labor intensive.

Community Resources

Schools, service clubs, and faith organizations may contact the care team for assistance. Members of the health care team must remember that family permission is required before sharing confidential information. Without the family's permission to share specific information regarding the ill child, the health care professional may share only information that is commonly known or reasonably applicable to other similar situations.

Assisting ill children and their classmates in the school setting is important. Hospice or palliative care involvement should be available to the school beginning from the time the child is diagnosed with a life-threatening condition. The classroom teacher may look for guidance in sharing information with classmates regarding the diagnosis, treatment, possible return to school, and the potential for death. Teachers do not always feel competent to address these areas of concern with their students. Discomfort with the subject matter may prevent some teachers from addressing the subject at all, leaving the child's classmates to wonder and worry alone. Specific issues to address may also include the question of transmissibility, classmates' concern that they may have done something to cause the child's illness, permission to ask questions and express fears, and conversation about visiting their ill classmate and making "get well" or "thinking of you" cards. The interdisciplinary team can also provide assistance to the teacher and principal in drafting a letter to the classmates' parents (with permission from the ill child's parents) sharing pertinent information about how to contact the family and child, where to send correspondence, and any assistance the family may be open to receiving. Team members may visit the school and give presentations about significant disease or illness courses, answer students' questions in a classroom setting, or meet with the faculty to better inform and support them.

Another important role the interdisciplinary team serves is to assist the school when the ill child may be preparing to return. This transition for hospitalized children is frequently facilitated by child-life specialists. However, children receiving care in their home do not always receive such help. Hospice and palliative care programs must develop strategies to assist children healthy enough to return to school, even if only for a partial school day. Part of the psychosocial assessment must include questions regarding the child's desire to return to school and his or her physical capacity to do so.

Returning to school is not always an easy process for the affected child. The interdisciplinary team can help, using clinical interventions that vary according to the individual child's chronological and development level as well as his or her physical status. At a minimum, the counselor must address issues of social and behavioral adjustment. For the homebound child, all school-based activities are at a standstill. For his or her classmates, there has been no such interruption in school life; relationships have continued, and new friendships have been cultivated. The ill child may have missed, or been unaware of, many school-based activities and events. For the homebound child, it can be quite difficult to understand and accept that friendships may have changed in response to the lack of shared experience and activity. Moreover, the ill child's priorities and values may have evolved because of his or her own unusual experiences.

Olson and colleagues (1993) conducted a study measuring overall functioning of children with cancer, using the children's teachers and parents as respondents. The study finds that 55 percent of the children had little or mild impairment when returning to school, 30 percent were moderately impaired, and 15 percent had marked impairment. Impairment was noted primarily in behavioral problems and social competence. For some children, the impairment was great enough to affect their ability to reintegrate into the classroom. Other studies show less conclusive evidence that the child with cancer has difficulty integrating into the classroom. It has been theorized that teachers and other school personnel may be overly sympathetic to the ill child and overlook or make excuses for behavior that may be symptomatic of poor integration (Noll et al. 1999).

It is not enough to prepare the ill child for return to the classroom. If successful integration is to be ensured, the classmates and teacher also need time to prepare. Assisting the ill child in a successful return to school requires providing assistance to the other children in the classroom. If the classmates and teachers are not prepared to accept the ill child back into the classroom, the reintegration process will fail. There are many factors to consider when working with schoolmates and classmates. There will be some concerns specific to the chronological and developmental ages of the children. As noted above, students of all ages may wonder or worry about "catching" the returning student's illness, or if they were somehow responsible for their classmate's illness. The returning child's physical appearance may be altered. Some children may be frightened about how their classmate looks and ignore the child because of their fear.

The interdisciplinary team should be prepared to spend some time working with the teacher and classmates before the homebound student's first day back. Ideally, the counselor will talk first with the child's parents, inquiring about what confidential information may be shared with their child's teacher and classmates. An important tenet of hospice or palliative care holds that the patient and family (in this case, the ill child and parents) are at the center of the care. They serve to direct the plan of care, and the care team serves to implement the care. The parents must be active participants in the decision-making process, as the psychosocial counselor cannot make the decision about what information is shared with the school. The parents may want to meet with the school principal, guidance counselor, teacher, and other staff before their child returns to school. It would be appropriate, if the parents so request, for the psychosocial counselor from the palliative care team to attend that meeting. At this meeting, decisions are made regarding the development of an implementation plan.

The psychosocial factors that influence siblings are also evident in the school setting and must be addressed within that environment. During the school meeting it is important to address any issues or concerns that may affect siblings who attend the same school. If the siblings attend another school, it would be helpful for the parents to initiate and maintain the same level of involvement at that school. The sibling's classmates may also have questions, and may also benefit from clinical intervention throughout the ill child's illness, not just when he or she is returning to school. Given that good hospice or palliative care is family focused, it is important to develop school-based interventions that support the entire family. Classmates of the healthy sibling may feel uncomfortable and uncertain about how to communicate concern. This discomfort may lead classmates to avoid the sibling, further increasing the healthy sibling's sense of isolation and abandonment. Sibling issues and concerns are vast and are discussed in chapter 6 of this volume.

This same level of involvement within the school setting should continue throughout the course of hospice or palliative care. The psychosocial counselor would again be in a position to provide school-based intervention when the child dies. This intervention may include visiting the classroom to facilitate discussion, preparing classmates who may choose to attend a funeral, viewing, or other religious ritual related to the death, and meeting with individual classmates (with their parents' or guardians' permission) who may be more emotionally affected than others.

Other school-based activities include group support. Hospice or palliative care programs and schools have a wonderful collaborative opportunity to provide group support for students during the school day. Some comprehensive hospice or palliative care programs currently provide such group support free of charge. These programs are financially supported by donations.

Many ill children and their siblings are also part of a religious or faith-based community. They may be active in a synagogue, church, or mosque youth group. As the child becomes ill, progressively more peers in their faith community struggle with the same questions, concerns, and anxieties as the ill child's classmates. Comprehensive hospice or palliative care programs will be able to address these concerns within the faith-based community. The psychosocial services provided by pediatric hospice and palliative care programs must integrate with and will complement the support provided by the community's religious or spiritual leader. Psychosocial counselors can most effectively meet with the ill child's peers in religious school classes, after worship services, and during youth group service projects.

Another sphere of influence for children is service groups such as Boy Scout and Girl Scout programs and athletic leagues. Service groups, in particular, may wish to do something to assist the ill child and his or her extended family. Service groups can approach a family and offer to assist with yard work, child care, and food drives. The psychosocial counselor can serve as the contact and coordinate between the service groups and the affected family. It is a basic human reaction to feel helpless during times of great stress and uncertainty; children feel especially helpless. Providing guidance and assistance in channeling uncertain feelings into action is an important role of the psychosocial counselor.

Societal Needs

If remaining in the hospital increases the risk of unwanted medical testing and interventions and is emotionally, physically, and financially burdensome to the child, the family, and society, why is there such a paucity of private or government insurance coverage for palliative or hospice services? Why are there so few trained pediatric home care or hospice personnel and so few programs structured to facilitate care in the home from the time of diagnosis? What are the costs and benefits of home care as compared with the costs and benefits of an acute care hospital stay? How can the current care dilemma be resolved when hospice programs may not have or wish to have home care licenses and are limited by criteria for admission based on an adult model that is not relevant to children? How can home care agencies provide the comprehensive care required by children and their families when reimbursement is limited by a narrow vision of "medical necessity" and fee-for-service models?

Unfortunately, most home care and hospice regulations were not developed with children in mind. The nature of pediatric chronic and life-threatening illness has changed dramatically, and many children survive today who twenty years ago would have lived much shorter lives (Ries et al. 1999; Feudtner, Christakis, and Connell 2000). Furthermore, there remains the problem of prognostication with rare disorders. How long does a child with a rare metabolic disorder live? Children do not die according to formulas—making the hospice entry criterion of six months' life expectancy an even greater impediment to access to palliative care for them than for adults. Even when reasonable estimates of prognosis exist, they are unlikely to be shared accurately with or understood by families (Wolfe, Grier, et al. 2000). When the child outlives the prognosis, hospices may be at risk of being accused of fraud and thereby face legal jeopardy.

Invasive or disease-modifying comfort measures, such as chemotherapy, radiotherapy, artificial hydration and nutrition, and blood product support, fall outside the spectrum of typically provided hospice services, despite their capacity to improve the quality of life. Children already receiving life-sustaining technologies that require continuous or scheduled in-home nursing care are at a particular disadvantage, as under current regulations hospice services are seen as a duplication of service. The child and his or her family must often make a difficult choice. Should they maintain established relationships with the skilled nurses and caregivers that are providing respite and ongoing care to the child and family? Must they abandon these services to engage with strangers who can provide interdisciplinary care for their emotional and spiritual needs and see to ongoing bereavement support after the child has died?

For these reasons, many children requiring such therapies and nursing services have no access to hospice care. The extraordinary challenge for non-hospice home health providers, therefore, is to attempt to provide the necessary psychospiritual care these children and families need and deserve, despite lack of trained personnel and support and continuing education for in-home providers.

Although unique programs exist around the world that attempt to combine the best of home health, hospice, acute care, and community resources (Levetown 2000), they are all hampered by the lack of financial stability in the absence of regulations that acknowledge the need for such programs and provide reimbursement for services. Some such arrangements, particularly bridge programs between home health and hospice care within the same company, may be under close scrutiny by regulators to detect "impropriety," despite the obvious benefit to children and families.

Most community-based services are not currently reimbursable, and so some hospice or palliative care programs are barred from providing such services. An ill child is part of a larger system, a system that includes all spheres of influence in the child's life. Withholding care and treatment in some of these spheres prevents the hospice or palliative care team from providing comprehensive and optimally effective service to the child and his or her family. Hospice and palliative care programs can explore several avenues to find funding for community-based services. Hospice and palliative care state associations may choose to lobby their state legislatures and work on legislative changes to the reimbursement structure, as well as to participate in demonstration programs such as the Program for All-Inclusive Care for Children (www.chionline.org/programs/about.phtml).

Until reimbursement standards for palliative home care are changed, most support for services will continue to come from philanthropy. Many hospices and palliative care programs have foundations that serve as the fundraising component of the program and have been very successful in raising funds for children's programs. Hospice and palliative care programs may wish to develop grant initiatives with partners in their community, such as the local school system. Community foundations, church and civic groups, and service organizations such as the Junior League can also become reliable sources of support for programs. National groups with local chapters, such as Candlelighters, the American Cancer Society, the Leukemia and Lymphoma Society, and Compassionate Friends, offer information, resources, and support to families.

The issue of do-not-resuscitate orders for children in the home is also important. In many states, children do not have the protection of state law recognizing the validity of in-home do-not-resuscitate status for children (Sabatino 1999). Parents and providers outside of hospice, fearing legal action, face difficult decisions about putting their children at risk for unwanted resuscitation. This issue is particularly troublesome in the school setting (American Academy of Pediatrics 2000). In all situations, a letter from the child's attending physician verifying the diagnosis, life-threatening or terminal nature of the condition, and the joint decision made by the parents, physician, and, when age appropriate, the child, not to provide resuscitative or life-extending interventions should be available for parents to give to emergency medical services personnel and hospital emergency department staff.

Conclusion

Despite numerous barriers, comprehensive and compassionate palliative care for children in the home, school, and community is possible and should be part of a unified plan of care beginning at the time of diagnosis of a life-threatening condition. In the future, education for providers of community-based palliative care, development of standards for eligibility for palliative care services for children, the integration of palliative care specialists into home care teams and services, and new models of health care reimbursement for life-threatened children will need to be addressed. It will not be possible to break through the barriers to widespread access to effective community-based palliative home care and hospice, especially for children in rural and underserved areas, until these issues have been resolved. Research rigorously demonstrating the benefits of care for the dying child in the community is also needed.

References

American Academy of Pediatrics, Committee on School Health and Committee on Bioethics. 2000. Do not resuscitate orders in schools. *Pediatrics* 105:878–79.

Carr-Gregg, M. R. C., S. M. Sawyer, C. F. Clarke, and G. Bowes. 1997. Caring for the terminally ill adolescent. *Med J Aust* 166:255–58.

Collins, J., M. Byrnes, I. Dunkel, J. Lapin, T. Nadel, H. Thaler, T. Polyak, B. Rapkin, and R. Portenoy. 2000. The measurement of symptoms in children with cancer. *J Pain Symptom Manage* 19:353–77.

Collins, J., T. Devine, G. Dick, E. Johnson, H. Kilham, C. Pinkerton, M. Stevens, H. Thaler, and R. Portenoy. 2001. The measurement of symptoms in young children with cancer: the validation of the Memorial Symptom Assessment Scale (MSAS 7–12) in children aged 7–12. *J Pain Symptom Manage* 23:10–16.

Collins, J. J., M. M. Stevens, and P. Cousens. 1998. Home care for the dying child: a parent's perception. *Aust Fam Physician* 27:610–14.

Feudtner, C., D. A. Christakis, and F. A. Connell. 2000. Pediatric deaths attributable to complex chronic conditions: a population-based study of Washington State, 1980–1997. *Pediatrics* 106:205–9.

Levetown, M. 2000. *Compendium of pediatric palliative care.* Alexandria, Va.: National Hospice and Palliative Care Organization.

Neale, A., B. Hodgkins, and R. Demers. 1992. The home visit in resident education: program description and evaluation. *Fam Med* 24:36–40.

Noll, R., M. Gartstein, K. Vannatta, J. Correll, W. Bukowksi, and D. Hobart. 1999. Social, emotional, and behavioral functioning of children with cancer. *Pediatrics* 103:71–77.

Olson, A., W. Boyle, M. Evans, and L. Zug. 1993. Overall function in rural childhood cancer survivors: the role of social competence and emotional health. *Clin Pediatr* 32:334–42.

Owens, M., G. McConvey, D. Weeks, and L. Zeisberg. 2000. A pilot program to evaluate pain assessment skills of hospice nurses. *Am J Hospice and Palliat Care* 17:44–48.

Ries, L., M. Smith, J. Gurney, M. Linet, Y. Tamra, J. Young, and G. Bunin, eds. 1999. *Cancer incidence and survival among children and adolescents: United States SEER program, 1975–1995.* NIH publication 99-4649; Bethesda, Md.: National Cancer Institute.

Sabatino, C. 1999. Survey of state EMS-DNR laws and protocols. *Journal of Law* 27:297.

Seligman, P., E. Massey, R. Fink, P. Nelson-Marten, and P. VonLobkowitz. 1999. Practicing physicians' assessments of the impact of their medical-school clinical hospice experience. *J Cancer Ed* 14:144–47.

Sirkia, K., U. Saarinen, B. Ahlgren, and L. Hovi. 1997. Terminal care of the child with cancer at home. *Acta Paediatr* 86:1125–1130.

Utah Department of Health. 2001. *Conversations with parents who lost a child to a life-threatening illness: promoting HOPE for Utah children.* Salt Lake City: Utah Department of Health.

Wolfe, J., H. Grier, N. Klar, S. Levin, J. Ellenbogen, S. Salem-Schatz, E. Emanuel, and J. Weeks. 2000. Symptoms and suffering at the end of life in children with cancer. *N Engl J Med* 342:326–33.

Wolfe, J., N. Klar, H. E. Grier, J. Duncan, S. Salem-Schatz, E. J. Emanuel, and J. C. Weeks. 2000. Understanding of prognosis among parents of children who died of cancer: impact on treatment goals and integration of palliative care. *JAMA* 284:2469–75.

13

The Child with a Genetic Condition

Sara Perszyk, R.N., B.S.N., and Anthony Perszyk, M.D.

"Katy is just part of what makes us a family. She is so much more than what we thought she could ever be, based on what we know about leukodystrophy.

"Within the first two weeks after Katy was born, we knew things were not right with her. She did not startle at loud noises—ever. We called our pediatrician's office and were told not to worry. We attempted to startle her ourselves. I think we did this more out of a need to prove to ourselves that nothing was wrong. We decided the problem had to be related to her hearing. We began trying to get her pediatrician to send her to an audiologist. After several visits to the doctor, we were again told not to worry, because she was a big baby, and sometimes they developed more slowly. We noticed that Katy did not move around as much as she had as a newborn, and she seemed to still be sleeping an awful lot. Finally, at about six months, the pediatrician decided that Katy might have a hearing problem.

"An audiologist tested Katy's hearing and said there was no problem with her hearing. We went back to the pediatrician when Katy was 7 months old. When they measured her head, the circumference was off the growth chart. They sent us to a neurologist at the children's clinic. An MRI was done and diagnosed Katy with leukodystrophy. Our lives were like a story out of *Reader's Digest* at this point. It was like being in a dream. I was watching my life unfold, but it didn't seem real to me at this point. We cried a lot. We prayed a lot.

"Coordinating regular checkups, sick patient visits, and therapies can be a logistical nightmare for a child with a rare condition. Emergency room visits are the worst. We try to avoid them at all costs because Katy has been subjected to unnecessary invasive testing in the emergency room when an attending refused to contact her primary physician upon our request. We have since learned not to be so passive. Katy can spike a fever and in three hours it will be gone, leaving us wondering what is going on with her. On the other hand, a cold can develop into pneumonia overnight.

"We tend to overlook the obvious. When Katy was 3 years old, she was very ill. She kept spiking fevers and just could not seem to get better. She was admitted to the hospital because she was dehydrated and running a fever. About the second day, they decided she had some sort of lung virus she had caught in the hospital. She was given breathing treatments several times a day. After about the fourth day, I knew she was not getting any better. I told Katy's pediatrician I thought I could take her home and give her breathing treatments myself. They sent me home with a nebulizer. I watched her at home, and as long as I gave her acetaminophen and ibuprofen every four hours, she could sleep some, but she was not well. I called her geneticist and told him that Katy was not getting better and that she was going to end up in the emergency room again if we didn't do something. He told me to bring her in; he looked in her ears and discovered a raging ear infection. Everyone had been so caught up in Katy's labored breathing (which is normal for her) that they forgot that she might have a typical childhood illness that could be easily treated.

"We did not think she would be able to respond much to the environment around her. We thought she would be homebound and unable to go on family outings. We have learned from her to take one day at a time. We have had many more good days than bad, and God has given us the grace and mercy necessary to make it through every single one of them. Some of our distant family members look at Katy and our family and pity her and pity us. They have no concept of what life with her is like. They think we just sit around and cry or stay depressed all the time. They cannot see how Katy could be anything but a burden. We feel sorry for them.

"We are not actively pursuing another pregnancy. We are in fact using preventive measures to keep from becoming pregnant again.

However, birth control is not foolproof, and should we become pregnant again, we would not abort that child even if we knew he or she had leukodystrophy. Children are a gift from God, and each life is important and valuable.

"I cannot imagine my life without Katy. She has become such an important part of our family and has been the catalyst that has caused us to become better people. We don't take too many things for granted. We have become aggressive when it comes to choosing what is right for Katy. We have become more adaptable. We just look at the day and what we have to do and get creative in how we might accomplish what needs to be done. We believe we have learned what is really important and have thus adjusted our priorities. Katy is our second child. She is lovely and fun. She gives pleasure to our family and brings much joy to us."

Katy's parents have survived earth-shattering news that their second-born daughter has Canavan leukodystrophy, a rare inherited disorder in which spongy degeneration of the central nervous system leads to progressive mental deterioration. Katy has experienced increased muscle tone, poor head control, megalocephaly, and blindness. Her parents and sister have ridden the roller coaster of Katy's degenerative illness, with its inexorable decline in abilities. In spite of her condition, or perhaps because of it, her family members feel they have changed for the better. They clearly display many of the strategies parents adopt over the course of their child's life-altering illness:

- They have routinized Katy's treatment-related tasks, including gastrostomy feedings, nebulizer treatments, and trips to the doctor.
- They have redefined what is "normal" for their family.
- They have reassessed their priorities in life.
- They have reconceptualized the future. They unconditionally love their daughter and revel in the irreplaceable child she is (Bluebond-Langner 1996).

Children with life-threatening genetic conditions and their families present distinctive challenges to the palliative care team. Frequently, these children have rare conditions that are unfamiliar to the family and their healthcare providers. How do these families cope with caring for a child with a rare condition? What approach should the health care professional take when working with such a family? For many of these conditions, there is no cure; palliative care is the only option. Inherited conditions can cause overwhelming feelings of guilt in parents. Considerations of future childbearing may generate intense angst. How can the health care professional support the family in dealing with parental guilt for having "passed down" an incurable genetic condition to their present and perhaps future children? Parents and other family members deal with profound existential questions and may question why their God would allow an innocent baby to die before being born or permit a child to be born with a condition for which there is no cure.

The diagnosis of a life-threatening genetic condition may come "out of the blue" with an amniocentesis, ultrasound, or the birth of an affected baby. On the other hand, some children possess genetic conditions that are diagnosed long after the parents first suspect a problem, and some conditions will not be diagnosed until a second child is born with the same disorder. What methods are effective in assisting families to cope with the uncertainties of their child's condition, treatment, and future? Because palliative care is the only option for some children, their parents may turn to unproven therapies, such as special vitamin mixtures. Given the rarity of many of these conditions, families may seek out information and support from the Internet. How can families' Internet searches be guided to provide quality results? Walking side-by-side with these families as they navigate the life-altering and often unknown journey of their child's illness requires knowledgeable, compassionate, and dedicated professional care.

Background

INCIDENCE OF LIFE-THREATENING GENETIC CONDITIONS IN CHILDREN

In 1997 forty-three thousand infants died in the United States. Almost two-thirds of these deaths occurred during the first month of life (Guyer et al. 1998), many owing to congenital abnormalities and genetic conditions. Birth defects remain the leading cause of infant mortality in the United States. The genetic conditions that afflict children range from common disorders, such as Down syndrome, neurofibromatosis, and fragile X syndrome, to a wide range of rare conditions, including nonketotic hyperglycinemia, spinal muscular

Table 13.1. Incidence and mode of inheritance of life-threatening rare genetic conditions in children

Disease category	Genetic condition	Incidence	Mode of inheritance
Dysmorphic syndromes	Anencephaly	1:1,000	Autosomal and X-linked recessive
	Arthrogryposis multiplex congenita	1:100,000	Usually not hereditary
	Asphyxiating thoracic dystrophy	1:120,000	Autosomal recessive
	CHARGE[a] association	1:25,000	Most often sporadic
	DiGeorge syndrome	1:10,000	Sporadic, familial
	Meckel syndrome	1:9,000 to 1:140,000	Autosomal recessive
	Osteogenesis imperfecta	1:20,000 to 1:50,000	Most common form autosomal dominant
	Potter syndrome	1:7,000	Sporadic
	Smith-Lemli-Opitz syndrome	170 cases recorded	Autosomal recessive
	Spondyloepiphyseal dysplasia congenita	1:100,000	Autosomal dominant
	Trisomy 13	1:12,000	Sporadic
	Trisomy 18	1:5,000 to 1:7,000	Sporadic
	Trisomy 21	1:800	Sporadic
	VACTERL[b] association	Very rare	Sporadic
Inborn errors of metabolism	Adrenoleukodystrophy, childhood	1:100,000	X-linked
	Adrenoleukodystrophy, neonatal	1:100,000	Autosomal recessive

312

	Citrullinemia	Fewer than 1,000 diagnosed	Autosomal recessive
	Fabry	Fewer than 2,500 diagnosed	X-linked
	Glycogen storage diseases	1:150,000	Autosomal recessive
	Hunter syndrome (MPS II)	1:100,000	X-linked
	Hurler syndrome (MPS I)	1:100,000	Autosomal recessive
	Niemann-Pick	Rare	Autosomal recessive
	Menkes	1:35,000 to 1:100,000	X-linked recessive
	Nonketotic hyperglycinemia	1:250,000	Autosomal recessive
	Pompe disease	1:40,000	Autosomal recessive
	Sanfilippo syndrome (MPS III)	1:50,000	Autosomal recessive
	Tay Sachs	1:50,000	Autosomal recessive
	Zellweger syndrome	1:100,000	Autosomal recessive
Neurological disorders	Batten disease	3:100,000	Autosomal recessive
	Duchenne muscular dystrophy	1:4,000	X-linked
	Krabbe leukodystrophy	1:40,000	Autosomal recessive
	Lissencephaly	Very rare	Autosomal recessive
	Metachromatic leukodystrophy	1:100,000	Autosomal recessive
	Spinal muscular atrophy, type 1	1:1,000,000	Autosomal recessive

[a]Combination of coloboma, heart defect, atresia, renal anomalies, genital hypoplasia, and ear anomalies.
[b]Combination of vertebral, anorectal, cardiac, tracheo, esophageal, renal, and limb abnormalities (absent radius).

atrophy, type 1, and citrullinemia. Table 13.1 illustrates the incidence and mode of inheritance of selected life-threatening genetic conditions in children.

CHILDREN WITH CHROMOSOMAL DISORDERS

The chromosomal anomaly conditions are individually rare, and each has many unique features, but collectively they constitute a sizable portion of the genetic disorders seen in young infants and children. Multiple organ involvement is the rule, yet some individuals have few external abnormalities. Up to one-half of the individuals born with chromosomal abnormalities do not have any obvious physical differences. The impact of a chromosomal disorder is significant; cardiac and brain anomalies result in a shortened life span. Although some are exceedingly rare, the common thread of comparable problems seen in children leads to common support systems and groups. Feeding problems, failure to thrive, gastroesophageal reflux, seizures, and vision and hearing problems are encountered. Yet the uniqueness of each child and family situation and values does not lend itself to universal treatment decisions.

Chromosomal conditions often result in an assortment of static deficiencies. If surgical correction is feasible for a particular defect, such as a malformed heart or blocked intestine, the child may do well, physically and medically, for a period of time. Irreversible cognitive developmental defects are usually present, however.

CHILDREN WITH INBORN ERRORS OF METABOLISM

Metabolic conditions are numerous and complex. Many acute life-threatening conditions can complicate the daily routine of a child and be exacerbated when that child has surgery or encounters a stressor such as fever, vomiting, or diarrhea. Hypoglycemia, seizures, and lethargy are common sequelae of a deranged metabolic process.

A growing awareness of metabolic disorders has increased the case reports of these conditions. Hypoglycemia can occur in a fasting state as a result of inadequate release of stored sugars or fats. Sometimes the diagnosis is made at autopsy, following the first life-threatening event. Interventions for these groups of disorders can be both promising and time consuming. If the metabolic disease cannot be adequately controlled, the likely consequence is the child's death. Even if the child's condition is viewed as stable, guilt may surface with each hospitalization or setback. Treatment and management of the disease may be feasible, but these disorders often prove unpredictable, following a roller-coaster course that stresses most families.

There is a large group of rare disorders with the collective outcome of degeneration of the brain. These can involve groups of enzymes, as is the case in lysosomal or peroxisomal disorders, or the mitochondrial energy pathways. There are many additional genes, however, yet to be fully understood. In some cases, the only clear findings are the changes seen on serial brain scans. Diagnosis of a large number of conditions still requires invasive diagnostic tests, such as nerve or muscle biopsy. Support provided for these families is based on assisting them in recognizing that the changes taking place are not caused by parental neglect or the lack of nutrition (for example, secondary to recurrent vomiting). Rather, these changes are rooted in the deterioration the child is experiencing as a result of the disease. The rate of progression of the child's condition affects the child's ability to hold up during illnesses and other stressors.

With medical interventions, the affected child's life span can be extended, but the rate of disease progression is not slowed. Supportive, life-prolonging care can benefit the family as it allows time for them to actually see the disease progression, have more time with their child, and gain support from their friends and relatives. When a child experiences a rapid decline or sudden loss of life, the family does not have sufficient time to prepare for the death, and their grief is thus more complex. Table 13.2 illustrates symptoms, treatments, and life expectancy for selected life-threatening genetic conditions.

Neurodegenerative conditions come in a variety of forms. The gradual process of degeneration, starting with loss of skills, slowly changes the direction of care from motor or nutritional concerns to daily care and then to supportive measures. Frequent visits are needed after the initial diagnosis and test results. The child and family need support and open, honest discussion. Common conditions are Batten disease, Duchenne muscular dystrophy, Krabbe leukodystrophy, lissencephaly, metachromatic leukodystrophy, and spinal muscular atrophy, type 1. Other less common disorders include Zellweger syndrome and nonketotic hyperglycinemia. The common pattern of decline with these disorders is progressive neurologic involvement. Some children have a period of normal or near-normal functioning. However, many have had minor problems along the way before the major problems are recognized. Different degrees of functional limitations and respiratory and feeding problems develop with time. Parents and family can recognize their child's

Table 13.2. Presentation, treatment, and life expectancy in selected life-threatening genetic conditions

Genetic condition	Signs and symptoms	Treatment	Life expectancy
Anencephaly	Poor feeding, low muscle tone, head size often small but may be large. Initial signs may be subtle; seizures or lack of social responsiveness is often a helpful tip-off. Some children have obvious spasticity.	Antiseizure medications, supportive care. In longer-lived individuals, therapies will benefit. Seizures, if not present initially, often develop by three to four months.	Minutes, days, a few weeks or months in 90 percent; a few live for many years.
Arthrogryposis multiplex congenita (more than fifty types)	Abnormal joint positions in the womb; fixed joints both distal and proximal; may involve the facial musculature. Amyoplasia type is often compatible with long-lived outcome and normal intelligence.	Casting or surgeries to correct malpositioning; supportive care; tube feedings. Some may have seizures; some may have progression of symptoms.	If on ventilator at thirty days, long-term survival not expected. Some mild forms respond well to orthopedic therapies.
Asphyxiating thoracic dystrophy	Severe restriction of chest size; may initially not need respiratory support in 10–20 percent. Five subtypes, some with additional organ cysts in liver or kidney, clefting, and so on. New types are being found.	Attempts to enlarge rib circumference have been moderately successful, but long-term complications and other organ involvement still make it a lethal condition for the most part.	Usually months; those who survive infancy have kidney failure later in life.

CHARGE association (can be variable with regard to the anomalies and specific combination present)	Coloboma (iris or retina or both); heart defect (ventriculoseptal defect, transposition of the great arteries); atresia of the coanal nasal passages (stenosis or partial blockage); renal anomalies (dysplastic or missing); genital hypoplasia; ear anomaly (with or without deafness); small birth weight and facial asymmetry.	Surgical care to correct anomalies. Poor postnatal growth is common. Often chromosome abnormality is found, and this changes outcome prediction.	Depends on the severity of the anomalies. Long-term survival is at least 75 percent.
DiGeorge syndrome	Classic features include heart anomaly, hypocalcemia, and immune deficit. Facial dysmorphic features may be subtle and easily overlooked. Many children have severe feeding problems and dysphagia and gastroesophageal reflux. Others may have cleft palate.	Surgery to correct heart defects. Prophylactic antibiotics for possible immunodeficiency. Monitor and treat hypocalcemia, especially when under stress.	Severe cardiac defects; little immune function; shortened life span. Most children affected with mild to moderate severity. Survival to two years indicates probable long-term survival.
Potter syndrome	Any number of defects can lead to blockage of kidneys or little or no amniotic fluid (oligo-hydramnios). Long-standing oligohydramnios, causes lung hypoplasia. Death occurs in the womb, or shortly after birth from respiratory failure.	Features of compression and deformation on the limbs, torso, and face are diagnostic and occur secondary to the lack of fluid around the baby.	There are no surgical interventions to correct lung hypoplasia. Supportive tube feedings can be attempted.

(continued)

Table 13.2. (continued)

Genetic condition	Signs and symptoms	Treatment	Life expectancy
Trisomy 13[a]	These babies are small and have tight limbs. Poor feeding is common. Many babies look very good, and most look like other family members.	Supportive measures may include oxygen per nasal cannula and a feeding tube to meet nutritional needs and sometimes surgery. With assistance, family can care for child at home.	Many babies survive for a few days or weeks.
Trisomy 18[a]	These babies are small and have tight limbs. Poor feeding is common. Many babies look very good, and most look like other family members.	Most heart conditions are not immediately life threatening. Supportive care in the home is common.	Several weeks to months. Respiratory and cardiac failure are commonly seen. Other babies develop poor growth patterns and get the "dwindles."

[a]Trisomy 13 and 18 are sometimes seen in children born alive. These conditions are lethal, yet at the start the children with either of these trisomy conditions may be relatively fit babies who feed well and go home from the hospital. Time and again the prediction that the baby will die during childbirth does not come true. The parents often need to plan that the baby will do well for a while and then be prepared to keep the baby comfortable with support. These children can be more responsive to their caregivers than experts often predict.

habits, routines, likes, and dislikes. The personality of the child is often endearing, even if the child is not able to communicate verbally.

Patients' and Families' Needs

Who we are as human beings is more than just our DNA. Nonetheless, our genetic heritage is an essential part of who we are and who we will become. For children with life-threatening genetic conditions, their flawed paired bases of adenine and thymine and guanine and cytosine propel them and their loved ones on a journey that can be filled with sadness, devastated dreams, and anguished mourning for the perfect child who could have been. Nonetheless, many of these families ultimately find love, joy, and delight in the special and unique human being who is their child.

Bluebond-Langner (1996) describes the "natural history of the illness" as the series of events, from diagnosis to death, that mark critical changes in the social and emotional life of the family as well as in the clinical status of the child. The natural history of the illness closely parallels, but is not identical to, the clinical course. The needs of the family of a child with a life-threatening genetic condition will fluctuate as the child and family move through this progression of events. Accordingly, the palliative care interventions essential to support this child and family will vary with time.

FAMILY NEEDS OVER THE COURSE OF THE CONDITION

"The impetus for living things to reproduce and create offspring who will survive them is so basic to life that it is one of the fundamental truths of our world, like gravity or the sun. Through it, continuity and a kind of immortality are achieved. The human impetus to reproduce and create offspring embraces both the biological and the symbolical. People both create life and give meaning to that life as part of existence and self-preservation" (Rubin and Malkinson 2001, 220). Given the biologic imperative to produce, care for, and protect our young, the requirements placed on the parents of a child with a life-threatening genetic condition are especially onerous.

Diagnosis. When a fetus, baby, or child is diagnosed with a life-threatening condition, the parents' world, both present and future, is rocked to its core. Sensitive, intelligent, and knowledgeable communication can make a difference in how the family copes with this initial trauma. The parents will carry the memory of this conversation with them for the rest of their lives:

while they most likely will not recall all the details, they will remember the tone of the discussion and how caring or brusque the physician was. Results of the genetic workup, such as amniocentesis, uterine ultrasound, or DNA results, should never be given over the phone. The parents should be informed together, if at all possible. The physician should avoid the use of any medical jargon, especially since genetics can be confusing for lay people to understand. Sufficient detail should be provided to the parents so that they understand what is wrong with their child but are not overwhelmed by the information. It is desirable for the physician and family to have a series of conversations over time, so that as the family moves out of shock and denial, they can begin to grasp the particulars of the condition and its treatment. A plan for further workup, treatment, or follow-up should always be presented with the initial discussion. This plan confers some sense of control on the family and furnishes them with a focal point for their actions in the near future. That something can be done is reassuring to the family, especially when cure is not an option.

Once the diagnosis is confirmed, the family may rush to the Internet for information and support, especially when a rare condition is diagnosed. Since the quality of the medical information available on the Internet is highly variable, the family may come away with erroneous information and perhaps false hope. On the other hand, the family may also receive tremendous support from other families with children similarly affected. The parents may engage in an e-mail or instant messaging relationship with one or more families to compare their children's development and treatment. For example, the mother of an infant with spinal muscular atrophy, type 1 logs on to AOL every night after her daughters go to bed to chat with other mothers of babies with the condition. Among all that she gleans from these conversations, she learns about the typical do-everything treatment map for spinal muscular atrophy. She now understands the progression from gastrostomy to in-exsufflator to BiPAP to tracheostomy to ventilator, well before her child requires any of these interventions, and can begin to mull over the ramifications of this course of action for her child and her family. She and her husband have numerous discussions over time about all this and are better prepared to make these difficult decision when their daughter's weight begins to drop precipitously and a feeding gastrostomy is proposed. Because so many families turn to the Internet for information and support, it is prudent to discuss the use of the Internet early on in the course of the relationship to steer their searches toward quality websites (see the appendix to this volume for website listings).

Family Needs during the Illness. Depending on the genetic condition, the child may experience a period of relative tranquillity after diagnosis. The family may settle into a routine of treatments, medications, therapies, and doctor's appointments. Some semblance of normal life is attained. If the child is doing relatively well, parents may begin to engage in a strategy that Bluebond-Langner (1996, 168) labels "redefinition of normal." This process involves expanding the realm of normal to encompass the ill child's condition and family situation. The nebulizer treatments, nighttime gastrostomy feedings, and physical therapy visits all become part of the everyday life of the family.

As time goes on, the ramifications of the child's illness become more apparent. The reality of the nature and quality of their child's future existence and the impact this has on the whole family system comes into clearer focus. This can be discouraging and depressing for the family. Some of the parents' initial hopes may be quashed. The family will require additional support from the entire professional caregiving team at this time. Palliative care professionals must find a delicate balance in acknowledging the "new" reality of the child's condition and at the same time preserving the family's hopes and dreams for their child. If the health care team errs too much on the side of reality, the family may turn away from them. It is common for parents to shun anyone who jeopardizes the foundation of their hopes. Among all the parents' anxieties and fears for the future, they need to retain "threads of optimism" (Bluebond-Langner 1996)—optimism for a newly found cure, a miracle, or a longer life than the doctors predict. Their hopes and threads of optimism help the parents get through each and every day.

Complications and Deterioration. As the child's condition deteriorates, the family may begin a phase that many identify as a roller coaster, with exacerbation in condition followed by recovery, each time without quite returning to the previous baseline. For example, the child with Menke disease undergoes a series of aspiration pneumonia episodes. With each incidence of pneumonia, the child's overall condition is weakened; the child loses weight and ultimately is unable to withstand the next pneumonia. At some point in this process the family may reassess their priorities. In two-career families, one of the parents may be forced into full-time caregiving responsibilities.

There are no curative options for many genetic conditions. For this reason, a number of families with children with life-threatening genetic conditions will turn to unproven therapies, from oil mixtures to vitamin preparations.

Purveyors may guarantee outright cure or some substantial benefit, such as enhanced or normal intelligence in a mentally retarded child. The family may be proffered this miracle cure from other families caring for a child with the same condition, or they might unearth these therapies on the Internet. Many websites for such treatments include testimonials and before-and-after photographs illustrating how much healthier or smarter the treated child appears. If the family fervently believes in the therapy, it may be best not to attempt to dissuade them from using it unless it has been proved ineffective or harmful or is extraordinarily expensive. The relationship between the parents and the palliative care professional can be adversely affected if the professional pushes too hard on this issue.

DEATH AND BEREAVEMENT

Once the child with a life-threatening genetic condition dies, the real work of the family begins. The experience they have had during the final chapter of their child's life can affect the family's abilities to cope with this devastating loss. The twin extremes of sudden death (such as a stillbirth) or a lingering expected death (such as from adrenoleukodystrophy or Canavan leukodystrophy) can overwhelm and erode the strengths and resilience of the child's parents. Given the magnitude of the entire experience, their ability to process the loss may be impaired. For many parents of young children, this loss meets them at a point at which they are engaged in the responsibilities of raising a family, juggling work and family obligations, and trying to establish themselves as adults (Gilbert and Smart 1992). Many parents of young children are barely adults themselves. Any healthy coping mechanisms they possess may not be well established, and their support systems may well be nonexistent. These families will be best served by comprehensive long-term bereavement services provided by pediatric bereavement counselors.

The death of a baby in the perinatal period, through spontaneous miscarriage or abortion, or in the immediate neonatal period, through extreme prematurity, birth injury, or congenital or genetic conditions, presents additional challenges for the palliative care team. The demise of a young child during pregnancy or shortly thereafter represents the loss of the hopes, dreams, and expectations invested in the hoped-for child (Rubin and Malkinson 2001). According to Riches and Dawson (2000), when a mother has chosen to abort her baby with a genetic condition, her grief can be complicated by the social stigma of the nature of the loss, an inability to share her grief or experiences with others, the possibility of lack of support from the baby's father, and ongoing ambivalence about the decision she has made. The sense of isolation and loneliness felt by women who have undergone abortions may be seen by others as totally illegitimate, and the daydreams they may have over how their baby might have grown up are rarely shared by anyone (Riches and Dawson 2000).

If the diagnosis was in doubt when the baby or child died, the family's grief may be complicated. Some families must wait up to six months for the entire autopsy to be completed, and the results may come in when the family is reaching the nadir of their grief. Presenting these autopsy results to the family at this time can be a complex but essential task for the physician involved. This information may aid the family in making sense of what transpired clinically with their child during his or her life and may facilitate the family's grief work. For some children who die, no firm diagnosis was ever made. This uncertainty can create appreciable hurdles for the family as they move through the grief process.

FAMILY NEEDS FOLLOWING MISCARRIAGE OR STILLBIRTH

The family who suffers miscarriage or stillbirth needs an understanding that the process of data collection on such losses takes time. In the eyes of the mother and father, the wait for these results can seem interminable. The parents cannot see any good reason for the process to take so long. During this time, it is important that the couple come in and meet with the doctor to review the details and discuss the workup in progress. The best approach is to make periodic phone contacts and follow up until all the studies are completed. It is desirable to give control to the parents and allow them to call as often as they feel necessary for results or to review the details of the discussions and plans.

CHILDBEARING ISSUES

Childbearing issues may have been discussed and dealt with during the course of the child's illness, particularly at the time of the initial diagnosis, and may resurface during the grief and bereavement phase. When the child's life-threatening genetic condition is autosomal recessive or linked to the X chromosome, the parents are faced with a 25 to 50 percent chance of having another affected child. Some families may decide this risk is too high, particularly if their religious tenets preclude prenatal testing if abortion will be the outcome for an affected fetus. However, prenatal testing can also be used to psychologically prepare for the ill child or to provide adequate time to make a definitive diagnosis for rare disorders. Prenatal testing is not an option for some genetic conditions, although the number of conditions that can be diagnosed in utero is increasing every year. Suggesting that parents have another child as a "substitute" for the lost child is inadvisable as a means of avoiding grief for many reasons, not the least of which is the possibility of confused boundaries between the deceased and the subsequent child (Rubin and Malkinson 2001).

As a result of parental guilt for having borne an imperfect child, the couple may experience difficulties demonstrating affection to each other. Especially if the recurrence risk is understood to be high, the couple may do everything in their power to avoid a chance of an accidental pregnancy, including sterilization or, in extreme cases, even abstinence. Gentle inquiries about the health of the marital bonds is appropriate.

DECISION-MAKING ISSUES

Differences in the distribution of the cause of death by age have important implications for the kind of end-of-life decisions that are made and by whom those decisions are made. Many infants and younger children die of birth-related, congenital, or genetic conditions. These children may never be healthy in the way their cohorts in the general population are. This situation raises complex quality-of-life issues. The parents are obliged to determine their child's best interests in the absence of information about the individual child's perceived life satisfaction (Sahler et al. 2000). Thus quality-of-life concerns can be thorny for the family of a child with a life-threatening genetic condition. Because often the child is neurologically impaired and cannot participate in consent or assent, and because there are often no curative treatment options for the child's condition, the burden is placed on the family to decide what to do.

Parents are often asked to make life-or-death decisions for their child at a time when they have just been confronted with the earth-shattering news of his or her diagnosis. They may be asked, for example, to make decisions about whether to intubate (or extubate) their child or to place a nasogastric or gastrostomy tube for feedings. The parents might have precious little practical information about the implications of this decision and may have no concept of what that child's life (and subsequently what their own lives) will be like. They most likely have never met a child with the condition their child has. Given the rarity of many genetic conditions, the physician, too, may have limited or no experience in dealing with the child's condition, the illness trajectory, and palliative care. Thus the family, who is most likely in a state of shock and disbelief, may be forced to make life-or-death decisions about their child, guided by a physician who knows little more than they do.

Often, multiple subspecialists are involved in the care of the child with a genetic condition. The child may be followed by pediatric specialists in genetics, neurology, pulmonology, cardiology, gastroenterology, surgery, otorhinolaryngology, orthopedics, nephrology, and other specialties. These specialists may offer widely varying predictions of prognosis, may propose treatment plans that conflict with one another, and may communicate poorly, if at all, with one another or with the family, especially when dealing with rare conditions. Deciding what to do with all these opinions can be confusing and upsetting for parents. Conflicting information from caregivers constitutes a form of fragmented care (Hilden et al. 2000, 161–98); parents report significant distress resulting from this seemingly avoidable but all too common occurrence.

The geneticist can unify the various subspecialists' opinions and discuss the input of the other doctors with the family. The geneticist can give parents a forum in which their questions about the various ideas are answered and the different "realities" are discussed. The parents must balance their need to know with the need to care for their child. Not every test needs to be done, just for the sake of pinning down a particular diagnosis. Far too often the discussions are focused only on what test to perform or what lab work to run. The family needs someone who will take into account the baby as a whole person, as a member of their family, and not just another case to "pick at" until the diagnosis is found. Genetic testing is often essential to diagnosing the condition with certainty and the ability to quote accurate recurrence risks. However, the discussions should focus on the category of the disease and statements about the certainty of disease trajectory for that group of conditions. There may be several possible diagnoses that all have the same disease trajectory and outcome. If the outcomes are variable, this uncertainty should be pointed out.

The focus of this discussion should be on how the patterns will reveal themselves, in the sense that the steps of the dying process can be predicted even if the exact cause is somewhat uncertain. Most families will at some point say they have learned enough to come to terms with the situation or to have sufficient understanding. They can then begin to move ahead with this knowledge and leave behind all the possible "what ifs." (For example, parents might query whether their exposure to a vapor from some chemicals, or having a flu shot last fall, or exposure to an unknown agent during the Persian Gulf war could have created cellular changes leading to the demise or stillbirth of the baby.)

GUILT

Parental guilt is a prominent feature of families with a child diagnosed with a life-threatening condition. Most parents will question to varying degrees what they might have done wrong during the pregnancy. Almost every family will feel some degree of guilt, even if the condition is determined to be the result of a sporadic mutation. This can range from a transient sense of guilt experienced before the actual diagnosis is confirmed to incapacitating, lifelong guilt felt irrespective of any careful explanations of inherited causality. Parental guilt for sick young children may be exacerbated by an unclear disease process. Until the diagnosis is known with certainty, some parents may feel this heightened sense of self-blame.

Careful, thorough explanations of the genetics involved in the child's condition may ameliorate some parental guilt. Medical jargon should be avoided. Simple words and sentences that both parents can understand are important; since the parents are in a state of shock, it is likely that only the broad strokes of the discussion will be remembered. It is essential to engage in a series of conversations over time to reiterate the information. Eventually, the information will "sink in," and the parents' guilt will be assuaged to varying degrees.

Feelings of blame or guilt are not always obvious. Sometimes the mother is a supermom who seems to cope well and take every event in stride. That the parent passed on a genetic factor to the child, resulting in his or her suffering, can indeed be the factor that drives the parent (mother or father) to provide optimal care and to lessen the child's suffering as much as possible. Such parents seek affirmation by asking about other families and how well other children with the illness or condition have done. They need to know they have had a positive influence on the course of their child's disease.

The parent may strive to prove the doctor wrong. Parents may take pride in their child's having outlived a predicted life span. Various manifestations of parental guilt must be recognized. Families may insist on doing "everything" to prolong the life of their child, or the family might dress the child in nice outfits or give the child lavish toys they would not otherwise have considered buying. Some parents will spend an inordinate amount of time with the affected child, including performing complex daily procedures at home and attending numerous doctor visits and therapy sessions while neglecting themselves, their marriage, and their other children. It is valuable to include a few questions about how the other children are coping and the ways in which they help out with their sibling as a part of each routine follow-up visit.

The reality of the disease becomes clearer as the suffering continues. Families begin asking more questions at their visits, possibly indicating a desire to discuss changing goals of care or indicating new worries about their ability to manage as the child's condition deteriorates. Asking the family when they want to return to the clinic gives them a sense of control. It also acknowledges that they can change their mind and return sooner or later, as changes in the child's condition warrant. Palliative care professionals must work to empower parents as their child's true care managers.

Sometimes guilt is experienced by one parent more than the other. This can occur even if a condition is autosomal recessive and both parents have contributed genetically to the child's condition. This discrepancy in the mind-sets of the parents can create problems in their relationship. If these feelings go unexpressed, the partners may begin to feel estrangement from each other. This intensifies the stress the couple is already experiencing.

Health Care Providers' Needs

PROFESSIONAL APPROACH TO THE CHILD WITH A LIFE-THREATENING GENETIC CONDITION

Developing an ongoing relationship with a family whose child has a life-threatening genetic condition is a challenging undertaking for the health care provider. The physician and other professionals working with the family may not be knowledgeable about the child's particular condition, especially if it is rare. Families with rare conditions, first and foremost, would prefer a physician who is an expert on their child's condition, but in lieu of that ideal, they readily accept physicians who demonstrate a consistent caring approach. Honesty about their lack of experience with this particular condition is desirable. The physician can suggest to the family that his or her past experience with similar conditions can provide the knowledge base necessary to allow proper medical management. The physician can seek out expert medical opinions and inform the family that he or she has done so. This will not undermine the parents' trust in the physician's care but rather will strengthen the family's trust in their physician.

The ideal psychological outcome for parents of a child with a life-threatening genetic condition is to move from the initial grief for the loss of the perfect child they envisioned to acceptance for the imperfect, albeit unique, child they have created. For most parents, this is a difficult and challenging journey, and they require a tremendous amount of professional support during this time. The fundamental approach of the palliative care professional to the child can make a substantial difference in the parents' reaching acceptance. Many of these children have physical deformities that affect their appearance. In this case, the child will inevitably be the object of numerous stares by strangers when the family is out in public. From the first encounter with the child and family, the physician and other palliative care professionals can demonstrate that despite the child's physical deformities and mental deficiencies, he or she will not be treated any differently. The child should not be left in the parent's lap or on the exam table but should be talked to, held, and touched by the physician. Normal or attractive features, positive developmental gains, and good behavior should be pointed out to the family. For example, a child born with massive hydrocephalus and an extensive bilateral cleft lip and palate may have beautiful, long, perfect fingers. Remarking on this can give tremendous comfort to the parents. The physician and other palliative care professionals can also note ways in which the child is distinctive and unique and maybe even better than the average child. For instance, some genetic conditions, such as Williams syndrome or Coffin-Lowry syndrome, are associated with pleasant, outgoing personalities.

The importance of the professional's approach to the child during the office visit cannot be overemphasized. In addition to the basic exam, it is beneficial, whenever possible, to take the time to examine the child out of his or her wheelchair and to remove any braces the child may be wearing. A better assessment of muscle tone and functional ability can be done by touching and holding the child. The structured steps of the neurological exam can best be done on the exam table, but some parts should be done in whatever way is most comfortable for the child. This includes sitting and holding the child on the examiner's lap or getting down on the floor with blanket and blocks to assess the child's abilities and skills.

Once a diagnosis is reached and the family realizes they have limited time with their child, a new set of medical concerns arises. The family's needs change from the immediate need to know the diagnosis and the reason for the condition to the care of the child in their home. The physician may find little to discuss once the diagnosis is made. The opposite is true for the family, because as they come to grips with the reality of the situation they often need more time and attention from the professional team. The team's assessment ought to include not only the child's physical needs but also feeding issues, pain control, and measures to prevent and control infection.

UNIQUE REACTIONS TO MEDICATIONS

Many genetic conditions limit the brain in its responses to medications and to painful stimuli. The use of strong opioid medications for pain control must be cautiously approached and in some pediatric conditions should be totally avoided.

Children with lysosomal disorders and "brain reduction" conditions, such as lissencephaly or holoprosencephaly, should not be prescribed morphine postoperatively. For example, the postoperative pain sensations experienced by a child with a lysosomal condition, such as metachromatic leukodystrophy, after gastrostomy tube placement may be beneficial in maintaining the child's respiratory drive. Giving an opioid-naïve child with this condition a strong opioid often results in apnea, thus necessitating intubation and a stay in the intensive care unit. No long-term effect is noted in such children, and as the disease progresses, the child can, without risk of apnea, and should be prescribed strong opioids, as pain is most often the predominant problem experienced by a child with one of these disorders.

Community Resources

Over the past twenty years, the Internet has made the search for information about rare genetic conditions less complicated. However, since a good percentage of the information found on the web is of questionable quality and accuracy, health care professionals working with children with life-threatening genetic conditions should steer parents toward long-standing websites sponsored by reputable organizations. Family goals of an Internet search include finding accurate information on their child's condition and seeking out other families with children with the same or a similar condition. The appendix at the end of this book lists recommended websites for both professionals and families.

Conclusion

Birth defects, including those stemming from premature delivery, account for the majority of childhood deaths. Parental feelings of guilt and blame are common in this setting, and it is critical for the survival of the family that they receive clear and empathic explanations, in a staged manner as well as affirmation that they did not intend for their child to be ill and did not cause his or her suffering. Means of accomplishing this goal include helping parents find community resources and locate accurate information on the Internet and providing ongoing care to relieve the child's and family's distress. Parents may individually perceive differing amounts of guilt or blame, and counseling to assist them to accept each other's reactions may be helpful.

There are commonalities among these rare disorders. Patterns emerge that enable the astute clinician who is willing to reach out for consultative services to effectively assist families keep their ill children in their communities, where both child and family are most likely to receive support from family and friends. Families who receive care in tertiary care centers are likely to receive conflicting information from a number of consultants. The geneticist or other qualified physician should serve as captain of the ship, streamlining the information and helping families think through their goals and treatment options. In this manner, the needs of families facing the deterioration and death of their child from a rare metabolic, degenerative, or developmental disease can be met, and the clinician will have the privilege of the amelioration and prevention of suffering of a fellow human being.

References

Bluebond-Langner, M. 1996. *In the shadow of illness: parents and siblings of the chronically ill child.* Princeton, N.J.: Princeton University Press.

Gilbert, K. R., and L. S. Smart. 1992. Grief on the individual level: the grieving process. In *Coping with infant or fetal loss: the couple's healing process,* ed. K. R. Gilbert and L. S. Smart, 27–49. New York: Brunner/Mazel.

Guyer, B., M. F. MacDorman, J. A. Martin, K. D. Peters, and D. M. Strobino. 1998. Annual summary of vital statistics, 1997. *Pediatrics* 102:1333–49.

Hilden, J. M., B. P. Himelstein, D. R. Freyer, S. Friebert, and J. R. Kane. 2000. Report to the National Cancer Policy Board: pediatric oncology end-of-life care. Washington, D.C.: National Academies Press.

Riches, G., and P. Dawson. 2000. *An intimate loneliness: supporting bereaved parents and siblings.* Maidenhead, Berkshire, U.K.: Open University Press.

Rubin, S. S., and R. Malkinson. 2001. Parental response to child loss across the life cycle: clinical and research perspectives. In *Handbook of bereavement research: consequences, coping and care,* ed. M. S. Strobe, R. O. Hansson, W. Stroebe, and H. Schut, 219–40. Washington, D.C.: American Psychological Association.

Sahler, O., G. Frager, M. Levetown, F. G. Cohn, and M. A. Lipson. 2000. Medical education about end-of-life care in the pediatric setting: principles, challenges, and opportunities. *Pediatrics* 105:575–84.

14

The Child with HIV Infection

Brian S. Carter, M.D., F.A.A.P., James Oleske, M.D., M.P.H., Lynn Czarniecki, M.S.N., C.N.S., and Sam Grubman, M.D.

Infection from HIV-1 (human immunodeficiency virus) is an unpredictable disease in infants, children, and adolescents, with multisystem involvement resulting in a chronic and complex illness. It is a multigenerational disease because usually other family members, especially parents, are also infected and have varying symptoms and substantial psychosocial problems.

At the onset of the HIV-1 epidemic, most perinatally infected infants died before they reached 4 years of age. With the advent of routine prenatal screening for HIV-1 and the use of antiretroviral treatment in mothers and infants, a marked reduction in vertical transmission has occurred over the past decade. In 2001 it was estimated that fewer than two hundred children in the United States had contracted HIV-1 (Sullivan and Luzuriaga 2001). This is in stark contrast to the approximately one thousand new cases occurring annually during the first fifteen years of the HIV-AIDS (acquired immunodeficiency syndrome) epidemic in this country (Davis et al. 1995). With improvements in antiretroviral therapy, prophylaxis for opportunistic infections, and good supportive care, many infected children are now long-term survivors living well into the teen years and beyond, and many with multiorgan system disease (United Nations 1991; Grubman et al. 1995).

Recall the case of Anna, presented in chapter 9 of this volume.

Anna, an 8-month-old infant with perinatally acquired HIV, has been hospitalized repeatedly with a variety of HIV-related health problems, including opportunistic infections, recurrent fever and sepsis, thrombocytopenia, impaired myocardial function, chronic diarrhea, encephalopathy, failure to thrive, and developmental delay. Six weeks ago, she was admitted to the hospital with respiratory distress, poor oxygenation, and failure to thrive. Her respiratory compromise worsened, and she was electively intubated and placed on mechanical ventilation. Her liver and spleen were greatly enlarged, her myocardial function diminished secondary to cardiomyopathy. Over the next week, she required maximal ventilatory support and oxygen supplementation and was unable to wean from the ventilator. She also experienced pain from muscle aches, mouth sores, candidiasis, hepatosplenomegaly, and frequent painful procedures.

When Anna was 5 months old, her 19-year-old mother died of AIDS-related complications. Anna had been placed in foster care as a newborn because of her mother's age and history of drug abuse and Anna's positive toxicology screen at birth. Anna's grandmother was unable to care for her because of her own history of schizophrenia and because she was the focus on an active protective service case for child neglect. Because no other relatives were available to assume her care, Anna became a ward of the state. She was initially cared for by her specially trained foster mother, but as Anna's condition worsened, it became necessary to admit her to a chronic care facility for children. (Adapted from Rushton et al. 1993)

Anna's case raises a number of issues common in palliative care of children infected with HIV:

- When should palliative care be incorporated into the overall care of an infant born to an HIV-infected mother?
- How does one explain to an HIV-positive parent that life-extending care may be pursued for their child and, without dashing hope, realistically note the need for pursuing palliative care?
- What role does informing an older HIV-infected pediatric patient have in determining an appropriate care plan?
- What do patients, families, caregivers, and the community need to do in order that the best support possible is provided for the child, at any age, with HIV infection?

Approximately ten thousand to twelve thousand children in the United States are currently HIV infected (Sullivan and Luzuriaga 2001). Relative to a decade ago, children with HIV are living longer and requiring greater support in every facet of their lives, from pain and symptom management to school performance and psychosocial needs. These facts help to illuminate new measures of support that can and should be provided, such as nutritional therapies, psychosocial support for the patient and caregiver, and improved communication among all involved persons. In many ways, children living with HIV infection have more in common with children living with other chronic illness rather than with those who are terminally ill. Palliative care provisions should take all of these issues into consideration when comprehensive care plans are made for pediatric HIV-AIDS patients.

Guiding Principles of Palliative Care and Hospice Services

Palliative care is comprehensive and multidisciplinary and includes physical, psychological, social, and spiritual care. Palliative care for children with chronic, multisystem, and life-limiting disease, such as HIV, should ensure the child's comfort and maximum function through the course of their illness. The use of palliative care within the context of other forms of medical treatment should not be reserved for the end of life (Frager 1996; Frager and Shapiro 1998). For children with HIV disease, palliative care is an important aspect of a comprehensive treatment program from the time of diagnosis (Boland, Burr, and Harvey 1995; Ferris and Flannery 1995; Oleske and Ruben-Hale 1995). The application of the principles of palliative care improves the quality of life of the child living with a chronic life-limiting illness. Quality of life, defined in large part by the patient and his or her family, includes the child's ability to carry on the activities of daily life with the minimum discomfort while receiving treatment for the illness. The quality of life of patients should be the main concern of any physician and the driving force throughout treatment of chronic illness (Fleischman et al. 1994; Lewis, Haiken, and Joyt 1994; Walco, Cassidy, and Schechter 1994; Attig 1996; Liben 1996; Robinson et al. 1996).

Patients' Needs

The continuum of palliative care for children infected with HIV-1 begins from the time an HIV-infected woman becomes pregnant through the course of disease and the eventual death of her child. For the well-being of the infant and the mother, all pregnant women should receive comprehensive prenatal care. For HIV-infected children, all care should be aggressive; during the course of illness some types of restorative care are also the best palliative care. For example, the prevention of Pneumocystis carinii pneumonia with co-trimoxazole oral prophylaxis is compatible with a continuum of palliative care that provides comfort by avoiding the substantial morbidity of this infection.

MANAGEMENT OF PAIN AND SYMPTOMS

Pain and other adverse symptoms need to be assessed at each patient encounter and treated vigorously. Recent reports of the prevalence and complications of pain in pediatric HIV-AIDS–affected children note that roughly one out of five will experience persistent pain (Gaughan et al. 2002). Typical risk factors include female gender, length of disease, patient age greater than 5 years, and low CD4 counts. Given the ramifications of persistent pain on the developing psyche of the child patient, interpersonal dynamics with caregivers, and performance in school (Fundaro et al. 1998), pain management is fundamental in the care of HIV-infected infants and children.

ANTIBIOTICS AND ANTIRETROVIRAL AGENTS

Other treatments for complications of HIV-1 disease that improve quality of life for the individual patient include antiretroviral therapy (except at the end of life), treatment and continuing prophylaxis of selected opportunistic infections (Pneumocystis carinii, mycobacterium avium complex [MAC] infection, cryptococcal meningitis, toxoplasmosis, cytomegalovirus retinitis, and herpes simplex), and the prevention of recurrent bacterial infections. The use of antiretroviral therapy has a significant impact on quality of life by improving survival, prolonging the time free of opportunistic infection, and improving and maintaining immunologic health. However, at end-stage disease, decisions relating to the continuation of antiretroviral therapy must balance the benefits against side effects of the medications and the ultimate futility of current treatment.

NUTRITION

Nutrition is an important part of supportive care and is considered by some as a form of treatment (Butensky 2001). It is a critical component in health maintenance and also adds to the patient's quality of life (Oleske 1995; Oleske, Rothpletz-Puglia, and Winter 1996; Paris and Schrieber 1996).

Although children infected with HIV-1 can show great variability in the clinical course of their disease, end-stage disease is characterized by the progression to the Centers for Disease Control and Prevention's class-C3 disease (severe clinical disease with substantial immune suppression). HIV-1 encephalopathy and wasting syndrome, which may be associated with cytomegalovirus infection, cryptosporidiosis, and atypical mycobacterial infection, are commonly part of this progression. End-stage disease is also associated with the development of HIV-1-specific malignant disease, such as leiomyosarcoma and central-nervous-system lymphoma. Multiple organ failure is evident in end-stage disease, and despite aggressive antiretroviral therapy, high HIV-1 RNA load persists with progressive loss of CD4 lymphocytes.

At this stage there is a shift from restorative care to more supportive care; the physician and the family therefore need to recognize when end-stage disease is present and hospice care becomes an appropriate option (Czarniecki, Boland, and Oleske 1993; American Academy of Pediatrics 1994; Attig 1996; McQuillan and Finlay 1996; Institute of Medicine 1997). Appropriate clinical management during the terminal phases of the child's illness should involve a coordinated plan of care developed with the family and the child. Spiritual care needs particular attention at this time (Meyers 1989).

The initial phases of terminal care usually begin when the issue of medical futility is raised by the patient, the family, or a member of the health care team and then acknowledged by the others (Nelson and Nelson 1992). Professionals should be alert to a patient's or a family's need to begin this discussion. The newness and unpredictability of HIV can cause uncertainty about the course and prognosis. This uncertainty can lead to ambivalence about the best plan of care. It can also mean that patients and families move back and forth between their needs for aggressive care and comfort care. Clinicians must recognize that this is a process and be patient.

A complete discussion between the family and the health care team of the child's medical status and prognosis should occur as frequently as the patient and family need. A plan should be jointly developed by the family and health care team that recognizes the family's need for some sense of control and ensures a painfree death. Hospice and other terminal care options should be discussed. This plan should be carefully documented in the medical record. One recent study advocates the use of a values-history and interview process within the clinical setting in which an appropriate advance directive might be obtained (Wissow, Hutton, and Kass 2001). While results may presently be considered preliminary, the ascertainment of values-history topics (such as disabilities that would make life not worth living, tolerance of pain and risk, personal preferences for end-of-life care, and spirituality) from the ten families, including three children aged 10 to 16, revealed essential components of the necessary dialogue between caregivers, patients, and health care professionals.

The family and health care team should review and revisit this plan at designated intervals to ensure that the family's wishes and the patient's needs are being addressed. The plan should be communicated to hospice and terminal care providers to ensure that the care accords with the child's and family's wishes. If the patient is in the hospital, the plan should be well documented in the patient's medical record and communicated to all hospital staff members caring for the patient and his or her family.

To ensure appropriate medical management that complies with the patient's and family's wishes, specific aspects of death and dying need to be discussed with the family, including the following:

- description and components of the meaning, procedure, and limitations of do-not-resuscitate orders
- treatments to be continued and withdrawn
- reassurance regarding supportive interventions, including pain management, hydration, and nutritional support
- plan of approach to emergency room visits and service calls
- the process of dying, including signs and pronouncement
- the role of autopsy

The United Nations Convention on the Rights of Children (United Nations 1991) should be followed with appropriate encouragement of the child's participation in his or her own health care. When possible, some form of memorial or living legacy could be encouraged. In families in which a parent also has HIV-AIDS, a discussion of the family's wishes around parent death is important, especially as related to guardianship.

PSYCHOSOCIAL SUPPORT

Psychosocial supports, specifically around issues of terminal care, are critical to the child's and family's comfort and ability to cope during the terminal phase of the child's illness. There should be an age-appropriate discussion with the child about death and dying, with opportunities for continued discussion as requested. The hospital staff or the health care team should remain informed of the child's and the family's understanding. Support in discussing death and dying should be available to staff members. Counseling should be provided as needed and desired by the family or child. The counselor's familiarity with issues of death and dying and HIV-AIDS is important.

During the end stage of disease, children can benefit from knowing that they are dying and should be given the opportunity to discuss their fears with their loved ones. Similarly, families of a dying child also need to be knowledgeable, supported, and active participants in decisions about end-of-life care for their child. Health care providers need to recognize the multiple difficulties and feelings experienced by children and their families during this time, including ambivalence, fear, isolation, anger, loss of control, helplessness, and sadness. Members of the health care team need to maintain a compassionate physical presence. In so doing, they may more adequately recognize the need to relieve the multiple causes of pain and suffering while balancing the need for restorative care (disease-specific management with aggressive antiretroviral therapies and prophylaxis and treatment of opportunistic infections) and supportive care (nutrition, pain management, and other aspects of palliative care).

Families' Needs

COMMUNICATION

Repeatedly, the literature attests to parental difficulties with disclosure of their child's diagnosis to the child—and when or how this should take place (Grubman et al. 1995; Flanagan-Klygis et al. 2001). While the American Academy of Pediatrics (1999) has found no apparent evidence to support the fear that disclosure of HIV infection to children will negatively affect the parent-child relationship, many parents, and even their child's health care providers, do not know how best to proceed. Gerson and colleagues (2001) provide a staged conceptual framework for addressing this issue over a continuum of time. Five stages are noted:

- Information gathering and trust building, characterized by the establishment and maintenance of a trust-based working relationship between the caregiver and the health care professional.

- Education, beginning with initial assessments of caregiver and child knowledge and attitudes (including cultural and religious beliefs) and continuing through a gradual full disclosure to the child. This may take weeks to years.
- Determining when the time is right for disclosure, a process that must include changes in the child's health status, parental health or relationship, and perhaps the initiation of experimental, risky, or more burdensome treatments.
- The actual disclosure event, which may be accomplished by the caregiver in the presence of the health care professional.
- Monitoring postdisclosure coping and disclosure-related bumps in the road, such as direct or indirect observations of behavior, school performance, and peer relationships, and facilitating acceptance and adjustment with behavioral health professional consultation as needed.

Responsible health care providers will help parents, families, and in-home caregivers work through this essential communication task. Communication needs remain fundamental throughout the course of HIV-related illness.

PSYCHOSOCIAL SUPPORT

As with any chronic illness, HIV infection will introduce a strain on interpersonal relationships. The adaptability of parents dealing with a chronically ill child is quite varied. While much has been written about the potential for marital, sibling, or other interfamilial discord experienced within these families (see chapters 6 and 8), little information specific to the adaptive needs of families caring for an HIV-infected child is available. Perhaps this reflects the previously noted prevalence of maternal-fetal acquisition, and the death of the mother to HIV, in the early years of the HIV-AIDS epidemic in this country. Nonetheless, psychological adjustment and parenting stress have been noted among fathers (Wiener, Vasquez, and Battles 2001), families in general, aging adolescents with HIV (Battles and Wiener 2002), and all caregivers (Bachanas et al. 2001). The coexisting stresses of poverty, disorganized living environments, and limited coping skills may also contribute to perceived stress. Well-integrated and interdisciplinary support through community agencies, in-home caregiver networks, faith communities, social services, and nursing and behavioral health professionals may all be required to ensure an optimal outcome for the child living with HIV infection and his or her family.

HOSPICE CARE

The guiding ethical principles of palliative care include autonomy, beneficence, nonmalfeasance, and justice (see chapters 2 and 5 in this volume). When the process of shared decision making is used, the family and child are full partners with the health care team in management decisions. The child's best interests are paramount, and care is provided in an atmosphere of kindness in which access to appropriate palliative care is made available (American Academy of Pediatrics 1994, 1995a, 1995b; Grothe and Brody 1995; Welch et al. 1998). Coordinated, broad support for children and families during all phases of the illness is critical to providing physical, psychosocial, and spiritual comfort throughout the course of the disease and, at the end, death with dignity for children.

Hospice care is a philosophy of care that promotes dying with comfort and dignity. It is care that incorporates the principles of palliative care used in earlier stages of illness but with an enhanced emphasis on easing the burden of end-of-life care for the patient and family. The focus is on comfort care, while limiting or withdrawing life-prolonging measures. Hospice care is most often provided in the home setting but can also be offered in hospitals, nursing homes, and freestanding facilities. As part of the continuum of palliative care, hospice services maximize patient dignity and allow for a transition to appropriate family and staff bereavement (American Academy of Pediatrics 1992; Attig 1996; Davies et al. 1996; Goldman 1996; Faulkner and Armstrong-Dailey 1997).

During the end stage of HIV-AIDS, hospice and terminal care services can typically provide the most comprehensive services to meet the needs of the child and family for medical and emotional support. Access to appropriate and flexible hospice and terminal care services needs to be expanded. The hospice paradigm includes the following:

- Careful discussion of the child's and family's wishes and assessment of present status are critical to determining the most appropriate hospice or terminal-care situation. When ideal services cannot be obtained, an understanding of family priorities is important in terminal care choices.

- Because traditional hospice care is not always appropriate or available, support for establishing new innovative services should be provided when possible.
- Innovative plans such as flexible home hospice plans, foster family hospice, and use of home health teams for hospice care should be considered.
- The definition of the partnership between hospital health care teams and hospice services is critical to coordination of services for the child and family.
- Hospital health care teams may need to redefine their roles with patients as they move to hospice care.
- After the child's death, support services for the family, and even the community, should continue as appropriate. Bereavement support has been found to be particularly critical in families affected by HIV-AIDS, and provision of these services should be facilitated.
- Practical planning, including funeral arrangements, is supportive for families at this time.
- Referral to community resources to replace the medical, resource, and emotional support provided by the health-care team is advisable.
- Discussion of future connections to the hospital team, as desired by the family, is necessary, so that families do not also experience the loss of important caregivers.
- Visits to the child's school, faith community, or extracurricular organization (Boy Scouts or Girl Scouts, for example) by trained bereavement support staff may be helpful.

Health Care Providers' Needs

Grief work for the staff is essential. Over the life of a pediatric HIV-AIDS patient, numerous health care professionals become involved in supporting the family as well as the child. When the child dies, staff members often grieve as part of the community of caregivers. While the terminal nature of HIV-AIDS may allow for preparatory measures to be taken to make accepting loss easier in these circumstances, it does not preclude the very human feelings brought to the surface when reckoning with the loss of an individual infant, child, or adolescent. Caregivers need support and allowance to grieve. Often, continued contacts with families may provide a measure of healing (see chapter 9 in this volume).

Community Resources

Few disease processes will challenge the community in its capacity to accept, respond to, and support a child as does HIV-AIDS. Providing comprehensive and individualized palliative, respite, and terminal care services for children with HIV and their families is unquestionably important, yet it presents a significant challenge to health care providers and social support systems. With AIDS, more rage, shame, fear, and unresolved grief are experienced, often associated with stigmatization and disenfranchisement. The multigenerational complexity of AIDS, social stigma, and fears of contagion can deprive children and families of critical community and extended family support. Care for children with HIV or AIDS involves multiple medical appointments, developmental services, complex home medical treatments, and frequent illness, at times requiring constant care. Providing care is often complicated by illness in multiple family members and inadequate financial and community resources. As there are no national guidelines for access, delivery, or eligibility of providers for pediatric palliative, hospice, and respite care, creativity in care provision is required (Lenker, Lubeck, and Vosler 1993; Armstrong-Dailey and Fair 1994). Innovative models for hospice and terminal care of children with HIV are required.

Owing to the unique needs of children with HIV and AIDS, hospice care for these children differs from traditional hospice care: prognosis is uncertain, and the medical course can be variable; multidisciplinary hospice services may be required for more extended periods of time; and children often require active as well as palliative treatment. Access to appropriate programs varies greatly in different geographical areas, and immediate health care support, a critical part of hospice services, is not available in some disadvantaged areas (Koocher and Gudas 1992). One of the goals to support palliative and end-of-life care for HIV-affected children and families is to strengthen access to these services.

Recommendations

Palliative, hospice, and respite care is important to a family's ability to cope with pediatric HIV-AIDS and to adhere to a treatment plan. Access to appropriate palliative, respite, and end-of-life care should be expanded.

- An assessment should be made of each family's need for various forms of palliative and respite care and hospice service support as well as the available family and community systems.
- Palliative and respite support plans will need modification with changes in family situations and the child's health status and requires monitoring at clinic visits.
- Palliative and respite services to be considered should include in-home services, with homemaker, sitter, or parent-trainer, as well as out-of-home services in family care, respite houses, or hospice centers.
- Families should have access to nursing, social service, therapeutic, and pastoral care services.
- Appropriate palliative and respite plans that are flexible in response to the changing health needs of developing children with HIV-AIDS may not be available. Sites should provide information on palliative and respite resources, AIDS information, and medical backup if community resources are to be established.

Children's emotional comfort and need for a sense of security require consistency in palliative, respite, and hospice arrangements, particularly in the context of concurrent losses. Palliative, hospice, and respite care should be considered for parents, other significant caregivers in the family's care system (often grandparents), foster parents, and siblings, as well as for the child with HIV or AIDS.

Conclusion

Quality of life is difficult to define because it varies with the individual and its subjective nature limits measurement. In the final analysis, the quality of life for anyone depends on the presence of others. For the child with HIV-AIDS, the presence of others necessarily includes health care professionals, all of whom should be familiar with palliative care principles. A decent quality of life for a child with HIV-AIDS includes the ability to dream about tomorrow; to wake up each day with purposes and goals while living, playing, and working as normally as possible in the home, school, or workplace; to be free of pain and other symptoms as much as possible through the progression of the disease; and finally, to be held and comforted by loved ones at the time of death.

A number of religious traditions and philosophies provide the historical imperative for the obligation to care for and relieve the suffering of others. The first principle of Buddha is "Look deeply into the nature of suffering to see the cause of suffering and the way out." The Prophet Mohammed tells us, "For every good deed there is a reward. But for taking care of a person in need the reward is God himself." Much can be learned from the oral traditions of the Native Americans: "Every moment that humans spend cherishing and worrying about the life around them is another spark added to the ocean of time. It drives back the darkness for just that much longer." According to the New Testament, Christ was a carpenter by trade, but throughout his ministry, he was a healer. His call "Suffer the little children to come unto Me" (Mark 10:14) admonishes us not just to hold a beautiful child but to heal and comfort the leper, the 16-year-old prostitute with HIV infection, and the 40-year-old gay man with AIDS. In the Jewish tradition, *pikuach nefish*—the saving of a life—supersedes and is more important than any other law or commandment.

Perhaps the strongest statement of our obligation to care and relieve suffering is found in the story of Elijah's second coming. Elijah said that when he returned to earth it would foretell the coming of the Messiah. When his students questioned him on how they would recognize the Messiah, Elijah told them they should "go to the city gates and look for the individual kneeling among the sick and injured changing their bandages. This would be the Messiah." All health care workers have the tremendous privilege of being like the Messiah in their activities as care providers, but with this privilege and trust comes the obligation to provide care and relieve suffering. In providing care to those with chronic life-threatening diseases, no act of kindness, no matter how small, is ever wasted. Sometimes in life, the little things we do, almost without thought, become our most important accomplishments.

Children with life-limiting illness, regardless of diagnosis, socioeconomic status, or geographic location, should receive a continuum of palliative care and have access to hospice services that maximize their quality of life and ease the burden of dying. William Wordsworth, in his poem "We Are Seven," asks, rhetorically, "A simple child / That lightly draws its breath, / And feels its life in every limb, / What should it know of death?" The simple answer is that the child should know that though death is near it will not be painful; that it will be faced not alone but in the company of those he or she loves.

References

American Academy of Pediatrics, Committee on Bioethics. 1994. Guidelines for forgoing life-sustaining medical treatment. *Pediatrics* 93:532–36.

——, Committee on Fetus and Newborn. 1995a. The initiation or withdrawal of treatment for high-risk newborns. *Pediatrics* 96:362–63.

——, Committee on Fetus and Newborn. 1995b. Perinatal care at the threshold of viability. *Pediatrics* 96:974–76.

——, Committee on Pediatric AIDS. 1999. Disclosure of illness status to children and adolescents with HIV infection. *Pediatrics* 103:164–66.

——, Committee on Psychosocial Aspects of Child and Family Health. 1992. The pediatrician and childhood bereavement. *Pediatrics* 89:516–18.

Armstrong-Dailey, A., and C. Fair. 1994. Respite and terminal care for children with HIV infection and their families. In *Pediatric AIDS: the challenge of HIV infection in infancy, childhood and adolescence*, ed. P. A. Pizzo and C. M. Wilfert, 829–38. Baltimore: Williams and Wilkins.

Attig, T. 1996. Beyond pain: the existential suffering of children. *J Palliat Care* 12:20–23.

Bachanas, P. J., K. A. Kullgren, K. S. Schwartz, J. S. McDaniel, J. Smith, and S. Nesheim. 2001. Psychological adjustment in caregivers of school-age children infected with HIV: stress, coping, and family factors. *J Pediatr Psychol* 26:359–61.

Battles, H. B., and L. S. Wiener. 2002. From adolescence through young adulthood: psychosocial adjustment associated with long-term survival of HIV. *J Adolesc Health* 30:161–68.

Boland, M., C. Burr, and D. Harvey. 1995. Pediatric AIDS revisited: family, social and legal issues. *Semin Pediatr Infect Dis* 6:40–45.

Butensky, E. A. 2001. The role of nutrition in pediatric HIV/AIDS: a review of micronutrient research. *J Pediatr Nurs* 16:402–11.

Czarniecki, L., M. Boland, and J. M. Oleske. 1993. Pain in children with HIV disease. *PAAC Notes* 5:492–95.

Davies, B., K. Cook, M. O'Loane, D. Clarke, B. Mackenzie, C. Stutzen, S. Connaughty, and J. McCormick. 1996. Caring for dying children: nurses' experiences. *Pediatr Nurs* 22:500–507.

Davis, S. F., R. H. Byers Jr., M. L. Lindegren, M. B. Caldwell, J. M. Karon, and M. Gwinn. 1995. Prevalence and incidence of vertically acquired HIV infection in the United States. *JAMA* 274:952–55.

Faulkner, K. W., and A. Armstrong-Dailey. 1997. Care of the dying child. In *Principles and practice of pediatric oncology*, ed. P. Pizzo and D. Poplack, 1349–51. 3d ed. Philadelphia: Lippincott-Raven.

Ferris, F., and J. Flannery, eds. 1995. *A comprehensive guide for the care of persons with HIV disease: module 4: palliative care.* Toronto: Mount Sinai Hospital–Casey House Hospice.

Flanagan-Klygis, E., L. F. Ross, J. Lantos, J. Frader, and R. Yogev. 2001. Disclosing the diagnosis of HIV in pediatrics. *J Clin Ethics* 12:150–57.

Fleischman, A. R., K. Nolan, N. N. Dubler, M. F. Epstein, M. A. Gerben, M. S. Jellinek, I. F. Litt, M. S. Miles, S. Oppenheimer, and A. Shaw. 1994. Caring for gravely ill infants and children. *Pediatrics* 94:433–39.

Frager, G. 1996. Pediatric palliative care: building the model, bridging the gaps. *J Palliat Care* 12:9–12.

Frager, G., and B. Shapiro. 1998. Pediatric palliative care and pain management. In *Psycho-oncology*, ed. J. C. Holland, 907–22. New York: Oxford University Press.

Fundaro, C., N. Miccinesi, N. F. Baldieri, O. Genovese, C. Rendeli, and G. Segni. 1998. Cognitive impairment in school-age children with symptomatic HIV infection. *AIDS Patient Care and STDs* 12:135–40.

Gaughan, D. M., M. D. Hughes, G. R. Seage III, P. A. Selwyn, V. J. Carey, S. L. Gortmaker, and J. M. Oleske. 2002. The prevalence of pain in pediatric human immunodeficiency virus/acquired immunodeficiency syndrome as reported by participants in the Pediatric Late Outcomes Study (PACTG 219). *Pediatrics* 109:1144–52.

Gerson, A. C., M. Joyner, P. Fosarelli, A. Butz, L. Wissow, S. Lee, P. Marks, and N. Hutton. 2001. Disclosure of HIV diagnosis to children: when, where, why, and how. *J Pediatr Health Care* 15:161–67.

Goldman, A. 1996. Home care of the dying child. *J Palliat Care* 12:16–19.

Grothe, T. M., and R. V. Brody. 1995. Palliative care for HIV disease. *J Palliat Care* 11:48–49.

Grubman, S., E. Gross, N. Lerner-Weiss, M. Hernandez, G. D. McSherry, L. G. Hoyt, M. Boland, and J. M. Oleske. 1995. Older children and adolescents with perinatally acquired HIV infection. *Pediatrics* 95:657–66.

Institute of Medicine. 1997. *Approaching death: improving care at the end of life.* Washington, D.C.: National Academy Press.

Koocher, G. P., and L. J. Gudas. 1992. Terminal and life-threatening illness in childhood. In *Developmental-behavioral Pediatrics,* ed. M. D. Levine, W. B. Carey, A. C. Crocker, and R. T. Gross, 327–36. Philadelphia: W. B. Saunders.

Lenker, S. L., D. P. Lubeck, and A. Vosler. 1993. Planning community-wide services for persons with HIV infection in an area of moderate incidence. *Public Health Reports: Hyattsville* 108:3850–93.

Lewis, S. Y., H. J. Haiken, and L. G. Joyt. 1994. Living beyond the odds: a psychosocial perspective of long-term survivors of pediatric human immunodeficiency virus infection. *J Dev Behav Pediatr* 15:S12–17.

Liben, S. 1996. Pediatric palliative medicine: obstacles to overcome. *J Palliat Care* 12:24–28.

McQuillan, R., and I. Finlay. 1996. Facilitating the care of terminally ill children. *J Pain Symptom Manage* 12:320–24.

Meyers, H. I. 1989. Spiritual care in pediatric hospice. *Am J Hospice Care* 6(May–June):12.

Nelson, L. J., and R. M. Nelson. 1992. Ethics and the provision of futile, harmful or burdensome treatments to children. *Crit Care Med* 20:427–33.

Oleske, J. M. 1995. *Preventing disability and providing rehabilitation for infants, children and youths with HIV/AIDS.* NIH publication 95-3850. Bethesda, Md.: U.S.

Department of Health and Human Services–National Institute of Child Health and Human Development, January.

Oleske, J. M., P. M. Rothpletz-Puglia, and H. Winter. 1996. Historical perspectives on the evolution in understanding the importance of nutritional care in pediatric HIV infection. *J Nutr* 126:2616S–19S.

Oleske, J. M., and A. Ruben-Hale. 1995. Enhancing supportive care and promoting quality of life: clinical practice guidelines. *Pediatr AIDS HIV Infect Fetus Adolesc* 6:187–203.

Paris, J. J., and M. D. Schrieber. 1996. Physicians' refusal to provide life-prolonging medical interventions. *Clin Perinatol* 23:563–71.

Robinson, W. M., S. Ravilly, C. Berde, and M. E. Wohl. 1996. End-of-life care in cystic fibrosis. *Pediatrics* 100:205–9.

Rushton, C. H., E. E. Hogue, C. A. Billet, K. Chapman, D. Greenberg-Friedman, M. Joyner, and C. D. Parks. 1993. End-of-life care for infants with AIDS: ethical and legal issues. *Pediatr Nurs* 19:79–83; 94.

Sullivan, J. L., and K. Luzuriaga. 2001. The changing face of pediatric HIV-1 infection. *N Engl J Med* 345:1568–69.

United Nations. 1991. *Convention on the rights of children.* New York: United Nations.

Walco, G. A., R. C. Cassidy, and N. L. Schechter. 1994. The ethics of pain control in infants and children. *N Engl J Med* 331:541–44.

Welch, K., P. Kessinger, R. Bessinger, K. Dascomb, A. Morse, and E. Gleckler. 1998. The clinical profile of end-stage AIDS. *AIDS Patient Care and STDs* 12:125–29.

Wiener, L. S., M. J. Vasquez, and H. B. Battles. 2001. Fathering a child living with HIV/AIDS: psychological adjustment and parenting stress. *J Pediatr Psychol* 26:353–58.

Wissow, L. S., N. Hutton, and N. Kass. 2001. Preliminary study of a values-history advance directive interview in a pediatric HIV clinic. *J Clin Ethics* 12:161–72.

15

Children and Adolescents with Cancer

*Joanne M. Hilden, M.D., Sarah Friebert, M.D., Bruce P. Himelstein, M.D., F.A.A.P.,
David R. Freyer, D.O., and Janice Wheeler, M.Ed.*

Pediatric oncology is a gratifying field, largely because so many children with cancer are cured and because providers enjoy long-term relationships with children and their families. Both of these facts can make the care of a child and family particularly challenging when the child does not survive cancer. What are the elements of care, and what skills are needed to make this part of practice go well for all?

> Valerie was an active 13-year-old when she was diagnosed with stage IV metastatic Ewing sarcoma with bone marrow metastasis. Chemotherapy commenced immediately, and radiation was delivered to the initial tumor site six months later, midway through the chemotherapy protocol. During her antitumor treatment, Valerie was a positive and cooperative patient, and she developed excellent relationships with the members of her treatment team. Valerie always participated in consultations, and her parents encouraged her to discuss her concerns with the team whenever there were decisions to be made or unanticipated procedures to be performed.
>
> After a year, Valerie was declared free of disease. She began to set short- and long-range goals for her physical recovery after treatment, and within a few months she was able to compete in a national softball tournament and begin high school. However, her reprieve was short lived. Seven months later, sharp back pains led to restaging scans and evaluation. Supported by her parents and her adult brother and his wife, Valerie learned in consultation with her oncologist that her cancer

had returned. A favorite nurse also was present. The oncologist, with much compassion and empathy, explained to Valerie that treatment options for recurrent Ewing sarcoma were limited. With bone marrow involvement, Valerie was ineligible for most trials.

Valerie was an important part of discussions about treatment choices; she decided she was not willing to undergo "just any old treatment." She and her parents discussed her fears, and her parents felt it especially important to emphasize that she would not face the treatments alone. One of the social workers mentioned hospice, but her family decided against this option. The pain management service at the hospital helped to manage Valerie's pain.

In family discussions, Valerie's father expressed anger, often misdirected at the oncologists, that nothing was available for Valerie to try. He wanted his wife to persuade Valerie to agree to some alternate therapies that had been offered (none of which promised cure). However, Valerie's mother was adamant that she would not try to "talk Valerie into anything."

As she fully absorbed the concept of "life-limiting illness," Valerie decided to pursue gene therapy treatment at the National Cancer Institute, fifteen hundred miles from home. She elected this trial because she believed it was the least intrusive treatment on offer and provided some promise for extending her life. Her father was pleased with Valerie's decision. However, the oncologists there explained that she was no longer a candidate for the gene therapy protocol. In fact, the doctors felt that Valerie might not survive more than a few days. Hospice was again offered, and this time Valerie's parents accepted, realizing they could not take care of her at home without help.

The pediatric palliative care team quickly established a good relationship with Valerie and gained her trust. Valerie's philosophy was to get up every day and make it a great day; she saw herself as a normal teenager with a limited life span. She dated, entertained friends, and traveled whenever she could. In restaurants, she always ordered dessert first. In the months that followed, Valerie was still able to pursue her talent in art—even when she could no longer study. Although Valerie frequently returned to the hospital for radiation treatments for pain control, she never spent another night away from her home and family. Blood transfusions were given to increase her energy level so that she could participate in activities to promote her overall quality of life.

Various members of the oncology team including her primary oncologist, made personal visits to Valerie as death grew nearer. A close circle of friends, along with immediate and extended family, also supported Valerie on her journey. Throughout the seven-month hospice experience, Valerie's pain was very well controlled. Valerie died peacefully at home with her parents and sister present.

The hospice bereavement coordinator kept in touch with Valerie's family, encouraging them to accept an invitation to a family bereavement camp offered by the pediatric hospice program. This experience seemed to be the pivotal event that helped the family begin to adjust to life without Valerie. The bereavement camp offered a mixture of group and family activities designed to help them look more deeply at their feelings and relationships. As her mother reflects, "We are changed forever, but we have not lost hope. We are going to be okay."

Now an ardent advocate for the widespread availability of pediatric palliative care, Valerie's mother realizes, "We were at the far end of the bell curve. We had an excellent oncology team, a pediatric-specific hospice program, a supportive community, and a strong family unit. That should be the goal for every child with a terminal illness."

Valerie had good symptom control, and she and her family enjoyed a continuous relationship with her oncology team throughout her illness. They had access to systematized information throughout her illness, which facilitated shared, informed decision making as things changed. The family made it a routine part of care to involve Valerie directly in important decision making. They had the help of a hospice team with pediatric experience. In addition, Valerie's family had community support and help with siblings.

Most children who die from cancer, however, experience uncontrolled symptoms and suffering (Collins et al. 2000; Wolfe et al. 2000), and their parents experience confusion about medical communication (Goldman 1999). This occurs despite the American Society of Pediatric Hematology/Oncology's recommendation that the pediatric oncology team include psychosocial support staff (including social workers, child-life therapists, and chaplaincy staff) and despite the availability of guidelines and algorithms for the treatment of pain (Arceci et al. 1998).

All of the services provided by such staff are recognized as crucial for good palliative care for children. How can the core components of good pediatric palliative care be systematized throughout the continuum of the pediatric cancer experience? How do we provide continuity of care, good symptom control, and help with siblings? Most important, how can we help parents make difficult decisions for and with their child in a way that minimizes suffering for all? How do we do so while still respecting the frequent need to proceed with phase I or other experimental therapies (Vickers and Carlisle 2000)?

Decision Making

ALWAYS DEFINE THE GOALS OF CARE

While decision making and defining the goals of care have been covered in earlier chapters, there are special considerations in this regard in oncology. These considerations challenge current concepts and definitions of palliative care. Perhaps the best way to promote quality palliative care for children with cancer is to introduce the concepts of palliation (with its attention to control of physical and psychosocial symptoms and interdisciplinary teamwork and assistance with decisions as a child's condition changes) as close to the time of diagnosis as possible. Even as physicians begin initial therapy for the child with cancer and the family has eased into comfort with the team, the phrase "palliative care" should be introduced, along with the word "cure."

By explaining that the goal of treatment is to seek cure while simultaneously providing palliative care, the doctors and nurses can present palliative care as an integral part of the services provided for the child with cancer. Another potential benefit is that the child and his or her parents will view palliative, or comfort, care as an integral part of good cancer treatment rather than as an indicator that all hope for cure has been extinguished.

The availability of phase I and phase II clinical trials for pediatric oncology patients with relapsed or recurrent disease offers continued cancer-directed therapy but only a small chance of life-prolonging benefit to the specific patient. To make the best individual decision, the child and parents will need detailed information regarding these therapies, including clearly explained hoped-for benefits, known burdens (side effects, procedures, time at the clinic or in the hospital), and how participation will contribute to the care of future patients. Research clearly demonstrates that patients and families prefer to be guided in these discussions by practitioners they trust (Whittam 1993; Frager 1996). Thus oncology teams will most often be the ones to help families with these decisions. Given the prognosis of children considered for phase I and II therapies, by current standards, at this time the team should also be discussing with the family palliative goals of care and, along with the oncology team, the simultaneous availability of palliative care and hospice professionals (American Academy of Pediatrics 2000; Field and Behrman 2002).

It is important to state clearly to patients and families that the scientific goal of phase I research is to determine the toxicity and maximum-tolerated dose of an investigational agent. Data indicate that only one-third of competent adult patients enrolled in a phase I trial were able to state the scientific purpose of the trial after the standard process of informed consent (Daugherty et al. 1995). The investigators also revealed that participants in phase I trials held strong beliefs in the hope of personal therapeutic benefit. However, the chance of tumor response (some degree of shrinkage) in phase I trials is low (4% to 6%), and remission or cure is even less common (Decoster, Stein, and Holdener 1990; Daugherty et al. 1995). The data for children are similar (Shah et al. 1998). It appears that in phase I investigational agent trials, physicians tend to communicate, or families tend to hear, more positive potential benefit from experimental chemotherapy than is justified (Daugherty et al. 1995). Furthermore, pediatric oncologists have historically deferred discussion of palliative goals of care to the time when there is "no viable therapy to offer," if the topic is mentioned at all (Hilden et al. 2001). Although these biases are not intentional, they may invalidate the informed consent process, raising further ethical questions about these trials (Emanuel 1995).

Thus in obtaining informed consent and helping families and children define the goals of care, all of the information noted in exhibit 15.1 should be imparted to the patient with advanced cancer and his or her family. In short, families need an informed and complete appreciation of the expected effects of treatment decisions in the physical, psychological, spiritual, and practical realms of care. This can clearly require multiple discussions.

The following actual case illustrates the effect of a decision by the oncology team to withhold information, depriving the family of informed consent.

The day after a mother learned that her teenage daughter had stage IV metastatic bone cancer, she asked the pediatric nurse for any books and information about cure rate for the disease. The nurse responded that there was no information available at the hospital for the parent to read, when in fact there were numerous articles and references on site. Not convinced, but also not having asked the other members of the

Exhibit 15.1. Information that should be imparted to the family and patient with advanced cancer

---

- All available treatment goals and options, including palliative goals
- Diagnosis and prognosis, including the likelihood of death
- Likely effects of the disease on the patient
- Likely effects of various treatment options on the patient, including probable hospitalization, clinic visits, and invasive procedures
- Any relevant physical or emotional problems likely to affect the child and family
- Uses and interactions of medications
- Availability of pharmacologic and nonpharmacologic interventions to ease suffering
- Availability of hospital, community-based, and national professional and non-professional resources to aid the family, including palliative care, symptom control, hospice, support groups, and practical assistance
- Predictable changes in the child's functional status and their anticipated time course
- Impact, as predictable, on the child's quality of life
- Impact on the family, including marital stress, sibling concerns, financial and practical concerns, and spiritual and grief-related issues
- What death will look and be like with and without artificial intervention
- Impact on school, peers, and community

---

team, the parent researched the public library and the Internet to find information. She learned that her child's chances for cure were less than 20 percent. Later, she discovered that the nurse had not furnished her this information because the nurse "did not think the mom could handle it." Although the mother pointed out that decisions regarding treatment would not have changed, this incident left her feeling that she could not rely on the care team to be honest and truthful. She followed up with her oncologist and said, "Don't allow your staff to make presumptions about what I can or cannot handle. Answer my questions honestly and frankly, and don't hide information from me. Your team's responsibility is to be the doctor, the nurse, the social worker, not my guardian. I have to take responsibility for how I respond to the truth."

SPECIAL CONSIDERATIONS FOR ADOLESCENTS WITH CANCER

Decision making for adolescents at the end of life can be particularly challenging because of certain ethical and legal considerations that pertain to this age group. As exemplified in the case of Valerie, the factors in decision making at this stage of illness include the adolescent's physical condition, his or her school, family, social relationships, and the emerging personal independence that normally seeks expression during these years. The most fundamental decision facing teenagers with advanced cancer is whether to discontinue active efforts to treat the underlying disease. In approaching this decision, most adolescents are in a position to draw upon the considerable medical experience accumulated since the initial diagnosis. Rarely, a teenager may be faced with a decision not to begin antineoplastic therapy at all, in light of a particularly dismal prognosis. More commonly, patients with advanced or recurrent disease will have experienced a medical course characterized by gradual debilitation resulting from prolonged attempts at curative therapy and disease progression. Because of their greater cognitive maturity compared with much younger patients, at each relapse informed adolescents will be aware of both their diminishing prognosis for cure and the benefits and burdens of continued treatment. How they weigh these considerations and to what extent their opinions hold sway in end-of-life decisions largely reflect their own developmental maturity, preexisting family dynamics, and the biases of the involved clinical personnel.

From an ethical and legal perspective, decision making for adolescents at the end of life hinges on the issue of capacity and competency. In the United States, legal competency is defined by having achieved the age of majority, 18 years. It is presumed that by this age individuals have the necessary mental capacity (ability to understand goals of care and benefits and burdens of therapy) to make medical decisions for themselves, including the decision to forgo life-prolonging treatment. The basis for this right is the ethical value of personal autonomy. To be exercised, autonomy has several preconditions, including the ability to comprehend relevant information and to grasp the consequences of the decision; the receipt of sufficient information pertaining to the choice to make an informed choice; and freedom from coercive influences (Beauchamp and Childress 1989). In large part, a patient's autonomy is protected by the process of informed consent. Thus properly informed patients aged 18 years or older may choose not to begin or continue treatment of their underlying disease or its complications. It follows that these patients also may choose when to begin exclusively palliative goals of care or which of its elements to use.

In contrast, adolescents under the age of 18 are not ordinarily considered legally competent to make medical decisions for themselves, including those pertaining to end-of-life care. However, many care providers for adolescents and older children have recognized that medically experienced patients of this age often demonstrate notable insight into their situations. This observation has led to attempts to clarify what cognitive elements are necessary for minor patients to demonstrate they are *functionally* competent (that is, they have intact decision-making capacity). King and Cross (1989) and Leiken (1989) have suggested that functional competence (capacity) requires the ability

- to reason (to consider multiple factors in predicting future consequences);
- to understand (to comprehend essential medical information);
- to choose voluntarily (in relation to authority figures, such as parents and physicians); and
- to appreciate the nature of the decision (the gravity, immediacy, and permanence of the choice).

Leiken (1989) also emphasizes the importance of a child's conceptualization of death for participating in end-of-life decisions.

Incorporating these considerations, a consensus emerging from pediatric health professionals, developmental psychologists, ethicists, and lawyers holds that adolescents as young as 14 years of age can be presumed, unless demonstrated otherwise, to have the functional competence to make binding medical decisions for themselves, including decisions to discontinue life-prolonging therapy (American Academy of Pediatrics 1994, 1995; Weir and Peters 1997). Because of the maturing effects of chronic illness, some experienced pediatric clinicians feel that terminally ill children substantially younger than 14 years, probably less than 10, often demonstrate attributes of functional competence and should have substantial input on major end-of-life decisions, including discontinuation of treatment (Freyer 1992; Nitschke et al. 2000). Caution must be taken that authority for medical decision making not be given to minors inappropriately, partly on the grounds that "long-term" or "future autonomy" might be sacrificed for "present-day autonomy" through premature loss of life (Ross 1997; Friebert and Kodish 1999). However, in the setting of terminal illness, the consensus noted above supports the presumption of decision-making capacity for chronically ill, intellectually intact patients in the adolescent age range of approximately 10 to 20 years, unless there is evidence to the contrary.

The legal status of end-of-life decision making by adolescents is inconsistent. As summarized by Traugott and Alpers (1997) and Weir and Peters

(1997), legal rights have been recognized for some adolescents making certain other personal medical decisions. Some states permit decisions by patients who are deemed to be "emancipated minors," on the basis of marriage and other circumstances. Some states have "minor treatment" statutes allowing minors to authorize treatment for conditions that might be left untreated if parental notification were required, such as treatment for sexually transmitted diseases. Other states have permitted judicial hearings to allow capable adolescents to override parents' wishes in certain medical decisions. But even recently, fewer than half of state legislatures had statutes specifically addressing end-of-life decisions by adolescents (Weir and Peters 1997).

Despite these legal inconsistencies, the ethical considerations previously discussed permit an approach that is satisfactory for most adolescent cancer patients needing to make end-of-life decisions. These individuals possess substantial medical experience and enjoy established relationships with their care providers. These facts are valuable for facilitating a decisional role. When approached in a sensitive and respectful way, many adolescents will share their feelings about impending death and their opinions about continued treatment. These expressions can have crucial "effects of moral persuasion," as termed by Weir and Peters (1997, 35). In response to them, adults can support an adolescent's decision-making role, irrespective of the patient's exact legal status.

How to support the minor's autonomy varies according to particular circumstances. Older adolescents who clearly possess functional competence should be given full decisional authority. In these cases, the decision to discontinue antineoplastic treatment is communicated to the legally responsible adult, who then executes the decision through a "modified substituted judgment" (the application of a minor's expressed preferences in a decision made on his or her behalf) (Freyer 1992). Substituted judgment is a legal concept normally invoked for decisions involving previously competent adults who have already revealed their treatment preferences. In considering the application of this doctrine for the benefit of minors (who are, by definition, "pre-legally competent"), it should be noted that its purpose is to apply the *minor's stated wishes*, not those of a responsible adult seeking decisional control. Advance directives also have been advocated for older adolescents (Weir and Peters 1997).

For younger patients who meet some but not all of the criteria for functional competence, serious account should be taken of their decisional preferences while reserving full authority for the responsible adult. In these situations, the notion of *assent,* rather than *consent,* has been suggested (American Academy of Pediatrics 1995). However, to avoid violating the very spirit of seeking assent, care must be taken that the child's preference, once solicited, be respected.

As discussed previously, inclusion of children in phase I and phase II studies raises important issues. This is also true for adolescents, particularly as it relates to the question of assent, which is not required by federal law for studies of investigational therapy offering the possibility of direct benefit to the patient (Code of Federal Regulations 1991). Exaggerated hope for clinical benefit without full acknowledgment of the risk for toxicity may lead to undue pressure for the adolescent to enroll in such a study. On the other hand, in the face of bleak odds, a highly motivated or altruistic adolescent may wish to continue treatment in the context of a phase I or phase II study but be discouraged from doing so by parents with faltering hopes for cure and alternative goals for the remaining time. Of course, such patients need to be counseled sensitively but honestly to temper their motivation with realism. In every case, it is critical that the adolescent's true desires be carefully distinguished from a natural tendency to please authority figures like parents, physicians, or other adults.

Whether assent is applied to choices involving research or clinical care, the critical element is respect for the minor's dignity and ability to choose in matters profoundly and intimately affecting them as individuals, their bodies, and feelings. For an adolescent with relapsed cancer, the central choice is whether to continue or forgo antineoplastic therapy—conventional chemotherapy, radiation therapy, or investigational therapy. Throughout the course of an adolescent's illness, numerous other choices present themselves concerning daily routines and the comfort measures discussed later in this chapter. At a minimum, these simpler but important choices permit meaningful involvement even by very young children and less mature adolescents. For more capable patients, such choices promote decision-making skills that help prepare them for the more profound choices that may await them.

It is essential to provide the adolescent and family with a forum that promotes acquisition of accurate information and decisional integrity. One successful means for this is the "final-stage conference" described by Nitschke and colleagues (2000, 268). The final-stage conference is a communication approach employed at the time of cancer relapse, with the goal of communicating essential information concerning the disease, treatment options, and possible course, including palliative care options. The child, even if very young, is routinely included in the conference (with parental permission). Nitschke et al. report numerous benefits of this approach, including optimal involvement of the child, improved intrafamily communication, and increased trust in the medical team. Older adolescents may wish to include significant peers in their conferences.

Palliative Care and Hospice Services in Pediatric Oncology

Parents of children with cancer most commonly feel the need to try all available life-prolonging therapies (Vickers and Carlisle 2000). Accordingly, so do their oncologists (Liben 1996; Hilden et al. 2001). This has resulted in delayed and at times total lack of attention to issues related to death and dying, such as anticipatory bereavement, and it has prevented appropriate and timely palliative care throughout the cancer experience. Children and parents rely on the health care team to prepare them for the worst as they hope for the best. As one bereaved parent has put it, "As parents of kids with serious illnesses, we know that death is a possibility from the beginning. You as health care providers push those thoughts to the back of our minds with your options and statistics. Then when things don't go right, you have to reintroduce the subject. Don't insult or patronize us—let us know that you're fighting as hard as you can but that you need to help prepare us in case we don't win."

The American Academy of Pediatrics (2000) and other groups recommend introducing palliative care principles, language, and staff early in the course of therapy (Children's International Project on Palliative/Hospice Services 2001). Families usually prefer that the oncology team with whom they are most familiar manage the child throughout the illness until death, if that occurs (Martinson 1995; James and Johnson 1997). Yet most providers are not well trained in interdisciplinary palliative care (Sahler et al. 2000; Hilden et al. 2001). Pediatric oncology groups may need a palliative care specialist, or team, if their own team does not have the expertise to manage the comprehensive needs of the patient and family, particularly for symptom management, community-based care, sibling needs, and bereavement aftercare. The solution is earlier integration of the palliative care–symptom management team, so that they are part of care early on and are familiar to the family. They can be brought in again later as needed, especially if the illness ends in death.

At the time of relapse or progression of disease despite therapy, even though it is most likely that curative therapy will be pursued, a palliative care or hospice referral should definitely be considered. It may very well not be accepted, but the mention of palliative care at this time can plant the first seeds of acceptance. If the concept of palliative care has been a part of treatment to this point in the disease, the child and parents will be less likely to associate it (or the use of hospice services) with loss of hope. They may benefit from the addition of services attentive to needs present throughout the illness, whether it ends in cure or death.

The role of a hospice team, what they can contribute, and when to involve them are confusing issues for pediatric providers. Professionals in the fields of hospice and palliative care have appropriately responded to the lack of access to their services because of the stigma of the word "hospice" by broadening their mission (and sometimes the name of their organizations) to "hospice and palliative care." Both providers and parents are sometimes unsure of what is at issue, and what sort of care is meant, when palliative care is discussed. Families are helped when the care team they trust can explain the added benefit such care provides.

Hospice is not a place; it is a philosophy of care that embodies palliative care but also focuses on promoting quality of life by helping people live until they die, fostering choice in end-of-life care decision making, and supporting effective grieving for patients and their families. This philosophy can be implemented anywhere a child is located—at home, in an alternative home setting, in the hospital, even in the intensive care unit. Hospice providers' expertise includes the management of patients who are actively dying, but most hospices care predominantly for adults, and some may have serious knowledge gaps when it comes to providing care for terminally ill children. On the other hand, some locations have long-standing pediatric palliative care teams who provide expert, comprehensive care for such children.

Families need to be supported, whatever they have chosen as the place for their child to die. Home is better for some; hospital is better for others. While it is true that many families will choose to have their child at home if they feel adequately supported, it is equally true that many will choose to remain in a familiar environment that has become a home away from home for them. What is right for each individual family is what must be facilitated; either can be done with the integration of a qualified (pediatric) hospice and palliative care team. The role of the hospice and palliative care team is not to replace the primary team. Rather, the additional personnel can augment the oncology team to provide holistic support to the entire family, including the community and the "forgotten grievers" touched by the life of the patient (siblings, grandparents, church groups, school classes, scout groups; see chapter 8 in this volume).

Optimal care of our oncology families must include close coordination between the primary oncology team and the hospice and palliative care team. Depending upon the care system, this may best be accomplished through a seamless transition from acute care to palliative and hospice care, so that families do not feel abruptly switched from one to the other. Alternatively, primary care team members may need additional training to smooth transitions of care and to remain as involved as possible, thus lessening the appearance of abandonment and the family's likelihood of refusing services.

Despite the growing number of hospice and palliative care programs in this country, fewer than 10 percent of dying children receive these services. Exact statistics are difficult to interpret because of differences in definitions of pediatric hospice or palliative care programs across the country and because lengths of stay for children can and do exceed one year. However, in the year 2000 (the most recent year for which data are available), approximately five thousand children were served by hospice programs (National Hospice and Palliative Care Organization 2003, annual data collection). Traditionally, oncology teams have been resistant to hospice referrals for their patients for a number of reasons, including the following:

- shortage of specialized pediatric hospice teams
- resistance on the part of hospices to enroll children who continue to receive any type of life-extending, invasive, expensive therapy, including total parenteral nutrition, palliative chemotherapy or radiation, and transfusion support
- reluctance to transition families to a new team of people to care for the child
- misunderstandings about hospice benefit rules and do-not-resuscitate requirements

Often, practitioners assume that families are not "ready" for hospice or that broaching the topic will indicate that the team is "giving up" on the child. Similarly, families may also feel that mentioning hospice they will appear to be "giving up" or will disappoint their oncologist. Alternatively, they may simply be unaware of the services available, since most of these families are young and have not had occasion to encounter hospice programs. Again, an honest conversation, in the context of reviewing goals of care, may clear up many of these bidirectional misconceptions. To have this conversation, however, practitioners must be aware of what hospice programs can provide and must be able to explain these services in nonthreatening ways. Sometimes this is best done together with the palliative care team so that myths and barriers to access can be broken down. Much as in a consultation from any other subspecialty service, the palliative care team may be best able to describe the care that will be offered. Here too, a concurrent model throughout treatment is likely to be most effective.

In 1997 the Institute of Medicine looked specifically at the reasons that most people who die do not receive hospice and palliative care. These factors were reiterated in the 2001 report issued by the National Cancer Policy Board, including a section on children (Hilden et al. 2001). The common barriers to excellent end-of-life care are many, including the following:

- *Financial.* Coverage for hospice care is poor, often tied to the six-month prognosis rule.
- *Educational deficiencies.* Health care providers are not traditionally taught how to care for dying patients or how to initiate difficult conversations with families about end-of-life issues.
- *Health care system fragmentation.* Care is often delivered in different systems by many providers, often with poor communication among them.
- *Difficulty with enrollment criteria.* Medicare coverage for hospice care has been limited to patients with a six-month prognosis for survival, which is very hard to determine accurately. This is especially so with children, since they tend to have healthier organ systems than adults and tend to "live until they die" rather than quietly dwindling away.
- *Patient and family issues.* Many patients see hospice care as "giving up," so they do not want to use it.

Across the country, a tremendous variation exists in hospice programs in terms of willingness to enroll children whose plan of care is more invasive and expensive than that of the traditional adult hospice patient. Hospice programs without a home health license are limited to a standard all-inclusive, per diem payment based on the child's level of care (inpatient or symptom control, $470); routine home care ($110); or residential (in an inpatient hospice or alternative home setting, $110). These payments are intended to cover nursing services, other personnel, pharmacy expenses, and durable medical equipment. For nonprofit hospices with small censuses, one patient receiving expensive treatment will seriously drain program resources and will limit the number of people who can be served. Larger hospices are often able to absorb more expensive plans of care for pediatric patients, but resource allocation, again, is the bottom line. Nevertheless, it is increasingly being recognized within the hospice community that the provision of excellent pediatric hospice care should be a priority and that traditional enrollment standards should not apply to most children.

Steps are being taken to amend these regulations. Hospice programs are able to do their best work with families when they are involved for much longer than a few days. It takes time to build rapport and to integrate the many services available through the program without overwhelming families early on. Short lengths of stay with families interfere with the team's ability to focus on prevention of unnecessary pain and other symptoms, effective communication, preparation for death, and orchestration of care to achieve the child's and family's goals (Children's International Project on Palliative/ Hospice Services 2001). In fact, one of the major goals of hospice and palliative care teams is to help families to prepare advance directives and to feel supported enough to forgo life-extending therapy when it becomes unduly burdensome. Therefore, if the requirement for hospice means that the family must already have chosen to forgo "cure-oriented" care, only those who have already done this difficult work will have access. This is where the integration of the hospice and palliative team and the oncology team is so crucial: preparation for these decisions should start well before the word "hospice" is mentioned. Most hospice programs do not require an agreement to forgo resuscitation before enrollment for their pediatric programs.

For practitioners, it is helpful to know what hospice programs exist in the area and whether they have expertise with pediatric patients. Hospice personnel are usually more than willing to visit oncology treatment centers to explain their services. It may also be beneficial to have the two programs walk in each other's footsteps, with oncology nurses spending a day with a pediatric hospice nurse and vice versa. This exchange of personnel and information goes a long way to clear up misconceptions and break down barriers. Oncology practitioners should also approach hospice programs on a case-by-case basis, rather than assuming that a particular child or family is not appropriate for the program. A simple phone call may reveal that a creative solution can be worked out.

For families, it is helpful to know that anyone can make a referral to a hospice program. Families often feel a great gulf between the wide array of services available at the hospital or clinic relative to the paucity of those available in the home. They may need help with concrete tasks such as shopping and light housework, or they may need interventions for the child's siblings that do not disrupt their routines even more by requiring them to spend time at the hospital or clinic. They may also need additional support to handle the barrage of relatives and friends who cannot understand the decisions being made and might benefit from talking with medical personnel about the issues. Oncology teams are busy, and families may feel that their additional needs are not as important as the needs of other children and families they encounter in the hospital. It may relieve them to know there are extra people available to provide support, people who work in concert with their primary team.

Finally, some practitioners are reluctant to refer because they are not aware of what a palliative care and hospice program can add to the care of a pediatric oncology patient at the end of life. When the child is receiving ongoing care in the clinic or hospital setting, nursing support and pediatric medical supervision may not be needed. However, palliative care includes psychosocial, spiritual, and volunteer support. Palliative care practitioners are expert communicators and can clarify confusing ideas. Psychosocial support to address the strain illness places on marriages, assistance with amending financial concerns, integration with community groups, and assistance with prevention and management of symptom distress are all added benefits. Additionally, most programs have expressive therapists (art, music, dance and movement) who can work with the child patient and his or her siblings. Most important, the benefit includes a minimum of thirteen months of bereavement support to families after the child has died. While many oncology teams can and do provide excellent care for the whole family during the dying process, often there is little or no follow-up after the family has left the acute care setting.

Psychosocial Support

A diagnosis of cancer strains a family's coping resources enormously. This strain is magnified greatly when it becomes likely that a child will not survive the disease.

While family coping patterns rarely change during stressful times, the transition to a palliative care approach does change family routine and increases demands on practical, financial, emotional, and spiritual resources, impacting everyone in the family individually as well as within their relationships.

Professional caregivers must be able to acknowledge these changes and direct families to appropriate resources to enhance their ability to cope. Similarly, health care professionals must also be able to recognize the need to support and enhance their own well-being and coping skills, as the strain of working with childhood death and chronic illness is cumulative.

The most important tool that oncology teams have at their disposal is an interdisciplinary approach. While boundary issues need to be respected, all team members can influence and facilitate a family's ability to cope. All members of the team need to communicate well to provide constructive support, which will enhance a family's sense of well-being. Team members also need to support one another in this difficult work. Interdisciplinary respect and face-to-face communication are essential to a well-functioning team.

In *A Practical Guide to Paediatric Oncology Palliative Care,* Dr. Helen Irving and her colleagues list what they call the "essential aspects" of good psychosocial support, which "form the foundation upon which all other aspects of palliative care are built." These are empowerment; trust, openness, and honesty; clear communication; emotional safety; respect for and understanding of the uniqueness of each family; and community perspective (Irving et al. 1999, 373–86). The oncology team is called on to systematize and integrate the involvement of their psychosocial staff for the child with advanced illness.

Once the decision has been made to incorporate palliative care strategies into the care plan, with or without continued treatment of the underlying disease, there once again can be special issues for the adolescent. Denial of impending death is accepted as universal, though it does evolve over time. Adolescents may speak and plan as if they have no doubt about their survival, despite discussions and obvious symptoms pointing to the contrary. (It is also occasionally true that adolescents, rather than their parents, may have the most realistic understanding of their fate.) Caregivers should be respectful of the need for time in an adolescent's gradual acceptance of death. Many adolescents will set proximate goals for survival, such as graduation, birthdays, or special trips. Cancer treatment is sometimes chosen specifically to enable them to reach these goals, which, when realized, contributes meaning to their remaining lives. A desire to participate in these activities does not usually signal denial but rather indicates an attempt to live as a normal teenager with a limited life span, as Valerie did. The adolescent's normal need for peer contact can be met by going home or by medical institutions' welcoming friends and offering participation in teen groups. Older teens and young adults may have committed relationships with partners of the opposite or same sex that are an important source of support. Acknowledgment of these relationships can be extremely valuable to the therapeutic relationship between clinician and patient.

Control of Pain and Other Symptoms

The work of Collins and colleagues (2000) and Wolfe and colleagues (2000) demonstrates that there are many underrecognized and undertreated symptoms from which children with cancer suffer. Although pain management should be part of good basic oncology care, it is often undertreated. Other physical symptoms such as nausea, dyspnea, anorexia, constipation, diarrhea, and mucositis may be difficult to manage. Infection and bleeding are two of the major risks for the terminally ill child with cancer, each with its unique symptomatic presentation. More subjective and difficult to measure symptoms such as fatigue, spiritual distress, anxiety, and depression may be ignored. Collins and colleagues (2000) further demonstrate the importance of considering the distress associated with cancer-related symptoms, not just the presence of the symptom itself. Wolfe and colleagues (2000) data also indicate a recognition gap, with parents reporting the presence of symptoms and related distress much more frequently than physicians.

Untreated symptoms cause suffering and isolation, unnecessary fear, and interference in relationships, not only for the child but also for the caregivers, health care providers, and extended community. With good symptom control, many children are able to truly "live until they die." This section that follows briefly addresses management of the most common symptoms. Several outstanding and more comprehensive resources on pain management in children are available (Yaster et al. 1997; World Health Organization 1998).

ASSESSMENT AND MANAGEMENT OF PAIN

Pain has been defined as "an unpleasant sensory and emotional experience associated with actual or potential tissue damage, or described in terms of such damage" (International Association for the Study of Pain 1979). The pain experience is affected by environmental, developmental, behavioral, psychological, familial, and cultural factors. Many children with cancer have pain at some time during the course of their illness, including both treatment-related and disease-related pain (Miser et al. 1987). How well pain is managed during the early illness phases will have a profound impact on the trajectory of terminal illness. Children with terminal cancer may suffer from somatic, visceral, or neuropathic pain, depending on the disease and its extent. Different therapies will be indicated based upon these factors. For example, metastatic bone pain may respond to steroids, nonsteroidal anti-inflammatory agents, opiates and radiopharmaceuticals, while neuropathic pain from nerve impingement might be best treated with anticonvulsants or tricyclic antidepressants. In planning palliative care approaches in pediatric oncology, it is often appropriate to consider using chemotherapy or radiotherapy (or both) as analgesics; even slight reductions in tumor burden can go a long way in treating pain.

Pain assessment for the child with cancer, as for any other, must be age and developmentally appropriate, if possible by self-report. Following the model of Collins et al. (2000), assessment should consider not only pain frequency and intensity but also how much distress is associated with the pain. Determination of the cause of pain and modulating factors will define the treatment course best suited to maintain comfort and quality of life. For example, localized abdominal pain from extensive intraperitoneal tumor spread may suggest a local approach such as a neurolytic block or intrathecal opiate administration, while disseminated bone and nerve pain associated with progressive sarcomas, for example, will require a more systemic approach. Untreated severe pain represents an emergency for the affected patient and should elicit a commensurate response from the clinician.

For children with cancer, the simplest, most effective, least painful route of administration of medication should be chosen. Despite occasional resistance and apprehension from home providers, children with central venous catheters should be offered the option of parenteral medications. Intramuscular injections are never indicated. Maintaining dignity, control, and choice in the dying process must be considered of great importance, particularly in the case of the older child. This is especially important when considering rectal administration of medication. Subcutaneous infusion, popular in adult hospice and palliative medicine, is possible in children. Unfortunately, pharmacodynamic data are sparse for many routes of medication administration in children; in the absence of data, treatment regimens are often extrapolated from adult data.

In treating cancer-associated pain, as-needed (PRN) scheduling should be avoided. In the PRN paradigm, the child must first experience pain in order to obtain relief. In most cancer-related pain, the pain is predictable enough to mandate around-the-clock dosing, with extra medication provided for breakthrough pain. There is no maximum dose for pure opioid analgesics.

The dose required is the dose effective in treating the pain without undue toxicity; treatment of severe pain may bring children close to dose-limiting toxicity, which can usually be managed symptomatically or by changing to an alternate opiate. While it is rarely relevant, the ethical principle of double effect holds that it is permissible to treat pain appropriately even if other untoward effects, such as respiratory suppression, supersede. However, pain is a powerful respiratory drive stimulant. Nevertheless, parents need to be counseled proactively about this principle, as well as about the differences between drug tolerance, dependence, and addiction, as many parents and older children fear addiction.

Preventing opiate-induced side effects is critical in providing for optimal quality of life for end-stage cancer patients. Constipation is universal; a prescription for a long-acting or chronically dosed opiate without a laxative regimen is poor pain management. Similarly, high-dose oral opiates are associated with nausea often enough that some form of therapy, be it an antihistamine or phenothiazine, should be available for PRN use. Other occasional side effects such as pruritis, hallucinations, or myoclonus should be treated symptomatically or by changing opiates.

Many children with cancer have been exposed to behavioral methods of pain control, especially children requiring frequent painful procedures such as bone marrow samplings. Behavioral techniques are effective and can be provided by parents and caregivers, increasing their sense of contribution to the well-being of the child (Kazak et al. 1998). Modalities to consider include deep breathing (blowing bubbles), relaxation, yoga, biofeedback, touch therapies including massage, transcutaneous electrical nerve stimulation (TENS), physical therapy, heat and cold therapy, acupuncture or acupressure, and cognitive modalities such as distraction through art, music, play, guided imagery, and hypnosis.

PALLIATIVE CHEMOTHERAPY AND RADIOTHERAPY

As mentioned above, many phase I and phase II chemotherapy and biologic response modifiers are currently available for children with progressive malignancy. Patients and families should be given rational explanations of such trials that artfully combine hopefulness for benefit with realism about poor prognosis. Any discussion about these trials must include issues of palliative care, quality-of-life management, and advance care planning. The discussion of the particular agents must not divert from the essential psychoemotional "work" necessary to prepare for the likelihood of the child's death.

Beyond phase I and phase II agents, many oncologists continue to offer children "off-label" parenteral and oral chemotherapy. Oral chemotherapy may be a particularly attractive option for families and children seeking low-technology therapy and is clearly preferred by adults for palliation (Liu et al. 1997). However, there is an absence of efficacy data for many of these agents. Some newer oral chemotherapies are available, including etoposide, irinotecan, idarubicin, capecitabine, and temozolamide, as well as older oral medications such as hydroxyurea, cyclophosphamide, mercaptopurine, or methotrexate, which may also have a palliative role (Ashley et al. 1996; DeMario and Ratain 1998; Royce, Hoff, and Pazdur 2000).

Although radiotherapy is often used in cancer palliation, there are few published data regarding its impact on quality of life near the end of life for children with progression of malignant disease. Anecdotally, it can be very helpful for pain control. Newer radiopharmaceuticals such as samarium (Serafini 2000) and ^{131}I MIBG (Tepmongkol and Heyman 1999) for bone metastases and neuroblastoma, respectively, are also showing promise in palliative care, but the resulting myelosuppression may require extensive blood-product support.

PALLIATION OF BONE MARROW
FAILURE IN THE HOME SETTING

Bone marrow failure often derives from primary malignancy such as leukemia or neuroblastoma in the bone marrow or from the toxic effects of medications. Progressive fatigue, risk of infection, and bleeding resulting from anemia, leukopenia, and thrombocytopenia, respectively, can all significantly and adversely impact the child's and family's quality of life. Decisions regarding interventions for these symptoms depend on the overall medical goals and psychospiritual well-being of the child and family.

Children with progressive leukemia, for example, might be maintained with combinations of palliative chemotherapy, including phase I or phase II investigational agents, blood product support, or expectant treatment of potential infection (or a combination of the three). For a child with protracted bleeding, severe infection, or other complications of end-stage cancer, these interventions might not be appropriate; prevention of suffering should be the paramount goal.

Red blood cell transfusions may be used to treat anemia-induced fatigue. Prophylactic platelet infusions may be appropriate; clinical titration with scheduled infusions may be easier on the child and family than awaiting a bleeding episode. Transfusions at home, if possible, are obviously appreciated by families trying to minimize hospital and clinic time. The availability depends heavily on regional regulations and staffing levels. Gentle oral hygiene with soft toothettes is necessary. Aminocaproic acid, tranexamic acid, desmopressin, and topical thrombin may all be useful treatments for mucosal bleeding and can be used at home. For massive hemorrhage, sedation may be necessary. For aesthetics reasons, it is important to have dark towels handy.

Decisions should be reached in advance with regard to the treatment of infection or fever in the immunocompromised child. Such decisions should hinge on the overall quality of life of the child. The active, school-attending child might clearly benefit from life prolongation with antibiotics, while the comatose child in renal failure might not. For children with central catheters, depending on available services, broad-spectrum antibiotics, such as ceftri-axone or ciprofloxacin, can be stored in the home to be used as needed. Alter-natively, plans for cultures with or without antibiotic administration can be made with local emergency rooms. Parents must be made aware of the risks of treatment failure, including death, in any of these situations.

FATIGUE

Fatigue is very common, difficult to measure, and difficult to treat in chil-dren dying of cancer. Symptoms may include weakness, irritability, sleep disturbance, asthenia, and decreased participation in activities of daily life. Some chemotherapeutics may cause fatigue and generalized weakness and may need to be stopped. Treatment should be directed at the medical, psy-chological, or emotional condition most likely associated with fatigue, for example, anemia or depression. Steroids, blood products, and methylphenidate (particularly for sedation associated with high-dose or rapidly escalating opi-ate therapy) may be tried.

NEUROLOGICAL SYMPTOMS

Seizures, headaches, and sleep disturbances occur frequently in children with cancer, particularly those with central nervous system malignancy. Seizures are often the result of primary or metastatic brain lesions, metabolic distur-bances, or the side effects of chemoradiotherapy or medications. Maintenance anticonvulsant therapy is likely to be appropriate for children with a seizure history. For those at risk, decisions should be made regarding prophylaxis or at a minimum the availability of anticonvulsants such as rectal diazepam in the home. Many other anticonvulsants, such as valproic acid, phenytoin, pentobarbital, lorazepam, phenobarbital and fosphenytoin, can be given by alternative routes at home.

Increased intracranial pressure may result in not only headache but also associated symptoms of suffering, including nausea, vomiting, photophobia, lethargy, transient neurological deficits, or severe irritability. Treatment options depend upon overall quality-of-life assessment and should always include early and aggressive use of analgesics, antiemetics, and often benzodiazepines. Steroids, radiotherapy, chemotherapy, and, less often, surgery may also have a role.

In children with progressive malignancy, sleep disturbance may be common, particularly if specifically addressed by the medical team. Undertreated symptoms such as pain, pruritis, anxiety, or dyspnea, for example, will lead to poor sleep. Medications such as corticosteroids may also contribute. Low-dose tricyclic antidepressants or hypnotics may be helpful if all other potential causes of sleeplessness have been addressed.

At the Time of Imminent Death

Preparing families for the signs and symptoms of impending death is important. In many cases, with good preparation, no specific medical interventions may be necessary. Changes in mental status or state of awareness, including restlessness or delirium, respiratory changes such as agonal, Cheyne-Stokes, or rattling patterns, changes in skin color and temperature, and preterminal bowel and bladder evacuation can all be frightening if unexpected. Honest explanations of these changes in advance may prevent some distress. Physicians should recognize that a single explanation of these signs and symptoms might not be sufficient. Parents faced with the stress and trauma of the loss of a child may need repeated consultation and clarification of end-stage signs and symptoms as well as discussion of relevant psychosocial and spiritual issues. Continued exploration of meaning and hope should always be part of terminal care, and the medical team must be willing to allocate the necessary time that such exploration demands.

References

American Academy of Pediatrics. 1994. Guidelines on forgoing life-sustaining medical treatment. *Pediatrics* 93:532–36.
———, Committee on Bioethics. 1995. Informed consent, parental permission, and assent in pediatric practice. *Pediatrics* 95:314–17.

————, Committee on Bioethics. 2000. Palliative care for children. *Pediatrics* 106: 351–57.

Arceci, R. J., G. H. Reaman, A. R. Cohen, and B. C. Lampkin. 1998. Position statement of the need to define pediatric hematology/oncology programs: a model of subspecialty care for chronic childhood diseases. *J Pediatr Hematol Oncol* 20:98–103.

Ashley, D. M., L. Meier, T. Kerby, F. M. Zalduondo, H. S. Friedman, A. Gajjar, L. Kun, P. K. Duffner, S. Smith, and D. Longee. 1996. Response of recurrent medulloblastoma to low-dose oral etoposide. *J Clin Oncol* 14:1922–27.

Beauchamp, T. L., and J. F. Childress. 1989. *Principles of biomedical ethics.* New York: Oxford University Press.

Children's International Project on Palliative/Hospice Services. 2001. *Compendium of pediatric palliative care.* Alexandria, Va.: National Hospice and Palliative Care Organization.

Code of Federal Regulations. 1991. Protection of human subjects: requirements for permission by parents or guardians and for assent by children. 45 CFR 46.409 (1991); 56 Fed. Reg. 28,032.

Collins, J. J., M. E. Byrnes, I. J. Dunkel, J. Lapin, T. Nadel, H. T. Thaler, T. Polyak, B. Rapkin, and R. K. Portenoy. 2000. The measurement of symptoms in children with cancer. *J Pain Symptom Manage* 19:353–77.

Daugherty, C., M. J. Ratain, E. Grochowski, C. Stocking, E. Kodish, R. Mick, and M. Siegler. 1995. Perceptions of cancer patients and their physicians involved in phase I trials. *J Clin Oncol* 13:1062–72. [Published erratum appears in *J Clin Oncol* 1995 13(1995):2476.]

Decoster, G., G. Stein, and E. E. Holdener. 1990. Responses and toxic deaths in phase I clinical trials. *Ann Oncol* 1:175–81.

DeMario, M. D., and M. J. Ratain. 1998. Oral chemotherapy: rationale and future directions. *J Clin Oncol* 16:2557–67.

Emanuel, E. J. 1995. A phase I trial on the ethics of phase I trials [editorial]. *J Clin Oncol* 13:1049–51.

Field, M. J., and R. E. Behrman. 2002. *When children die: improving palliative care and end-of-life care for children and their families.* Institute of Medicine report. Washington, D.C.: National Academies Press.

Frager, G. 1996. Pediatric palliative care: building the model, bridging the gaps. *J. Palliat Care* 12:9–12.

Freyer, D. R. 1992. Children with cancer: special considerations in the discontinuation of life-sustaining treatment. *Med Pediatr Oncol* 20:136–42.

Friebert, S. E., and E. D. Kodish. 1999. Kids and cancer: ethical issues in treating the pediatric oncology patient. In *Ethical issues in cancer patient care,* ed. P. Angelos, 99–136. Norwell, Mass.: Kluwer Academic.

Goldman, A. 1999. *Care of the dying child.* Oxford, U.K.: Oxford University Press.

Hilden, J. M., E. J. Emanuel, D. L. Fairclough, M. P. Link, K. M. Foley, B. C. Clarridge, L. E. Schnipper, and R. J. Mayer. 2001. Attitudes and practices among pediatric oncologists regarding end-of-life care: results of the 1998 American Society of Clinical Oncology survey. *J Clin Oncol* 19:205–12.

International Association for the Study of Pain, Subcommittee on Taxonomy. 1979. Pain terms: a list of definitions and notes on usage. *Pain* 6:249–52.

Irving, H., K. Liebke, L. Lockwood, M. Noyes, D. Pfingst, and T. Rogers. 1999. *A practical guide to paediatric oncology palliative care.* Brisbane, Australia: Royal Children's Hospital.

James, L., and B. Johnson. 1997. The needs of parents of pediatric oncology patients during the palliative care phase. *J Pediatr Oncol Nurs* 14:83–95.

Kazak, A., B. Penati, P. Brophy, and B. Himelstein. 1998. Pharmacologic and psychologic interventions for procedural pain. *Pediatrics* 102:59–66.

King, N. M., and A. W. Cross. 1989. Children as decision makers: guidelines for pediatricians. *J Pediatr* 115:10–16.

Leikin, S. 1989. A proposal concerning decisions to forgo life-sustaining treatment for young people. *J Pediatr* 115:17–22.

Liben, S. 1996. Pediatric palliative medicine: obstacles to overcome. *J Palliat Care* 12:24–28.

Liu, G., E. Franssen, M. I. Fitch, and E. Warner. 1997. Patient preferences for oral versus intravenous palliative chemotherapy. *J Clin Oncol* 15:110–15.

Martinson, I. M. 1995. Improving care of dying children. *West J Med* 163:258–62.

Miser, A. W., J. A. Dothage, R. A. Wesley, and J. S. Miser. 1987. The prevalence of pain in a pediatric and young adult cancer population. *Pain* 29:73–83.

National Hospice and Palliative Care Organization. 2003. Facts and figures on hospice care in America. Alexandria, Va. www.nhpco.org/files/public/facts_and_figures_0703.pdf (accessed February 24, 2004).

Nitschke, R., W. H. Meyer, C. L. Sexauer, J. B. Parkhurst, P. Foster, and H. Huszti. 2000. Care of terminally ill children with cancer. *Med Pediatr Oncol* 34:268–70.

Ross, L. F. 1997. Health care decisionmaking by children: is it in their best interest? *Hastings Cent Rep* 27:41–45.

Royce, M. E., P. M. Hoff, and R. Pazdur. 2000. Novel oral chemotherapy agents. *Curr Oncol Rep* 2:31–37.

Sahler, O., G. Frager, M. Levetown, F. G. Cohn, and M. A. Lipson. 2000. Medical education about end-of-life care in the pediatric setting: principles, challenges, and opportunities. *Pediatrics* 105:575–84.

Serafini, A. N. 2000. Samarium Sm-153 lexidronam for the palliation of bone pain associated with metastases. *Cancer* 88:2934–39.

Shah, S., S. Weitman, A. M. Langevin, M. Bernstein, W. Furman, and C. Pratt. 1998. Phase I therapy trials in children with cancer. *J Pediatr Hematol Oncol* 20:431–38.

Tepmongkol, S., and S. Heyman. 1999. [131]I MIBG therapy in neuroblastoma: mechanisms, rationale, and current status. *Med Pediatr Oncol* 32:427–31; discussion at 432.

Traugott, I., and A. Alpers. 1997. In their own hands: adolescents' refusal of medical treatment. *Arch Pediatr Adolesc Med* 151:922–27.

Vickers, J. L., and C. Carlisle. 2000. Choices and control: parental experiences in pediatric terminal home care. *J Pediatr Oncol Nurs* 17:12–21.

Weir, R. F., and C. Peters. 1997. Affirming the decisions adolescents make about life and death. *Hastings Cent Rep* 27:29–40.

Whittam, E. H. 1993. Terminal care of the dying child: psychosocial implications of care. *Cancer* 71:3450–62.

Wolfe, J., H. E. Grier, N. Klar, S. B. Levin, J. M. Ellenbogen, S. Salem-Schatz, E. J. Emanuel, and J. C. Weeks. 2000. Symptoms and suffering at the end of life in children with cancer. *N Engl J Med* 342:326–33.

World Health Organization. 1998. *Cancer pain relief and palliative care in children.* Geneva: World Health Organization.

Yaster, M., E. J. Krane, R. F. Kaplan, C. J. Cote, and D. G. Lappe. 1997. *Pediatric pain management and sedation handbook.* St. Louis, Mo.: Mosby–Year Book.

APPENDIX: WEBSITES, ORGANIZATIONS, AND OTHER RESOURCES

Websites for Pediatric and End-of-Life Care

American Academy of Pediatrics, Emergency Preparedness for Children with Special Health Care Needs: www.aap.org/advocacy/emergprep.htm

American Academy of Pediatrics, Policy Statement on Palliative Care for Children: www.aappolicy.aappublications.org/cgi/content/full/pediatrics;106/2/351

Association for Children with Life-Threatening or Terminal Conditions and Their Families (ACT): www.act.org.uk
A U.K. organization working to improve care and services for all children in the United Kingdom with life-threatening or terminal conditions and their families. The website is comprehensive in addressing palliative care for children.

Canadian Network of Palliative Care for Children: www.CNPCC.ca
A resource for those involved in palliative and end-of-life care of children in Canada.

Children's Hospice International: www.chionline.org
Information, books and other media, and a network of support and care for children with life-threatening conditions, their families, and health care professionals.

Children's International Project on Palliative/Hospice Services: www.nhpco.org/i4a/pages/index.cfm?pageid=3409

End-of-Life Care for Children: www.childendoflifecare.org
    Funded by the Texas Cancer Council, this website gives an overview of
    high-quality care promoting a family-centered approach.

The Footprints Program: www.footprintsatglennon.org
    Cardinal Glennon Children's Hospital Pediatric Palliative Care Project,
    St. Louis, Missouri.

Great Ormond Street Hospital for Children and the Institute of Child Health:
    www.ich.ucl.ac.uk
    Resources from the London-based hospital and institute; extensive links to
    other sites.

Growth House: www.growthhouse.org
    Terrific search engine and links to hundreds of end-of-life resources via the
    Internet.

Ian Anderson Continuing Education Program in End-of-Life Care:
    www.cme.utoronto.ca/endoflife/
    The University of Toronto's center, including a pediatric module on decision
    making.

Initiative for Pediatric Palliative Care: www.ippcweb.org
    Dedicated to facilitating improvement in the quality of care for children
    living with life-threatening conditions and their families. The website
    provides interdisciplinary and interactive educational resources that have
    been pilot tested at several of the nation's leading children's hospitals.
    Print materials can be downloaded free of charge from this website.

Innovations in End-of-Life Care: www.edc.org/lastacts
    International on-line journal written by leaders in palliative care. Includes
    editions addressing pediatric-specific issues.

Moyers on Dying: www.pbs.org/wnet/onourownterms/
    Four-part public television series hosted by Bill Moyers that addresses death
    and dying in the United States (videotapes may be purchased). Website
    includes a guide to children's grief written by Kenneth J. Doka.

National Academies Press, Washington, D.C.: www.nap.edu/catalog/10390.html
    *When Children Die: Improving Palliative and End-of-Life Care for Children
    and Their Families* is the Institute of Medicine's text on needs to address
    pediatric palliative care. Edited by Marilyn J. Field and Richard E. Behrman,
    Committee on Palliative and End-of-Life Care for Children and Their
    Families.

National Alliance for Children with Life-Threatening Conditions:
www.nacwltc.org/
A coalition of organizations and individual leaders serving as a unified voice
to improve quality of life for children with life-threatening conditions and
those who care for them.

National Center for Grieving Children and Families: www.dougy.org
Providing support materials, information, and publications on end-of-life
care, grief, and bereavement. A newsletter is available at request by contact-
ing the Dougy Center, by e-mail, at help@dougy.org.

National Hospice and Palliative Care Organization: www.nhpco.org

Paediatric Palliative Care List Service: www.act.org.uk/paedpalcare/
paedpalcare.
The ACT international discussion forum for those working with children
with life-limiting conditions. The aim of ACT is to promote palliative care
for children. To subscribe to the list-serve, send an e-mail to paedpalcare@
act.org.uk; type "subscribe" into the subject box. Frequently asked questions
and the list archive can be found at www.act.org.uk.

Project on Death in America: www.soros.org/death/index.htm

Websites of Organizations for Professionals

PALLIATIVE CARE

American Association of Hospice and Palliative Medicine: www.aahpm.org

Americans for Better Care of the Dying: www.abcd-caring.com

Children's Hospice International: www.chionline.org

Hospice Foundation of America: www.hospicefoundation.org

Last Acts: www.lastacts.org

Midwest Bioethics Center: www.midbio.org

National Alliance for the Cure of Children with Life-threatening Conditions:
www.nacwltc.org

National Hospice and Palliative Care Organization: www.nhpco.org

Promoting Excellence in End of Life Care: www.promotingexcellence.org/

Supportive Care of the Dying: www.careofdying.org

PAIN

Pediatric Pain: www.dal.ca/~pedpain/

Pediatric Pain Education: www.nursing.uiowa.edu/sites/pedspain/

World Health Organization (publications on palliative care):
www.who.int/bookorders/anglais/qsearch1.jsp?sesslan=1

ETHICS

Buddhism and Bioethics: www.changesurfer.com/Bud/BudBioEth.html

Center for Ethics in Health Care, Oregon Health Science University:
www.ohsu.edu/ethics/

Ethical Wills: www.ethicalwill.com

Ethics in Biomedicine (Internet links from the Karolinska Institutet University
Library, Stockholm, Sweden): www.mic.ki.se/Diseases/k1.316.html

National Reference Center for Bioethics Literature:
www.georgetown.edu/research/nrcbl/

Schlesinger Institute (Jewish Medical Ethics):
www.szmc.org.il/index.asp?id=94

St. Louis University Center for Health Care Ethics:
www.slu.edu/centers/chce/

University of Toronto Joint Centers for Bioethics: www.utoronto.ca/jcb/

CULTURE AND SPIRITUALITY

Beliefnet: www.beliefnet.com/index/index_700.html

Cross Cultural Health Care Program: www.xculture.org

Last Acts Diversity Resource Committee: www.lastacts.org/files/misc/
la_diversity.htm

EDUCATION

Association for Death Education and Counseling: www.adec.org

Education for Physicians in End of Life Care: www.ama-assn.org/
ama/pub/category/2910.html

End-of-Life Physician Education Resource Center: www.eperc.mcw.edu

Family Village: A Global Community of Disability Related Resources:
www.familyvillage.wisc.edu and www.familyvillage.wisc.edu/index.htmlx
The University of Wisconsin in Madison's Family Village website is a superb
source of information on rare conditions for both families and professionals.
Through its support network families can participate in chat rooms and can
hook up with other families in the mailroom. There are hundreds of well-
maintained links for rare and common diseases.

Family Village Same Diagnosis Bulletin Board:
www.familyvillage.wisc.edu/post.htm
Provides an excellent way for families to connect with others with the same
situation. Includes parent-to-parent connections for same diagnosis, same
procedure, condition undiagnosed, professionals, and general information.
Posting here can often result in responses from others who have found a
good support group; families can connect with others whose situations are
"closest" to their own.

Medical College of Wisconsin: www.mcw.edu/pallmed/

Mountain States Genetic Network: www.mostgene.org
This site includes educational materials and links to resources and networks
on the web.

National Organization of Rare Disorders (phone: 800-999-6673): www
.NORD-RDB.com/~orphan
Not comprehensive, but a good starting point for patient materials for the
truly rare conditions.

Parent to Parent: National Parent to Parent Organization Website: www
.netnet.net/mums
This website has a long list of diagnoses and is another way to connect to
others. It contains limited medical information; family support is the key to
information exchange here. Specific technical and medical information is not
well represented. Sharing from parent to parent is a good opportunity for
support, yet it is variable how much useful exchange comes from each
encounter.

PubMed, Entrez-PubMed: MEDLINE for the General Public:
www.ncbi.nlm.nih.gov/PubMed/index.html
The National Library of Medicine Entrez is a newer site. Several pages with
access for basic and advanced skills for searching the library's archives. You
can request a document to be delivered to the library nearest you through
the Loansome Doc feature and Inter-Library Loan program.

Rare Genetic Diseases in Children:
www.mcrcr2.med.nyu.edu/murphp01/homenew.htm
Another good website on rare conditions and diseases that affect children. Supported by the NYU Medical Center, this site focuses mainly on lysosomal diseases.

FAMILY SUPPORT / BEREAVEMENT

Children and Grief: Off-line resources:
www.shpm.com/articles/loss/lossoffc.html

Children Coping with Grief: www.grannyg.bc.ca/ckidbook/grief.html

Compassionate Friends: www.compassionatefriends.org

Coping with Grief, Bereavement, and Loss (multiple links to Internet sites):
www.bishops.ntc.nf.ca/ctilley/loss.htm

Dougy Center: www.dougy.org

Empowering Caregivers: www.care-givers.com

Growth House: www.growthhouse.org/natal.html
Devoted to issues around grief over perinatal death

Program for All-Inclusive Care for Children:
www.chionline.org/programs/about.phtml
Demonstration sites for the federal Centers for Medicaid and Medicare Services (CMS) waiver initiative to overcome barriers to providing pediatric palliative care

SHARE Pregnancy and Infant Loss Support: www.nationalshareoffice.com

Support Organizations for Families

For parents of children with cancer:
Candlelighters Childhood Cancer Foundation
1901 Pennsylvania Avenue N.W., Suite 1001
Washington, DC 20006
(202) 659-5136

For parents who have lost a child for any reason:
Compassionate Friends
P.O. Box 3696
Oakbrook, IL 60522-3696
(312) 990-0010

For parents who have lost a child through sudden infant death syndrome:
National SIDS Foundation
8200 Professional Place, Suite 104
Landover, MD 20785
(800) 212-7436

For parents who have a miscarriage, stillbirth, or neonatal death:
SHARE (Source of Help in Airing and Resolving Experiences):
www.NationalSHAREOffice.com
This is a self-help group of parents whose babies never came home (because of stillbirth, miscarriage, or neonatal death).
National S.H.A.R.E. Office
St. Joseph's Health Center
300 First Capitol Drive
St. Charles, MO 63301
(800) 821-6819

Referral service for self-help groups:
National Self-Help Center
1600 Dodge Avenue, Suite S-122
Evanston, IL 60201
(312) 328-0470

For names of counselors in parents' community:
Association for Death Education and Counseling
342 North Main Street
West Hartford, CT 06117-2507
(860) 586-7503

Books and Other Materials about Serious Illness and Death

PERINATAL LOSS

Cohen, M. D. *She Was Born, She Died: A Collection of Poems following the Death of an Infant.* Rev. ed. Omaha: Centering Corporation, 1996.

Davis, D. L. *Empty Cradle, Broken Heart: Surviving the Death of Your Baby.* Golden, Colo.: Fulcrum, 1996.

Davis, D. L. *Fly Away Home: For Bereaved Parents Who Turned Away From Aggressive Medical Intervention for Their Critically Ill Child.* Omaha: Centering Corporation, 2000.

Kohn, I., and P. L. Moffitt. *Pregnancy Loss: Guidance and Support for You and Your Family.* New York: Routledge, 2000.

Leon, I. G., and E. Furman. *When a Baby Dies: Psychotherapy for Pregnancy and Newborn Loss.* New Haven: Yale University Press, 1990.

Levy, Y. *Confronting the Loss of a Baby: A Personal and Jewish Perspective.* Hoboken, N.J.: KTAV Publishing, 1998.

Lothrop, H. *Help, Comfort and Hope after Losing Your Baby in Pregnancy or the First Year.* Tucson: Fisher, 1997.

Peppers, L. G., and R. J. Knapp. *How to Go On Living after the Death of a Baby.* Atlanta: Peachtree, 1985.

Vogel, G. E. *A Caregiver's Handbook to Perinatal Loss.* St. Paul, Minn.: A Place to Remember, 1996.

Wittwer, S. D. *Gone Too Soon: The Life and Loss of Infants and Unborn Children.* American Fork, Utah: Covenant Communications, 1994.

Woods, J. R., and J. L. E. Woods. *Loss during Pregnancy or in the Newborn Period.* Pitman, N.J.: Jannetti Publications, 1997.

FOR CHILDREN AND ADOLESCENTS

American Cancer Society. *Why Charlie Brown, Why?* Video cartoon. Hollywood, Calif.: Paramount Studio, 1995.

Breebart, J., and P. Breebart. *When I Die, Will I Get Better?* New York: Peter Bedrick, 1993.

Brown, L. K., and M. Brown. *When Dinosaurs Die: A Guide to Understanding Death.* Boston: Little, Brown, 1996.

Buscaglia, L. *The Fall of Freddie the Leaf.* 20th anniversary ed. Thorofare, N.J.: Henry Holt, 2002.

Dodge, N. C. *Thumpy's Story: A Story of Love and Grief Shared by Thumpy, the Bunny.* St. Charles, Mo.: SHARE Pregnancy and Infant Loss Support, 1984.

Greenlee, S. *When Someone Dies.* Atlanta: Peachtree, 1992.

Heegaard, M. *When Someone Very Special Dies.* Minneapolis: Woodland, 1988. [A workbook.]

Lazar, L., and B. Crawford. *In My World: Official Life Journal.* Omaha: Centering Corporation, 1999.

Mills, J. *The Gentle Willow.* Washington, D.C.: Magination, 1993.

Miner, J. C. *This Day Is Mine: Living with Leukemia.* Mankato, Minn.: Crestwood House, 1982.

Monroe, J. *The Facts about Leukemia.* Toronto: Crestwood House, 1990.

O'Toole, B., and D. O'Toole. *Facing Change.* Burnsville, N.C.: Compassion Books, 1995. [For adolescents.]

O'Toole, D., and K. L. McWhirter. *Aarvy Aardvark Finds Hope.* Burnsville, N.C.: Compassion Books, 1989.

Sanford, D. *It Must Hurt a Lot: A Child's Book about Death.* New York: Multnomah, 1986.

Schrauger, B. *Walking Taylor Home.* Nashville: W Publishing Group, 2001.

Varley, S. *Badger's Parting Gifts.* Repr. ed. New York: HarperTrophy, 1992.

Viorst, J. *The Tenth Good Thing about Barney.* New York: Aladdin Library, 1987.

White, E. B. *Charlotte's Web.* New York: Harper and Row, 1952.

Wiener, L. *Be a Friend: Children Who Live with HIV Speak.* Morton Grove, Ill.: Albert Whitman, 1996.

Wolfelt, A. D. *Healing Your Grieving Heart for Kids.* Fort Collins, Colo.: Companion Press, 2001.

FOR ADULTS

Adams, D. W., and E. J. Deveau. *Coping with Childhood Cancer: Where Do We Go from Here?* 3d ed. Hamilton, Ont.: Kinbridge, 1993.

Davis, D. *Loving and Letting Go: For Parents Who Decided to Turn Away from Aggressive Medical Intervention for Their Critically Ill Newborns.* Omaha: Centering Corporation, 2002.

Fitzgerald, H. *The Grieving Child.* Toronto: Fireside, 1992.

Frantz, T. T. *When Your Child Has a Life-Threatening Illness.* Washington, D.C.: Association for the Care of Children's Health, 1983.

Grollman, E. *Talking about Death: A Dialogue between Parent and Child.* Boston: Beacon, 1990.

Guthrie, N. *Holding On to Hope: A Pathway through Suffering to the Heart of God.* Wheaton, Ill.: Tyndale House, 2002.

Hamilton, J. *When a Parent Is Sick: Helping Parents Explain Serious Illness to Children.* Halifax, N.S.: Pottersfield, 2001.

Hilden, J. M., D. R. Tobin, and K. Lindsey. *Shelter from the Storm: Caring for a Child with a Life-Threatening Condition.* Cambridge, Mass.: Perseus, 2002.

Housden, M. *Hannah's Gift: Lessons from a Life Fully Lived.* New York: Bantam Doubleday Dell, 2002.

Johnson, J., S. M. Johnson, and B. Williams. *Why Mine? For Parents Whose Child Is Seriously Ill.* Omaha: Centering Corporation, 1981.

Martinson, I. M. *Home Care for the Dying Child: Professional and Family Perspectives.* New York: Appleton-Century-Crofts, 1976.

Mellonie, B., and R. Ingpen. *Lifetimes: A Beautiful Way to Explain Death to Children.* Toronto: Bantam, 1983.

Minnick, M. A., K. J. Delp, and M. C. Ciotti. *A Time to Decide, a Time to Heal: For Parents Making Difficult Decisions about Babies They Love.* 4th ed. St. John's, Mich.: Pineapple, 1992.

Schulman, J. L. *Coping with Tragedy: Successfully Facing the Problem of a Seriously Ill Child.* Chicago: Follett, 1976.

Stephens, S. *Death Comes Home.* New York: Morehouse-Barlow, 1973.

Zagdanski, D. *Something I've Never Felt Before: How Teenagers Cope with Grief.* Melbourne, Australia: Hill of Content, 1990.

FOR SCHOOL

Fox, S. S. *Good Grief.* Boston: New England Association for the Education of Young Children, 2000.

Goldman, L. *Life and Loss: A Guide to Help Grieving Children.* 2d ed. Philadelphia: Accelerated Development, 2000.

FOR ALL AGES, PARENT AND CHILD

Hanson, W. *The Next Place.* Minneapolis: Waldman House, 2003.

INDEX

Page numbers for entries occurring in exhibits are followed by an *e;* those for entries occurring in figures are followed by an *f;* and those for entries occurring in tables are followed by a *t.*

communication (*continued*)
final-stage conferences, 357–58
goals of, 121–22
between health care professionals
and family, 29, 70, 92
language used with children, 122–23
listening and, 127
model for decision making, 128–30,
131–34*e*, 135–38*e*
obstacles to good, 112
open-ended questions in, 127–28
parents' role in, 125
respect as basis of, 238
seven-step approach to, 126–27, 126*e*
styles of, 92
training in skills of, 113
veracity in, 114–18
See also bad news
communities
bereavement support resources in,
50, 216, 268
grief in, 196
needs of, 49, 142
palliative care in, 50–51, 294–96
pediatric home care services, 288, 295
resources for HIV-infected children,
342
service groups, 302–3
See also respite care; schools
compassion, 220, 239
Compassionate Friends, 298, 305
compassion fatigue syndrome, 228, 229
complementary and alternative
medicine (CAM)
discussion of, 146, 165, 165*e*
for genetic conditions, 321–22
in home, 297
increasing use of, 164
types of, 164–65
complex chronic conditions
as cause of death, 8, 11–12
definition of, 8
locations of deaths from, 13–14, 14*f*
maturing effects of, 354

number of deaths from, 11, 12, 12*f*
prevalence of, 11–13
survival into adulthood with, 11
types of health care received, 16–18
See also cancer; HIV, incidence of;
HIV-infected children
confidentiality, 118–20, 299, 301
continuity of care, 105–6, 106*e*
creative arts therapy
art therapy, 187–88, 189*f*, 190
based on child's age and
developmental level, 188–92
for bereaved siblings, 201
dance and movement therapy,
186–87, 188–90
in dying process, 186
in home, 297
music therapy, 188, 190–91
spiritual foundation for, 185–86
value of, 192
cultural values
associated with death, 93
of families, 92, 93*e*, 94*e*, 142, 147, 270
on full disclosure of information,
115–16, 117
of health care providers, 93–95

dance and movement therapy, 186–87,
188–90
death
appropriate, 214
cultural values and traditions
surrounding, 93
religious rituals associated with, 142
risk over time depending on
underlying condition, 4, 5*f*
See also bereavement support;
funerals; grief
deaths of children
acceptance of, 201–2
ages at death, 8
causes of, 8, 9–10*t*, 10*f*, 11, 198
difficulty of predicting time of, 47,
63, 303

effects on families, 196
at home, 13, 15–16, 50–51
locations of, 13–14, 14f, 15–16, 274
number in United States, 8, 45–46
preparing for, 197, 298, 357–58, 370
psychosocial impact of, 47
reactions of parents to, 199
societal perceptions of, 75–76
traumatic causes of, 11, 18, 198, 274,
283–84
deception, 115, 116, 117–18
decision making
by adolescents, 79, 80e, 353–58
capacity of children for, 94–96, 97e,
354
causes of disagreements in, 100
challenges of, 71–75
for children with genetic conditions,
324–26
on clinical trial participation, 83, 86,
351–52
communication model for, 128–30,
131–34e, 135–38e
conflict management in, 101–2, 105,
105e, 238, 254
consensus building in, 103, 267–68
cycle of, 92–106, 93f
educational module on, 71
evaluating options in, 100–102, 102e
families' perspectives on, 100, 102e
framing options for, 98–99, 99e
during illness trajectories, 73f, 83,
84–85t
importance of collaboration in,
33–34, 70
language for opening discussions,
97–98, 98e
legal issues in, 95, 354–56
in neonatal medicine, 253–57
as ongoing process, 75
parents' discomfort with, 103, 104e
participants in, 76–83, 77f, 97
physicians' perspectives on, 100, 102e
respect as basis of, 238

role of child in, 37, 76–79, 94,
146–47, 279, 281
roles of extended families in, 81–82
settings of discussions in, 96–97
by surrogates, 73–75, 81, 254, 324
timing of discussions in, 74, 96–97
types of decisions, 83–90
in urgent situations, 99, 100e
Declaration of Geneva, World Medical
Association, 114, 119
degenerative neurological or muscular
conditions, 315, 319
diagnosis
of cancer, 115
disclosure to HIV-infected children,
338–39
discussion of, 319–20
of genetic conditions, 311, 314,
319–20, 323–24, 325, 326
support for families at time of,
143–44
See also bad news
do-not-resuscitate orders
for children in home, 305
for children in school, 289, 305
discussion of, 33, 86
number issued for children, 17
in pediatric intensive care units, 18
See also resuscitation; withdrawal or
withholding of care

education. See schools
Education for Physicians on End-of-
Life Care (EPEC) program, 113,
126
education in pediatric palliative care,
51–52
accreditation, 60
auditing of existing practices, 60
in clinical settings, 53–54
on communication skills, 113
content of, 54–55, 55e
on decision making, 71
dimensions of, 56–59

education in pediatric palliative care
(*continued*)
  for home care, 298, 299
  in medical schools, 55
  methods of, 55–60
  objectives of, 53–55
  in residency programs, 52
Elijah, 344
emergency departments, 13, 198–99
emergency situations, 181–83
empathy, 54, 220, 223, 230
EPEC. *See* Education for Physicians on
    End-of-Life Care (EPEC) program
equifinality, 142
ethical issues
  acceptance of prognosis, 32–33
  articulate disagreement, 38–40
  avoidance or postponement of bad
    news, 28–29
  in clinical trials, 352
  in communication, 28–31, 114–21
  conflicts among values, 27, 29
  conflicts of interest, 121
  confusion, 36–38
  in decision making by adolescents,
    353–57
  denial of poor prognosis, 31–32
  dissension among health care
    providers, 34–36
  entrenched positions, 33–34
  hope of families, 32
  in palliative care, 27–28, 252–53
  poor communication, 30–31
  preferences of child patients, 37
  in research, 19
  thwarted agreement, 41–42
  values, 26–27
ethics codes, 114, 119
ethics committees, 38, 40
euthanasia, 35
extended families
  bereavement support for, 196–97
  informing about illness, 100, 101e
  needs of, 49, 81–82, 359–60

participation in decision making,
    81–82
  support for, 141–42
  See also families
extubation. *See* withdrawal or
    withholding of care

faith, 156, 157, 159. *See also* spirituality
families
  assessment of understanding of
    illness, 94, 95e
  communication styles of, 92
  communication with health care
    providers, 29, 70, 92
  coping strategies of, 310, 321, 327
  cultural values of, 92, 93e, 94e, 142,
    147, 270
  definition of, 141
  financial stress of, 152
  of HIV-infected children, 338–41,
    342–43
  hopes of, 32, 75
  maintaining normalcy, 184–85, 310
  needs of, 49
  practical needs of, 284
  psychosocial needs of, 15, 142, 266,
    339–40, 363–65
  reactions to illness, 151
  religious rituals of, 157–59
  spiritual needs of, 142, 266
  spiritual resources of, 156
  support during cure-oriented
    treatment, 144–45
  support groups for, 151–52
  support needed at time of diagnosis,
    143–44
  transition to palliative care, 145–46
  See also bereavement support;
    extended families; parents; siblings
fathers
  bereavement support for, 207–8
  grief of, 203–8
  of HIV-infected children, 339
  See also parents

Nouwen, Henri, 160
nurses
    compassion of, 230
    ethical issues for, 120–21
    reactions to neonatal deaths, 267
    self-care practices, 240
    suffering experienced by, 230
    training in pediatric palliative care,
        52, 59
    See also health care providers
nutrition
    artificial, 86–87, 177, 324
    for HIV-infected children, 335
    lack of appetite and, 176–77

O'Connor, Flannery, 159
oncology, pediatric, 348, 350. *See also*
    cancer
on-line support groups, 289, 320
opioids
    doses of, 170–72, 366–67
    major, 170–71
    myths about effects in children, 48
    regular administration of, 170
    relative potencies of, 172t
    responsiveness to, 168
    side effects of, 173, 178, 180, 367
    use in children, 48, 170–71, 173–74,
        281
    use in children with genetic
        conditions, 329
    use in infants, 262, 280
organ donations, from infants, 270

pain
    assessment of, 169, 258, 259t, 366
    breakthrough, 171, 366
    children's experience of, 166–67
    classification of, 167–68, 168t
    definition of, 365
    diagnosis of, 166–67, 169
    in nonverbal or preverbal children,
        166, 169, 258
pain management, 166

behavioral methods of, 367
in children with cancer, 15, 365–67
in children with genetic conditions,
    329
decision making in, 88–89
ethical guidelines for, 89e
in HIV-infected children, 335
in home, 296–97
improving quality of life with,
    169–70
for infants, 258, 260–61t, 262–63
medication forms for children, 170,
    172
medication types, 170, 175
myths about effects of medication
    in children, 48
in pediatric intensive care units,
    279–81
procedure-related pain, 184, 262
QUEST mnemonic, 167
reluctance to use medications for,
    41, 48
undertreatment in, 365
WHO pain ladder, 170, 171f
See also opioids
palliative care
    advocacy to improve, 60–64
    boundaries with curative care, 5–7,
        6f, 41
    continuity of care in, 105–6, 106e
    coordination of care, 153–54
    costs of, 19, 42
    definition of, 163
    delayed referrals to, 145
    goals of, 23–25, 334
    integrated model of, 143–44, 294,
        304, 358, 360, 362
    interdisciplinary, 25, 295–96
    introductory discussions of, 74,
        90–92, 97–98, 98e, 145, 358–59
    need for, 4, 5
    obstacles to children's access to,
        41–42, 44–49, 358
    readiness for, 91